The **BIOMEDICAL ENGINEERING** Series

Series Editor Michael R. Neuman

Analysis and Application of Analog Electronic Circuits to Biomedical Instrumentation

Robert B. Northrop

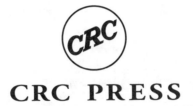

CRC PRESS

Boca Raton   London   New York   Washington, D.C.

Library of Congress Cataloging-in-Publication Data

Northrop, Robert B.
  Analysis and application of analog electronic circuits to biomedical instrumentation / by
Robert B. Northrop.
    p. cm. — (Biomedical engineering series)
  Includes bibliographical references and index.
  ISBN 0-8493-2143-3 (alk. paper)
  1. Analog electronic systems. 2. Medical electronics. I. Title. II. Biomedical engineering
series (Boca Raton, Fla.)

  TK7867.N65 2003
  610′.28—dc22   2003065373

Visit the CRC Press Web site at www.crcpress.com

© 2004 by CRC Press LLC

No claim to original U.S. Government works
International Standard Book Number 0-8493-2143-3
Library of Congress Card Number 2003065373
Printed in the United States of America 1 2 3 4 5 6 7 8 9 0
Printed on acid-free paper

Dedication

I dedicate this text to my wife and daughters: Adelaide, Anne, Kate, and Victoria.

Preface

Reader Background

This text is intended for use in a classroom course on analysis and application of analog electronic circuits in biomedical engineering taken by junior or senior undergraduate students specializing in biomedical engineering. It will also serve as a reference book for biophysics and medical students interested in the topics. Readers are assumed to have had introductory core courses up to the junior level in engineering mathematics, including complex algebra, calculus, and introductory differential equations. They also should have taken an introductory course in electronic circuits and devices. As a result of taking these courses, readers should be familiar with systems block diagrams and the concepts of frequency response and transfer functions; they should be able to solve simple linear ordinary differential equations and perform basic manipulations in linear algebra. It is also important to have an understanding of the working principles of the various basic solid-state devices (diodes, bipolar junction transistors, and field-effect transistors) used in electronic circuits in biomedical applications.

Rationale

The interdisciplinary field of biomedical engineering is demanding in that it requires its followers to know and master not only certain engineering skills (electronics, materials, mechanical, photonic), but also a diversity of material in the biological sciences (anatomy, biochemistry, molecular biology, genomics, physiology, etc.). This text was written to aid undergraduate biomedical engineering students by helping them to understand the basic analog electronic circuits used in signal conditioning in biomedical instrumentation. Because many bioelectric signals are in the microvolt range, noise from electrodes, amplifiers, and the environment is often significant compared to the signal level. This text introduces the basic mathematical tools used to describe noise and how it propagates through linear systems. It also describes at a basic level how signal-to-noise ratio can be improved by signal averaging and linear filtering.

Bandwidths associated with endogenous (natural) biomedical signals range from dc (e.g., hormone concentrations or dc potentials on the body surface) to hundreds of kilohertz (bat ultrasound). Exogenous signals associated with certain noninvasive imaging modalities (e.g., ultrasound, MRI) can reach into the tens of megahertz. Throughout the text, op amps are shown to be the keystone of modern analog signal conditioning system design. This text illustrates how op amps can be used to build instrumentation amplifiers, isolation amplifiers, active filters, and many other systems and subsystems used in biomedical instrumentation.

The text was written based on the author's experience in teaching courses in electronic devices and circuits, electronic circuits and applications, and biomedical instrumentation for over 35 years in the electrical and computer engineering department at the University of Connecticut, as well as on his personal research in biomedical instrumentation.

Description of the Chapters

Analysis and Application of Analog Electronic Circuits in Biomedical Engineering is organized into 12 chapters, an index, and a reference section. Extensive examples in the chapters are based on electronic circuit problems in biomedical engineering.

In Chapter 1, *Sources and Properties of Biomedical Signals*, the sources of bioelectric phenomena in nerves and muscles are described. The general characteristics of biomedical signals are set forth and we examine the general properties of physiological systems, including nonlinearity and nonstationarity.

In Chapter 2, *Models for Semiconductor Devices Used in Analog Electronic Systems*, we describe the mid- and high-frequency models used for analysis of *pn* junction diodes, BJTs, and FETs in electronic circuits. The high-frequency behavior of basic one- and two-transistor amplifiers is treated and the Miller effect is introduced. This chapter also describes the properties of photodiodes, photoconductors, LEDs, and laser diodes.

In Chapter 3, *The Differential Amplifier*, this important analog electronic circuit architecture is analyzed for BJT and FET DAs. Mid- and high-frequency behavior is treated, as well as the factors that lead to a desirable high common-mode rejection ratio. DAs are shown to be essential subcircuits in all op amps, comparators, and instrumentation amplifiers.

In Chapter 4, *General Properties of Electronic Single-Loop Feedback Systems*, we introduce the four basic kinds of electronic feedback (positive/negative voltage feedback and positive/negative current feedback) and describe how they affect linear amplifier performance.

Chapter 5, *Feedback, Frequency Response, and Amplifier Stability*, presents Bode plots and the root-locus technique as design tools and means of predicting closed-loop system stability. The effects of negative voltage and current feedback, as well as positive voltage feedback, on an amplifier's gain and bandwidth, and input and output impedance are described. The design of certain "linear" oscillators is treated.

In Chapter 6, *Operational Amplifiers*, we examine the properties of the ideal op amp and how its model can be used in quick pencil-and-paper circuit analysis of various op amp circuits. Circuit models for various types of practical op amps are described, including current feedback op amps. Gain-bandwidth products are shown to differ for different op amp types and circuits. Analog voltage comparators are introduced and practical circuit examples are given. The final subsection illustrates some applications of op amps in biomedical instrumentation.

In Chapter 7, *Analog Active Filters*, we illustrate three major architectures easily used to design for op amp-based active filters. These include the Sallen and Key quadratic AF, the one- and two-loop biquad AF, and the GIC-based AF. Voltage and digitally tunable AF designs are described and examples are given; AF applications are discussed.

In Chapter 8, *Instrumentation and Medical Isolation Amplifiers*, we describe the general properties of instrumentation amplifiers (IAs) and some of the circuit architectures used in their design. Medical isolation amplifiers (MIAs) are shown to be necessary to protect patients from electrical shock hazard during bioelectric measurements. All MIAs provide extreme galvanic isolation between the patient and the monitoring station. We illustrate several MIA architectures, including a novel direct sensing system that uses the giant magnetoresistive effect. Also described are the current safety standards for MIAs.

In Chapter 9, *Noise and the Design of Low-Noise Amplifiers for Biomedical Applications*, descriptors of random noise, such as the probability density function; the auto- and cross-correlation functions; and the auto- and cross-power density spectra, are introduced and their properties discussed. Sources of random noise in active and passive components are presented and we show how noise propagates statistically through LTI filters. Noise factor, noise figure, and signal-to-noise ratio are shown to be useful measures of a signal conditioning system's noisiness. Noise in cascaded amplifier stages, DAs, and feedback amplifiers is treated. Examples of noise-limited signal resolution calculations are given. Factors affecting the design of low-noise amplifiers and a list of low-noise amplifiers are presented.

Digital Interfaces, Chapter 10, details these particular interfaces, as well as derivation of aliasing and the sampling theorem. Analog-to-digital and digital-to-analog converters are described. Hold circuits and quantization noise are also treated.

In Chapter 11, *Modulation and Demodulation of Bioelectric Signals*, we illustrate the basics of modulation schemes used in instrumentation and biotelemetry systems. Analysis is conducted on AM; single-sideband AM (SSBAM); double-sideband suppressed carrier (DSBSC) AM; angle modulation including phase and frequency modulation (FM); narrow-band FM; delta modulation; and integral pulse frequency modulation (IPFM) systems, as well as on means for their demodulation.

In Chapter 12, *Examples of Special Analog Circuits and Systems in Biomedical Instrumentation*, we describe and analyze circuits and systems important in biomedical and other branches of instrumentation. These include the phase-sensitive rectifier; phase detector circuits; voltage- and current-controlled oscillators, including VFCs and VPCs, phase-locked loops, and applications; true RMS converters; IC thermometers; and four examples of complex measurement systems developed by the author.

In addition, the comprehensive references at the end of the book contain entries from periodicals, the World Wide Web, and additional texts.

Features

Some of the unique contents of this text are:

- Section 2.6 in Chapter 2 describes the properties of photonic sensors and emitters, including PIN and avalanche photodiodes, and photoconductors. Signal conditioning circuits for these sensors are given and analyzed. This section also describes the properties of LEDs and laser diodes, as well as the circuits required to power them.

- Chapter 8 gives a thorough treatment of the design of instrumentation amplifiers and medical isolation amplifiers. Also described in detail are current safety standards for MIAs.

- A comprehensive treatment of noise in analog signal conditioning systems is given in Chapter 9.

- Chapter 10 on digital interfaces examines the designs of many types of ADCs and DACs and introduces aliasing and quantization noise as possible costs for going to or from analog or digital domains.
- Chapter 11 illustrates the use of phase-locked loops to generate or demodulate angle-modulated signals, including phase and frequency modulation as well as AM and DSBSCM signals.
- Chapter 12 describes an applications-oriented collection of analog circuit "building blocks," including: phase-sensitive rectifiers; phase detectors; phase-locked loops; VCOs and ICOs, including VFCs and VPCs; true RMS converters; IC thermometers; and examples of complex biomedical instrument systems designed by the author that use op amps extensively.
- Many illustrative examples from medical electronics are given in the chapters.
- Home problems that accompany each chapter (except Chapter 1, Chapter 8, and Chapter 12) stress biomedical electronic applications.

Robert B. Northrop
Chaplin, Connecticut

The Author

Robert B. Northrop was born in White Plains, New York in 1935. After graduating from Staples High School in Westport, Connecticut, he majored in electrical engineering at MIT, graduating with a bachelor's degree in 1956. At the University of Connecticut, he received a master's degree in control engineering in 1958. As the result of a long-standing interest in physiology, he entered a Ph.D. program at UCONN in physiology, doing research on the neuromuscular physiology of molluscan catch muscles. He received his Ph.D. in 1964.

In 1963, Dr. Northrop rejoined the UCONN electrical engineering department as a lecturer and was hired as an assistant professor of electrical engineering in 1964. In collaboration with his Ph.D. advisor, Dr. Edward G. Boettiger, he secured a 5-year training grant in 1965 from NIGMS (NIH) and started one of the first interdisciplinary biomedical engineering graduate training programs in New England. UCONN currently awards M.S. and Ph.D. degrees in this field of study.

Throughout his career, Dr. Northrop's areas of research have been broad and interdisciplinary and have centered around biomedical engineering. He has conducted sponsored research on the neurophysiology of insect and frog vision and devised theoretical models for visual neural signal processing. He also performed sponsored research on electrofishing and, in collaboration with Northeast Utilities, developed effective working systems for fish guidance and control in hydroelectric plant waterways on the Connecticut River using underwater electric fields.

Still another area of Dr. Northrop's sponsored research has been in the design and simulation of nonlinear adaptive digital controllers to regulate *in vivo* drug concentrations or physiological parameters such as pain, blood pressure, or blood glucose in diabetics. An outgrowth of this research led to his development of mathematical models for the dynamics of the human immune system, which were used to investigate theoretical therapies for autoimmune diseases, cancer, and HIV infection.

Biomedical instrumentation has also been an active research area: an NIH grant supported Dr. Northrop's studies on use of the ocular pulse to detect obstructions in the carotid arteries. Minute pulsations of the cornea from arterial circulation in the eyeball were sensed using a no-touch, phase-locked ultrasound technique. Ocular pulse waveforms were shown to be related to cerebral blood flow in rabbits and humans.

Most recently, he has been addressing the problem of noninvasive blood glucose measurement for diabetics. Starting with a Phase I SBIR grant,

Dr. Northrop developed a means of estimating blood glucose by reflecting a beam of polarized light off the front surface of the lens of the eye and measuring the very small optical rotation resulting from glucose in the aqueous humor that, in turn, is proportional to blood glucose. As an offshoot of techniques developed in micropolarimetry, he developed a magnetic sample chamber for glucose measurement in biotechnology applications; the water solvent was used as the Faraday optical medium.

Dr. Northrop has written six textbooks that address analog electronic circuits; instrumentation and measurements; physiological control systems; neural modeling; signals and systems analysis in biomedical engineering and instrumentation; and measurements in noninvasive medical diagnosis. He was a member of the electrical and computer engineering faculty at UCONN until his retirement in 1997; throughout this time, he was program director of the biomedical engineering graduate program. As Emeritus Professor, he still teaches courses in biomedical engineering, writes texts, sails, and travels. He lives in Chaplin, Connecticut, with his wife, cat, and smooth fox terrier.

Table of Contents

1

Sources and Properties of Biomedical Signals

1.1   Introduction

Before describing and analyzing the electronic circuits, amplifiers, and filters required to condition the signals found in clinical medicine and biomedical research, it is appropriate to describe the sources and properties of these signals (i.e., their bandwidths, distribution of amplitudes, and noisiness). Broadly speaking, biomedical signals can be subdivided into two major classes: (1) endogenous signals that arise from natural physiological processes and are measured within or on living creatures (e.g., ECG; EEG; respiratory rate; temperature; blood glucose; etc.) and (2) exogenous signals applied from without (generally noninvasively) to measure internal structures and parameters. These include but are not limited to ultrasound (imaging and Doppler); x-rays; monochromatic light (e.g., two wave lengths used in transcutaneous pulse oximeters); fluorescence from fluorophore-tagged cells and molecules stimulated with blue or near UV light; optical coherence tomography (OCT); laser Doppler velocimetry (LDV) used to measure blood velocity; and applied magnetic fields used in NMR). Other examples of exogenous signals can be found in the text by Northrop (2002).

The following section examines the properties of endogenous bioelectric signals used in medical diagnosis, care, and research.

1.2   Sources of Endogenous Bioelectric Signals

The sources of nearly all bioelectric signals are transient changes in the transmembrane potential observed in all living cells. In particular, bioelectric signals arise from the time-varying transmembrane potentials seen in nerve cells (neuron action potentials and generator potentials) and in muscle cells, including the heart. The electrochemical basis for transmembrane potentials in living cells lies in two phenomena: (1) cell membranes are semipermeable, i.e., they have different transmembrane conductances and permeabilities for different ions and molecules (e.g., Na^+, K^+, Ca^{++}, Cl^-, glucose, proteins, etc.) and (2) cell membranes contain ion pumps driven by metabolic energy (e.g., ATP). The ion pumps actively transport ions and molecules across cell membranes against energy barriers set up by the transmembrane potential and/or concentration gradients between the inside and outside of the cell. In the steady state, ions continually leak into a cell (e.g., Na^+) or out of a cell (e.g., K^+) and ongoing ion pumping restores the steady-state concentrations.

In squid giant axons, the steady-state, *internal* concentrations are $[Na^+]_i = 50$ mM, $[K^+]_i = 400$ mM, $[Cl^-]_i = 52$ mM. The steady-state *external* concentrations (in extracellular fluid) are $[Na^+]_e = 440$ mM, $[K^+]_e = 20$ mM, $[Cl^-]_e = 560$ mM, and $[A^-]_i = 385$ mM (Kandel et al., 1991). $[A^-]$ is the equivalent concentration of large, impermeable protein anions in the cytosol. Ion concentration data exist for the neurons and muscles of a variety of invertebrate and vertebrate species (Kandel et al., 1991; West, 1985; Katz, 1966).

The steady-state transmembrane potential can be modeled by the Goldman–Hodgkin–Katz equation (Guyton, 1991):

$$V_{mo} = -\frac{RT}{F} \ln \left\{ \frac{[Na^+]_i P_{Na^+} + [K^+]_i P_{K^+} + [Cl^-]_i P_{Cl^-}}{[Na^+]_e P_{Na^+} + [K^+]_e P_{K^+} + [Cl^-]_e P_{Cl^-}} \right\} \tag{1.1}$$

where T is the Kelvin temperature; R is the MKS gas constant (8.314 J/mol K); F is the Faraday number, 96,500 Cb/mol; and P_X is the permeability for ion species, X. The resting transmembrane potential of neurons, V_{mo}, varies with species, neuron type, ionic environment, and temperature; it can range from 60 to 90 mV (inside negative with respect to outside). Muscle fibers, too, have a transmembrane potential of approximately $80 < V_{mo} < 95$ mV, inside negative.

1.3 Nerve Action Potentials

Nerve action potentials (APs) are in general the result of transient changes in specific ionic conductances and permeabilities induced electrically (or chemically by neurotransmitters) in the nerve cell membrane. In excitable neuron membranes, an *increase* in sodium permeability leads to a depolarization of the transmembrane potential (i.e., sodium ions flow rapidly into the neuron down a concentration gradient and electric field). The inrush of Na^+ causes the V_m to go positive, which is a depolarization.

When the excitable nerve membrane voltage reaches a depolarization threshold on the order of a few millivolts, the permeability events that lead to a propagating action potential or nerve spike occur. First, there is a further, "all-or-nothing," large transient increase in sodium permeability causing a strong transient inrush of Na⁺ ions. This inrush causes a large, fast depolarization so that V_m actually goes positive by tens of millivolts, generally in less than a millisecond. Immediately, permeability to K⁺ ions also increases, but at a slower rate, which causes an outward J_{K^+}, making V_m decrease from its positive peak to its negative resting value after a slight, transient undershoot (hyperpolarization). The total duration of the positive nerve action potential spike is on the order of 2 MS.

Once initiated, an action potential propagates down a neuron's axon at a velocity that depends on a number of physical and chemical factors, including the diameter of the axon. One of the earliest mathematical models for nerve impulse generation was given by Hodgkin and Huxley in 1952. The H–H model now appears to be somewhat oversimplified with its description of a single type of potassium channel, but is still valid and a useful model to teach about the dynamics of nerve impulse generation. Figure 1.1 illustrates the result of a computer simulation of the H–H model using Simnon™ (Northrop, 2001). Shown are the transmembrane voltage, the time-varying conductances for Na⁺, K⁺, and "leakage anions." Readers interested in pursuing the molecular and ionic details of neurophysiology should consult Kandel et al. (1991); West (1985); Guyton (1991); and Northrop (2001).

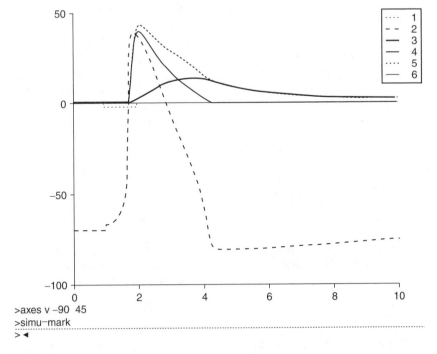

FIGURE 1.1
Results of a Simnon™ simulation of the Hodgkin–Huxley 1952 mathematical model for nerve action potential generation. Traces: (1) J_{in} ($\mu A/cm^2$). (2) $v_m(t)$ (transmembrane potential). (3) $g_K(t, v_m)$ mS/cm². (4) $g_{Na}(t, v_m)$ mS/cm². (5) $g_{net} = g_K + g_{Na} + g_L$ mS/cm². (6) J_{in}, $\mu A/cm^2$. (Northrop, R.B. 2001. *Introduction to Dynamic Modeling of Neuro-Sensory Systems*. CRC Press, Boca Raton, FL.)

Most neurons in the vertebrate CNS are too small to record their transmembrane potentials with glass micropipette electrodes directly. However, their action potentials can be recorded over long periods of time with extracellular, metal microelectrodes whose uninsulated tips are in the neuropile within several microns of axons or cell bodies. Action potentials from peripheral nerve bundles can be recorded with simple platinum hook electrodes, saline-filled suction electrodes, or saline-wetted wick electrodes coupled to silver–silver chloride electrodes. All extracellular recording techniques suffer from the problem that the electrodes pick up nerve spikes from active, adjacent, or neighboring neurons. This neural background noise is added to the desired unit's signal and, unfortunately, has the same bandwidth as the desired unit's spikes. In dissected peripheral nerve fibers, it may be possible to isolate single axons with hook, suction, or wick electrodes, thus greatly improving the recording SNR.

Because the nerve action potential is a traveling wave, it can be shown that an external electrode in close proximity to the outside surface of an axon will respond to the passage of the AP with an electric potential waveform that is in effect the second derivative of the transmembrane spike waveform (Plonsey, 1969) as shown in Figure 1.2. (The intracellular AP, V_m, is to scale, but its derivatives are not to scale.) The triphasic (second derivative) waveform of the AP recorded at a point near the axon comes from the fact that the AP is traveling along the axon with velocity, v. As the AP approaches the electrode, a weak, net *outward* J_{K+} causes a low positive voltage peak. When the AP has moved opposite the electrode, the electrode responds to the strong *inward* flow of J_{Na} with a large negative voltage peak. Then, as the AP passes the electrode, its potential again goes positive from the *outward* J_{K+} in the recovery phase of the AP. (The (–) terminal of the amplifier is connected to a Ag | AgCl reference electrode electrically far from the recorded neuron.)

In the author's experience, using fine platinum–iridium extracellular microelectrodes, which were glass insulated down to 6 to 12 μm of their conical tips, made it possible to record from single units in insect optic lobes and protocerebrum and frog tectum, with major spike amplitudes ranging from –50 to –500 μV. Midband gain for signal conditioning was 10^4 and signal conditioning bandwidth was 100 to 3×10^3 Hz (Northrop and Guignon, 1970).

Nerve APs recorded through the neuron membrane (in the cell body, base of dendrites, or axon) using glass micropipette electrodes can be approximately 100 mV or more peak to peak. A capacity-neutralized electrometer headstage used to couple the high-resistance microelectrode generally has a gain of 2 or 3; the second stage may gain from 5 to 30, so the overall gain can range from 10 to 90. Bandwidth is from dc to 3 to 5 kHz. The direct coupling is required because interest is usually in the neuron's resting potential, V_{mo}, or slow changes in V_m caused by incoming excitatory or inhibitory signals. If V_{mo} is not of interest, then it is technically simpler and less noisy to use external microelectrodes and band-pass filtering (e.g., 100 to 3 kHz). More gain will be required with external electrodes, however.

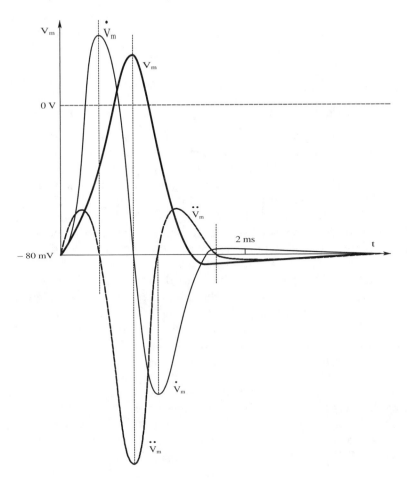

FIGURE 1.2

A nerve action potential and its first and second time derivatives (derivatives not to scale).

1.4 Muscle Action Potentials

1.4.1 Introduction

An important bioelectric signal that has diagnostic significance for many neuromuscular diseases is the electromyogram (EMG), which can be recorded from the skin surface with electrodes identical to those used for electrocardiography, although in some cases, the electrodes have smaller areas than those used for ECG (<1 mm²). To record from single motor units (SMUs) or even individual muscle fibers (several of which comprise an SMU), needle electrodes that pierce the skin into the body of a superficial muscle can also be used. (This semi-invasive method obviously requires sterile technique.) EMG recording is used to diagnose some causes of muscle weakness or paralysis, muscle or motor problems such as tremor or twitching, motor nerve damage from injury or osteoarthritis, and pathologies affecting motor end plates.

1.4.2   The Origin of EMGs

There are several types of muscle in the body, e.g., striated, cardiac, and smooth. Striated muscle in mammals can be further subdivided into fast and slow muscles (Guyton, 1991). Fast muscles are used for fast movements; they include the two gastrocnemii, laryngeal muscles, extraocular muscles, etc. Slow muscles are used for postural control against gravity and include the soleus; abdominal, back, and neck muscles; etc. EMG recording is generally carried out on both types of skeletal muscles. It can also be done on less superficial muscles such as the extraocular muscles that move the eyeballs, the eyelid muscles, and the muscles that work the larynx.

A particular striated muscle is innervated by a group of motor neurons that have origin at a certain level in the spinal cord. In the spinal cord, motor neurons receive excitatory and inhibitory inputs from motor control neurons from the CNS, as well as excitatory and inhibitory inputs from local feedback neurons from muscle spindles (responding to muscle length, x, and dx/dt), Golgi tendon organs (responding to muscle tension), and Renshaw feedback cells (Northrop, 1999; Guyton, 1991). Individual motor neuron axons controlling the contraction of a particular striated muscle innervate small groups of muscle fibers in the muscle called a *single motor unit* (SMU). Many SMUs comprise the entire muscle. The synaptic connections between the terminal branches of a single motor neuron axon and its SMU fibers are called *motor end plates* (MEPs). MEPs are chemical synapses in which the neurotransmitter, acetylcholine (ACh), is released presynaptically and then diffuses across the synaptic cleft or gap to ACh receptors on the subsynaptic membrane.

When a motor neuron action potential arrives at an MEP, it triggers the exocytosis or emptying of about 300 presynaptic vesicles containing ACh. (Approximately 3×10^5 vesicles are in the terminals of a single MEP; each vesicle is about 40 nm in diameter.) Some 10^7 to 5×10^8 molecules of ACh are needed to trigger a muscle action potential (Katz, 1966). The ACh diffuses across the 20 to 30 nm synaptic cleft in approximately 0.5 MS; here some ACh molecules combine with receptor sites on the protein subunits forming the subsynaptic, ion-gating channels. Five high molecular weight protein subunits form each ion channel. ACh binding to the protein subunits triggers a dilation of the channel to approximately 0.65 nm. The dilated channels allow Na^+ ions to pass inward; however, Cl^- is repelled by the fixed negative charges on the mouth of the channel.

Thus, the subsynaptic membrane is depolarized by the inward J_{Na} (i.e., its transmembrane potential goes positive from the approximately –85 mV resting potential), triggering a muscle action potential. The local subsynaptic

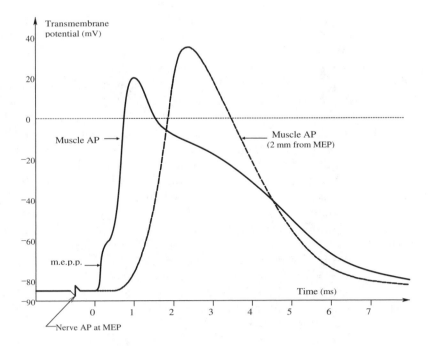

FIGURE 1.3

A typical single-fiber muscle action potential recorded intracellularly at the motor end plate and 2 mm along the fiber.

transmembrane potential can go to as much as +50 mV, forming an end plate potential (EPP) spike fused to the muscle action potential it triggers with a duration of approximately 8 MS, much longer than a nerve action potential. The ACh in the cleft and bound to the receptors is rapidly broken down (hydrolyzed) by the enzyme cholinesterase resident in the cleft, and its molecular components are recycled. A small amount of ACh also escapes the cleft by diffusion and is hydrolyzed as well.

Once the postsynaptic membrane under the MEP depolarizes in a superthreshold end plate potential spike, a muscle action potential is generated that propagates along the surface membrane of the muscle fiber, the sarcolemma. It is the muscle action potential that triggers muscle fiber contraction and force generation. Typical muscle action potentials, recorded intracellularly at the MEP and at a point 2 mm from the initiating MEP, are shown in Figure 1.3. A skeletal muscle fiber action potential propagates at 3 to 5 m/sec; its duration is 2 to 15 msec, depending on the muscle, and it swings from a resting value of approximately −85 mV to a peak of approximately +30 mV. At the skin surface, it appears as a triphasic spike of 20- to 2000-µV peak amplitude (Guyton, 1991).

To ensure that all of the deep contractile apparatus in the center of the muscle fiber is stimulated to contract at the same time and with equal strength, many transverse, radially directed tubules penetrate the center of the fiber along its length. These T-tubules are open to the extracellular fluid space, as is the surface of the fiber, and they are connected to the surface membrane at both ends. The T-tubules conduct the muscle action potential into the interior of the fiber in many locations along its length.

Running longitudinally around the outsides of the contractile myofibrils that make up the fiber are networks of tubules called the *sarcoplasmic reticulum* (SR). Note that the terminal cisternae of the SR butt against the membrane of the T-tubes. When the muscle action potential penetrates along the T-tubes, the depolarization triggers the cisternae to release calcium ions into the space surrounding the myofibrils' contractile proteins. The Ca^{++} binds to the protein troponin C, which triggers contraction by the actin and myosin proteins. (The molecular biophysics of the actual contraction process will not be discussed here.)

A synchronous stimulation of all of the motor neurons innervating a muscle produces what is called a *muscle twitch*; i.e., the tension initially falls a slight amount, rises abruptly, and then falls more slowly to zero again. Sustained muscle contraction is caused by a steady (average) rate of (asynchronous) motoneuron firing. When the firing ceases, the muscle relaxes.

Muscle relaxation is actually an active process. Calcium ion pumps located in the membranes of the SR longitudinal tubules actively transfer Ca^{++} from outside the tubules to inside the SR system. The lack of Ca^{++} in proximity to troponin C allows relaxation to occur. In resting muscle, the concentration, $[Ca^{++}]$, is about 10^{-7} M in the myofibrillar fluid (Guyton, 1991). In a twitch, $[Ca^{++}]$ rises to approximately 2×10^{-5} M and, in a tetanic stimulation, $[Ca^{++}]$ is about 2×10^{-4} M. The Ca^{++} released by a single motor nerve impulse is taken up by the SR pumps to restore the resting $[Ca^{++}]$ level in about 50 msec.

Just as in the case of the sodium pumps in nerve cell membrane, the muscles' Ca^{++} pumps require metabolic energy to operate; adenosine triphosphate (ATP) is cleaved to the diphosphate to release the energy needed to drive the Ca^{++} pumps. The pumps can concentrate the Ca^{++} to approximately 10^{-3} M inside the SR. Inside the SR tubules and cisternae, the Ca^{++} is stored in readily available ionic form, and as a protein chelate, bound to a protein, calsequestrin.

So far, the events associated with a single muscle fiber have been described. As noted earlier, small groups of fibers innervated by a single motoneuron fiber are called a single motor unit (SMU). In muscles used for fine actions, such as those operating the fingers or tongue, fewer muscle fibers, or, equivalently, more motoneuron fibers per total number of muscle fibers, are in a motor unit. For example, the laryngeal muscles used for speech have only two or three fibers per SMU, while large muscles used for gross motions, such as the gastrocnemius, can have several hundred fibers per SMU (Guyton, 1991). To make fine movements, only a few motoneurons fire out of the total number innervating the muscle and these do not fire synchronously. Their firing phase is made random in order to produce smooth contraction. At maximum tetanic stimulation, the mean frequency on the motoneurons is higher, but the phases are still random to reduce the duty cycle of individual SMUs. It is this asynchronicity that makes strong EMGs look like noise on a CRT display.

1.4.3 EMG Amplifiers

The amplifiers used for clinical EMG recording must meet the same stringent specifications for low-leakage currents as do ECG, EEG, and other amplifiers used to measure human body potentials (see Chapter 8). EMG amplifier gains are typically X1000 and their bandwidths reflect the transient nature of the SMU action potentials. An EMG amplifier is generally reactively coupled, with low and high −3-dB frequencies of 100 and 3 kHz, respectively. With an amplifier having variable low and high −3-dB frequencies, one generally starts with a wide-pass bandwidth, e.g., 50 to 10 kHz, and gradually restricts it until individual EMG spikes just begin to round up and change shape. Such an *ad hoc* adjusted bandwidth will give a better output signal-to-noise ratio than one that is too wide or too narrow.

EMGs can be viewed in the time domain (most useful when single fibers or SMUs are being recorded), in the frequency domain (the FFT is taken from an entire, surface-recorded EMG burst under standard conditions), or in the time–frequency (TF) domain (see Section 3.2.3 of Northrop, 2002). In the latter case, the TF display shows the frequencies in the EMG burst as a function of time. In general, higher frequency content in the TF display indicates that more SMUs are being activated at a higher rate (Hannaford and Lehman, 1986). TF analysis can show how agonist–antagonist muscle pairs are controlled to perform a specific motor task.

Still another way to characterize EMG activity in the time domain is to pass the EMG through a true RMS (TRMS) conversion circuit, such as an AD637 IC. The output of the TRMS circuit is a smoothed, positive voltage proportional to the square root of the time average of $x^2(t)$. The time averaging is done by a single time-constant, low-pass filter. For another time domain display modality, the EMG signal can be full wave rectified and low-pass filtered to smooth it.

1.5 The Electrocardiogram

1.5.1 Introduction

One of the most important electrophysiological measurements in medical diagnosis and patient care is that of the electrocardiogram (ECG or EKG). Because the heart is an organ essentially made of muscle, every time it contracts during the cardiac pumping cycle, it generates a spatio–temporal electric field coupled through the anatomically complex volume conductor of the thorax and abdomen to the skin, where a spatio–temporal potential difference can be measured. The amplitude and waveshape of the ECG depends on where the measuring electrode pair is located on the skin surface.

Before electronic amplification was invented, Willem Einthoven measured the ECG in 1901 using a magnetic string galvanometer. The galvanometer was connected to the patient by two wires connected to two carbon rods immersed in two jars of saline solution in which the patient placed either two hands or a hand and a leg (Northrop, 2002). With the advent of electronic amplification in 1928, it was quickly discovered that many interesting features of the ECG could be revealed by using different electrode placements (e.g., AV and precordial leads, and the Frank vector cardiography lead system) (see Chapter 10 through Chapter 12 in Guyton, 1991; Section 4.6 in Webster, 1992; and Section 4.4 in Northrop, 2002).

Figure 1.4 illustrates schematically the important pacemaker, cardiac muscle and conduction bundle transmembrane potentials in the normal human heart and their relation to the classic, Lead III ECG wave. Note that, following atrial contraction, excitation is conducted to the AV node and then to the ventricles by a complex network of specialized muscle cells forming the conduction bundle system. Propagation delay through the bundles and Purkinje fibers allows the ventricles to contract after the atrial contraction has had time to fill them with blood. The QRS spike in the ECG is seen to be associated with the rapid rate of depolarization of ventricular muscle just preceding its contraction. The P wave is caused by atrial depolarization and the T wave is associated with ventricular muscle repolarization.

1.5.2   ECG Amplifiers

Wherever recorded, the ECG QRS spike can range from a 400-μV to 2.5-mV peak. Its amplitude depends on the recording site and the patient's body type; thus the gain required for ECG amplification is approximately 10^3. ECG amplifiers are reactively coupled with standardized −3-dB corner frequencies at 0.05 and 100 Hz. If ECG bandwidth were not standardized, ECG interpretation would be difficult and confusing. Most ECG amplifiers allow the operator to switch in a 60-Hz notch filter to attenuate 60-Hz interference that can appear at the output in spite of differential amplification. The notch filter causes little distortion of the raw ECG output signal.

A further requirement of all ECG amplifiers is that they have galvanic isolation (see Chapter 8), which is required to protect the patient from electroshock accidents. Galvanic isolation places a very high impedance between the patient, the ECG electrodes, and ECG amplifier input ground, and the ECG amplifier output and output ground. This limits any current that might flow through the patient to the single microamps if the patient accidentally makes contact with the power mains while connected to the ECG system

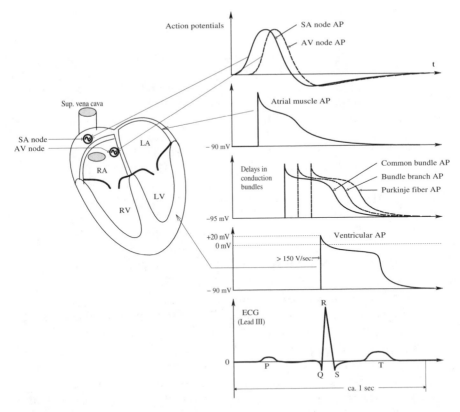

FIGURE 1.4
Schematic cut-away of a mammalian heart showing the SA and AV node pacemakers, as well as intracellular action potentials from different locations in the heart. Bottom trace is a typical lead III skin surface-recorded ECG waveform.

and otherwise not grounded. Other biopotential amplifiers used in a clinical or research setting with humans, such as for measurement of EEG, EMG, ERG, ECoG, etc., must also have galvanic isolation.

1.6 Other Biopotentials

1.6.1 Introduction

Many other biopotentials are measured for research and clinical purposes. These include the electroencephalogram (EEG); electroretinogram (ERG); electrooculogram (EOG); and electrocochleogram (ECoG) (Northrop, 2002). All of these signals are low amplitude (hundreds of microvolts at peak) and contain primarily low frequencies (0.01 to 100 Hz).

1.6.2   EEGs

The electroencephalogram is used to diagnose brain injuries and brain tumors noninvasively, as well as in neuropsychology research. Electroencephalograms are generally recorded from the scalp, which means the underlying, cortical brain electrical activity must pass through the *pia* and *dura mater* membranes, cerebrospinal fluid, skull, and scalp. Considerable attenuation and spatial averaging occurs due to these structures relative to the electrical activity, which can be recorded directly from the brain's surface with wick electrodes. The largest EEG potentials recorded on the scalp are approximately 150 μV at peak. In an attempt to localize sites of EEG activity on the brain's surface, multiple electrode EEG recordings are made from the scalp. The standard 10 to 20 EEG electrode array uses 19 electrodes; some electrode arrays used in brain research use 128 electrodes (Northrop, 2002).
EEGs have traditionally been divided into four frequency bands:

- Delta waves have the largest amplitudes and lowest frequencies (≤3.5 Hz); they occur in adults in deep sleep.

- Theta waves are large-amplitude, low-frequency voltages (3.5 to 7.5 Hz) and are seen in sleep in adults and in prepubescent children.

- The spectra of alpha waves lie between 7.5 and 13 Hz and their amplitudes range from 20 to 200 μV. Alpha waves are recorded from adults who are conscious but relaxed with the eyes closed. Alpha activity disappears when the eyes are open and the subject focuses on a task. Alpha waves are best recorded from posterior lateral portions of the scalp.

- Beta waves are defined for frequencies from 13 to 50 Hz and are most easily found in the parietal and frontal regions of the scalp. Beta waves are subdivided into types I and II: type I disappears and type II appears during intense mental activity (Webster, 1992).

EEG amplifiers must work with low-frequency, low amplitude signals; consequently, they must be low noise types with low $1/f$ noise spectrums. EEG amplifiers can be reactively coupled; their −3-dB frequencies should be about 0.2 and 100 Hz. Amplifier midband gain needs to be on the order of 10^4 to 10^5.

EEG measurement also includes evoked cortical potentials used in experimental brain research. A patient is presented with a periodic stimulus, which can be auditory (a click or tone), visual (a flash of light or a tachistoscopically presented picture), tactile (a pin prick), or some other transient sensory modality. Following each stimulus, a transient EEG response is added to the ongoing EEG activity. Very often this evoked response cannot be seen on a monitor with the naked eye. Because the pass band of the evoked response is the same as the interfering or masking EEG activity, linear filtering does not help in extracting transient response. Thus, signal averaging must be used to bring forth the desired evoked transient from the unrelated, accompanying noise (Northrop, 2002, 2003). Evoked transient electrical response can be recovered by averaging even when the input SNR to the averager is as low as −60 dB.

1.6.3 Other Body Surface Potentials

The electrooculogram (EOG), electroretinogram (ERG), and electrocochleogram (ECoG) are transient, low-amplitude, low-bandwidth potentials recorded for diagnostic and research purposes (Northrop, 2002). Each transient waveform is generally accompanied by unwanted, uncorrelated noise from EMGs and from the electrodes. The EOG is the largest of these three potentials, with a peak on the order of single millivolt. Thus, an ECG amplifier can be used with a 0.05 to 100 Hz −3-dB bandwidth and gain of 10^3. Averaging is generally not required.

The ERG, on the other hand, has a peak amplitude on the order of hundreds of microvolts and accompanying noise makes signal averaging expeditious. The ERG preamplifier generally has a band pass of 0.3 to 300 Hz, a gain of between 10^3 and 10^4, and an input impedance of at least 10 MΩ.

The electrocochleogram is the lowest amplitude transient, with a peak of only approximately 6 μV and waveform features of <1 μV. Signal averaging must be used to resolve the ECoG evoked transient. The signal conditioning amplifier has a midband gain of 10^4 and −3-dB frequencies of 5 and 3 kHz. The ECoG amplifier band pass is defined by 12 dB/octave (two-pole) filters.

1.7 Discussion

The preceding descriptions indicate that the frequency content of endogenous signals from the body ranges from near dc to about 3 kHz. These signals are accompanied by noise, which means that linear filtering to improve the SNR_{in} can often help. Some signals, such as ECoG and evoked brain cortical transients, require signal averaging for meaningful resolution. Endogenous signal peak amplitudes range from over 100 mV for nerve and muscle transmembrane potentials recorded with glass micropipette electrodes to less than a microvolt for evoked cortical transients recorded on the scalp.

1.8 Electrical Properties of Bioelectrodes

To record biopotentials, an interface is needed between the electron-conducting copper wires connected to signal conditioning amplifiers and the ion-conducting, "wet" environment of living animals. Electrodes form this interface. Some of the many kinds of electrodes are better than others in terms of low noise and ease of use. Early ECG electrodes were nondisposable, nickel–silver-plated copper, or stainless steel disks hard-wired to the amplifier input leads. Although conductive gel was used, this type of electrode had inherently high low-frequency noise due to the complex redox reactions taking place at the metal electrode surfaces. Still, acceptable ECG and EMG signals could be recorded.

Present practice in measuring ECG and EMG signals from the skin surface is to use disposable sticky patch electrodes. Patch electrodes use a silver│silver chloride interface to a conductive gel containing Na^+, K^+, and Cl^- ions. The gel makes direct, wet contact with the skin. Adhesive for the skin is found in a ring surrounding the electrolyte and AgCl. The copper wire makes contact with the Ag metal backing of the electrode, generally with a snap connector. More recently, skin electrodes have used Ag│AgCl deposited in a thin layer on an approximately 2.5-cm square of thin plastic film. The conductive gel and adhesive are combined in a layer all over the AgCl film. Contact with this inexpensive electrode is made with a miniature metal alligator clip on one raised corner.

Silver chloride is used with skin patch electrodes and many other types because the dc half-cell potential of the Ag│AgCl electrode depends on the logarithm of the concentration of chloride ions (Webster, 1992). Because the AgCl is in direct contact with the coupling gel, which has a high concentration of Cl^- ions, the dc half-cell potential of the electrode remains fairly stable and has a low impedance, thus low thermal noise.

Figure 1.5 illustrates the electrical characteristics of a pair of Ag│AgCl electrodes facing each other. The impedance measured as a function of frequency, $|2\,\mathbf{Z}_{el}(f)|$ suggests that each electrode can be modeled by a parallel R–C circuit in series with a resistance. Analysis of the impedance magnitude in this figure reveals that $R_G = 65\ \Omega$, $R_i = 1935\ \Omega$, and $C_i = 0.274\ \mu F$ for one electrode. The skin also adds a parallel R–C circuit to the electrode's equivalent circuit.

In general, it is desirable for the electrode $\mathbf{Z}$ to be as small as possible. Both resistors in the electrode model make thermal (white) noise. At low frequencies where the capacitive reactance is $\gg 1935\ \Omega$, one electrode's root noise spectrum is $\sqrt{4kT\,2000} = 5.76$ nV RMS/$\sqrt{Hz}$ — the same order of magnitude as an amplifier's equivalent short-circuit input noise. If the gel dries out during prolonged use, the $\mathbf{Z}_{el}$ will rise, as will the white noise from its real part.

Another type of electrode used in neurophysiological research is the saline-filled, glass micropipette electrode used for recording transmembrane potentials in neurons and muscle fibers. Because the tips of these electrodes are drawn down to diameters of a fraction of a micron before filling, their resistances when filled can range from approximately 20 to 10^3 MΩ, depending on the tip geometry, the filling medium, and the surround medium in which the tip is placed. Because of their high series resistances, glass micropipette electrodes create three major problems not seen with other types of bioelectrodes:

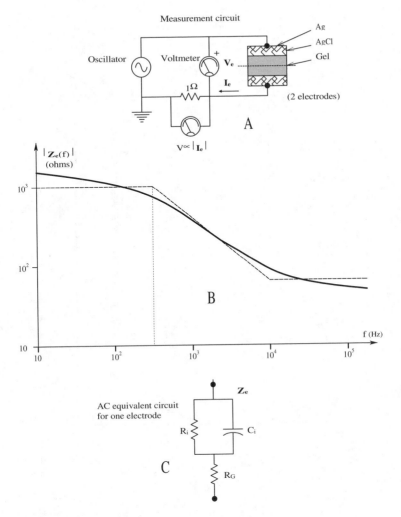

FIGURE 1.5
(A) Impedance magnitude measurement circuit for a pair of face-to-face, silver–silver chloride skin surface electrodes. (B) Typical impedance magnitude for the pair of electrodes in series. (C) Linear equivalent circuit for one electrode.

1. Because of their high series resistances, they must be used with special signal conditioning amplifiers called electrometer amplifiers, which have ultra-low, input dc bias currents. Electrometer input bias currents are on the order of 10 fA (10^{-14} A) and their input resistances are approximately 10^{15} Ω.

2. Glass micropipette electrodes make an awesome amount of Johnson noise. For example, a 200 MΩ electrode at 300 K, with a noise bandwidth of 3 kHz, makes $\sqrt{4kT \times 2 \times 10^8 \times 3 \times 10^3}$ = 99.68 µV RMS of noise.

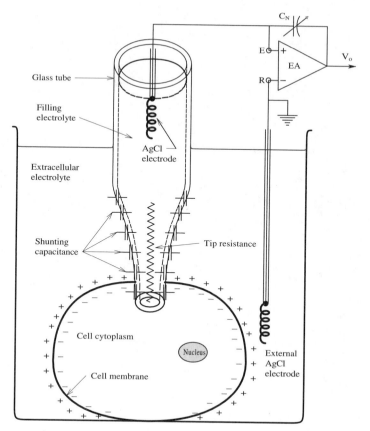

FIGURE 1.6

Schematic cross section (not to scale) of an electrolyte-filled, glass micropipette electrode inserted into the cytoplasm of a cell. Ag|AgCl electrodes are used to interface recording wires (generally Cu) with the electrolytes.

3. The tips of glass micropipette electrodes have significant distributed capacitance between the electrolyte inside and the electrolyte outside the tip (see Figure 1.6), which makes them behave like distributed-parameter low-pass filters, as shown in Figure 1.7(A).

This figure also illustrates the equivalent circuits of the Ag|AgCl coupling electrodes, the cell membrane, and the microelectrode tip spreading resistance and tip EMF. The distributed resistance of the internal electrolyte in the tip, R_{tip}, plus the tip spreading resistance, R_{tc}, plus the cell membrane's resistance, $1/G_c$, are orders of magnitude larger than the impedances associated with the AgCl coupling electrodes. Thus, they can be lumped together as a single R_μ and the distributed tip capacitance can be represented by a single, lumped C_μ in the simplified R–C LPF of Figure 1.7(B). V_{bio} is the bioelectric EMF across the cell membrane in the vicinity of the microelectrode tip. The break frequency of the B circuit is simply $f_b = 1/(2\pi R_\mu C_\mu)$ Hz.

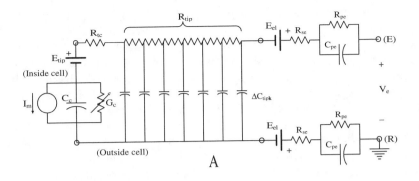

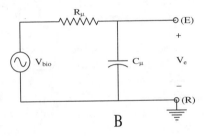

FIGURE 1.7
(A) Equivalent circuit of an intracellular glass microelectrode in a cell, including the equivalent circuits of the Ag|AgCl electrodes. Note the dc half-cell potentials of the electrodes and at the microelectrode's tip. The tip of the microelectrode is modeled by a lumped-parameter, nonuniform, R–C transmission line. (B) For practical purposes, the ac equivalent circuit of the glass micropipette electrode is generally reduced to a simple R–C low-pass filter.

Typical values of circuit parameters are $R_\mu \cong 2 \times 10^8\ \Omega$, $C_\mu \cong 1 \times 10^{-12}$ F. Thus $f_b \cong 796$ Hz. This is too low a break frequency to reproduce a nerve action potential faithfully, which requires at least a dc to 3-kHz bandwidth. To obtain the desired bandwidth, capacitance neutralization is used (capacitance neutralization is described in Section 4.5.2 of Chapter 4). As shown in Section 9.8.4 in Chapter 9, capacitance neutralization adds excess noise to the amplifier output.

1.9 Exogenous Bioelectric Signals

The preceding sections have shown that endogenous bioelectric signals are invariably small, ranging from single microvolts to over 100 mV. Their bandwidths range from dc to perhaps 10 kHz at the most. Signals such as ECG and EEG require approximately 0.1 to 100 Hz. Exogenous signals on the other hand, can involve modalities such as ultrasound, which can use frequencies from hundreds of kilohertz to tens of megahertz, depending on the application. Ultrasound can be continuous wave (CW) sinusoidal, sinusoidal pulses, or wavelets. The purpose here is not to discuss the details of how ultrasound is generated, received, or processed, but rather to comment on the frequencies and signal levels of the received ultrasound.

Reflected ultrasound is picked up by a piezoelectric transducer or transducer array that converts the mechanical sound pressure waves at the skin surface to electrical currents or voltages. Concern for damaging tissues with the transmitted ultrasound intensity (cells destroyed by heating or cavitation) means that input sound intensity must be kept low enough to be safe for living tissues, organs, fetuses, etc., yet high enough to give a good output signal SNR from the reflected sound energy impinging on the receiving transducer. Many ultrasound transducers are used at ultrasound frequencies below their mechanical resonance.

In this region of operation, the transducer has an equivalent circuit described by Figure 1.8. C_x is the capacitance of the transducer, which of course depends on thickness, dielectric constant of its material, and area of the metal film electrodes; C_x is generally on the order of hundreds of picofarads. G_x is the leakage conductance of the piezomaterial and also depends on the material and its dimensions. Expect G_x on the order of 10^{-13} S. The coaxial cable connecting the transducer to the charge amplifier has some shunt capacitance, C_c, which depends on cable length and insulating material; it will be on the order of approximately 30 pF/m. Similarly, the cable has some leakage conductance, G_c, which again is length and material dependent; G_c will be about 10^{-11} S. Finally, the input conductance and capacitance of the electrometer op amp are about $G_i = 10^{-14}$ S and $C_i = 3$ pF.

The circuit of Figure 1.8 is a charge amplifier, which effectively replaces $(C_x + C_c + C_i)$ and $(G_x + G_c + G_i)$ with C_F and G_F in parallel with the transducer's Norton current source. Thus the low-frequency behavior of the system is not set by the poorly defined $(C_x + C_c + C_i)$ and $(G_x + G_c + G_i)$ but rather by the designer-specified components G_F and C_F. (Analysis of the circuit is carried out in detail in Section 6.6.3 of Chapter 6.) Note that the Norton current source, i_x, is proportional to the rate of change of the ultrasound pressure waves impingent on the bottom of the transducer. The constant d has the dimensions of coulombs/newton. The charge displaced inside the transducer is given by $q = d\ F$. The Norton current is simply $i_x \equiv \dot{q} = d\ \dot{F} = d\ \dot{P}A$. If the op amp is assumed to be ideal, then the summing junction is at 0 V and, by Ohm's law, the op amp's output voltage is

$$V_o = \frac{dAsP(s)}{sC_F + G_F} \tag{1.2}$$

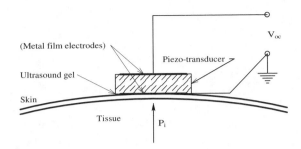

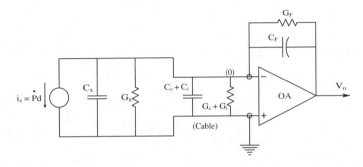

FIGURE 1.8
Top: Cross-sectional schematic of a piezoelectric transducer on the skin surface. The gel is used for acoustic impedance matching to improve acoustic signal capture efficiency. P_i is the sound pressure of the signal being sensed. Bottom: Equivalent circuit of the piezosensor and a charge amplifier. See text for analysis.

Written as a transfer function, this is

$$\frac{V_o}{P}(s) = \frac{dAsR_F}{sC_F R_F + 1} \tag{1.3}$$

At mid-frequencies, the gain is:

$$\frac{V_o}{P}(s) = \frac{dA}{C_F} \text{ volt/pascal} \tag{1.4}$$

The area A is in m^2. The parameter d varies considerably between piezo-materials and also depends on the direction of cut in natural crystals such as quartz, Rochelle salt, and ammonium dihydrogen phosphate. For example, d for X-cut quartz crystals is 2.25×10^{-12} Cb/N and d for barium titanate is approximately 160×10^{-12} Cb/N.

Now consider the mid-frequency output of the charge amplifier when using a lead–zirconate–titanate (LZT) transducer having $d = 140 \times 10^{-12}$ Cb/N, given a sound pressure of 1 dyne/cm^2 = 0.1 Pa; $A = 1$ $cm^2 = 10^{-4}$ m^2; and $C_F = 100$ pF.

$$V_o = \frac{PAd}{C_F} = \frac{0.1 \times 10^{-4} \times 140 \times 10^{-12}}{100 \times 10^{-12}} = 14 \ \mu V \qquad (1.5)$$

Thus, received voltage levels in piezoelectric ultrasonic systems are very low. Considerable low-noise amplification is required and band-pass filtering is necessary to improve signal-to-noise ratio. Not included in the preceding analysis is the high-frequency response of the charge amplifier, which is certainly important when conditioning low-level ultrasonic signals in the range of megahertz. (See Section 6.6.3 in Chapter 6 for high-frequency analysis of the charge amplifier.)

1.10 Chapter Summary

This chapter has stressed that endogenous biomedical signals, whether electrical such as the ECG or EEG, or physical quantities such as blood pressure or temperature, vary relatively slowly; their signal bandwidths are generally from dc to several hundred Hertz and, in the case of nerve spikes or EMGs, may require up to 2 to 4 kHz at the high end. All bioelectric signals are noisy — that is, they are recorded in the company of broadband noise arising from nearby physiological sources; in many cases (e.g., EEG, ERG, EOG, and ECoG), they are in the microvolt range and must compete with amplifier noise. In the case of a skin-surface EMG, the recorded signals are the spatio–temporal summation of many thousand individual sources underlying the electrodes, i.e., many muscle fibers asynchronously generating action potentials as they contract to do mechanical work. In the case of the scalp-recorded EEG, many millions of cortical neurons signal by spiking or by slow depolarization as the brain works, generating a spatio–temporally summed potential between pairs of scalp electrodes.

On the other hand, the electrical activity from the heart is spatially localized. The synchronous spread of depolarization of cardiac muscle during the cardiac cycle generates a relatively strong signal on the skin surface, in spite of the large volume conductor volume through which the ECG electric field must spread. Figure 1.9 illustrates the approximate extreme ranges of peak signal amplitudes and the approximate range of frequencies required to condition EOG, EEG, ECG, and EMG signals. Note that the waveforms that contain spikes or sharp peak transients (ECG and EMG) require a higher bandwidth to characterize.

Exogenous biomedical instrumentation signals, such as diagnostic and Doppler ultrasound and signals from MRI systems, were shown to require bandwidths into the tens of megahertz and higher. Amplifiers required for conditioning such exogenous signals must have high gain bandwidth products (f_T), and high slew rates (η), as well as low noise.

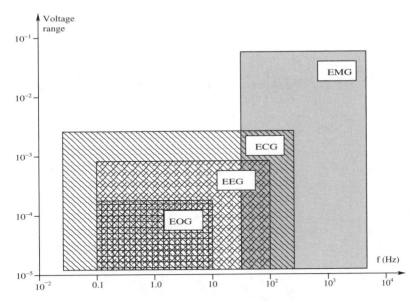

FIGURE 1.9

Approximate RMS spectra of four classes of bioelectric signals. Peak expected RMS signal is plotted vs. extreme range of frequencies characterizing the signal.

2

Models for Semiconductor Devices Used in Analog Electronic Systems

2.1 Introduction

This chapter will describe the properties and characteristics of the semiconductor components of analog integrated circuits (AICs). These include diodes, bipolar junction transistors (BJTs), and various types of field-effect transistors (FETs). Biomedical engineers probably will never be called upon to design circuits with or use discrete transistors, with the possible exception of power transistors. Instead, modern analog electronic systems use integrated circuits. To appreciate the behavior and limitations of ICs, however, it is necessary to understand the fundamental behavior of their semiconductor components. (The actual design of ICs is beyond the scope of this text.) One of the most ubiquitous analog ICs is the operational amplifier (op amp); op amps are used in many signal conditioning applications, including differential amplifiers; instrumentation amplifiers; active filters; true RMS converters; precision rectifiers; track-and-hold circuits; etc. Other commonly encountered ICs in biomedical engineering are dc voltage regulators, temperature sensors, phase-lock loops, synchronous rectifiers, analog multipliers, dc-to-dc converters, medical isolation amplifiers, analog-to-digital converters (ADCs), digital-to-analog converters (DACs), etc.

Specifically, the following sections will examine the salient circuit characteristics of *pn* junction diodes, light-emitting diodes (LEDs), laser diodes (LADs), *npn* and *pnp* small-signal BJTs, junction field-effect transistors (JFETs), and n- and p-MOSFETs. Large-signal and mid- and high-frequency small-signal models will be considered. The mid- and high-frequency behavior of IC "building blocks" that use two transistors will also be analyzed.

2.2 *pn* Junction Diodes

2.2.1 Introduction

There are several uses for *pn* junction diodes as discrete components and in ICs. As stand-alone components, power diodes are used to rectify ac to produce dc in power supplies. They are also used with inductive components such as relay coils, motor coils, and loudspeaker windings to clamp inductive voltage switching transients to prevent them from destroying the switching transistors. Small, discrete *pn* diodes are also used in op amp precision rectifier circuits, peak detectors, sample-and-hold circuits, logarithmic amplifiers, and exponential amplifiers. Diodes are used in IC designs for temperature compensation, to make current mirrors, and for dc level shifting (in the avalanche mode) (Millman, 1979).

2.2.2 The *pn* Diode's Volt–Ampere Curve

Figure 2.1 illustrates the static volt–ampere curve of a typical silicon *pn* signal diode (as opposed to power rectifier diode). Note the three major regions in the curve: (1) the forward conduction region in the first quadrant, the (2) blocking region, and the (3) avalanche breakdown (or zener) region in the third quadrant. The volt–ampere behavior of a diode's forward and blocking regions can be approximated with the well-known approximate mathematical model:

$$i_D = I_{rs} \left[\exp(v_D / \eta V_T) - 1 \right] \qquad (2.1)$$

v_D is the dc voltage across the diode, $V_T \equiv kT/q$, where T is the Kelvin temperature of the junction; q is the electron charge magnitude (1.6×10^{-19} Cb); k is Boltzmann's constant (1.38×10^{-23} J/K); and η is a bugger factor between 1 and 2 used to fit the diode curve to experimental data. $\eta \cong 2$ for silicon diodes; I_{rs} is the reverse saturation current (on the order of μA for signal diodes). I_{rs} is a strong increasing function of temperature and is taken to be non-negative. At 25°C, $V_T = 0.0257$ V. The crudeness of the model can be appreciated in the blocking region where the exponential argument is large and negative, so $i_D \cong -I_{rs}$. In reality, there is a strong ohmic (leakage) component to the reverse i_D, so the approximation, $i_D \cong -I_{rs} + v_D/\rho$, is more realistic for $v_D < 0$. ρ has the dimensions of resistance (ohms).

Avalanche occurs under reverse-biased conditions when minority carriers conducting the reverse i_D gain enough kinetic energy by accelerating in the strong electric field and, through collisions with the substrate atoms' electrons, create new electron–hole pairs. These new carriers in turn are accelerated in the high E-field and cause still more carriers to be formed. This avalanche process can be modeled by the empirical equation:

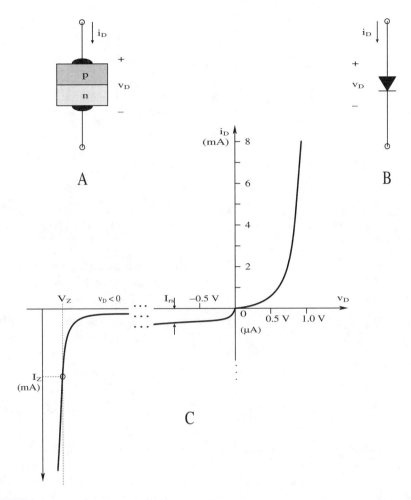

FIGURE 2.1
(A) "Layer cake" cross section of a silicon *pn* junction diode. (B) Diode symbol. (C) Typical I–V curve for a small-signal, Si diode, showing avalanche (zener) breakdown at reverse bias, $v_D = -V_z$.

$$i_D \cong \frac{-I_{rs}}{1 - \left| (v_D/V_z)^n \right|} \tag{2.2}$$

The exponent, n, can range from 3 to 6 and v_D lies between 0 and V_z. Depending on how the *pn* junction is doped (the density of donor atoms in the n material and acceptor atoms in the p material), V_z can range from approximately 3.2 to over 100 V.

Diodes operated in their avalanche regions can be used as voltage sources or references, and for dc voltage level shifting. Figure 2.2 illustrates an

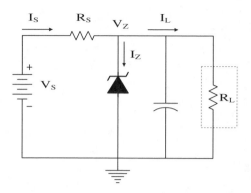

FIGURE 2.2
Use of an avalanche (zener) diode as a DC voltage source for R_L. The diode's zener resistance is neglected.

avalanche dc voltage source circuit. The tantalum filter capacitor is used to lower the source impedance of the avalanche supply at high frequencies. From Ohm's law:

$$I_L = V_Z/R_L \tag{2.3}$$

$$I_S = I_L + I_Z \tag{2.4}$$

$$R_S = \left(V_S - V_Z\right)/I_S = \frac{\left(V_S - V_Z\right)}{I_Z + V_Z/R_L} \tag{2.5}$$

Every avalanche (zener) diode has a preferred operating point, (V_Z, I_Z), given by the manufacturer, at which its dynamic impedance is low and power dissipation is safe. Thus in Equation 2.5 V_Z and I_Z are known and R_L is known (or I_L at V_Z), enabling one to find the required series R_S. The required power dissipated in R_S is simply $P_{R_S} = (V_S - V_Z)^2/R_S = I_S^2 R_S$ watts.

Excluding the avalanche region, the dc characteristics of a *pn* junction diode can be modeled by an ideal diode (ID) model, shown in Figure 2.3(A). For the ideal diode, $i_D = 0$ for $v_D < 0$, and $v_D = 0$ for $i_D > 0$. Figure 2.3(B) shows that, by adding a reverse-biasing voltage source, V_F, model diode volt–ampere curve can be shifted to the right by V_F. The model is made yet more real by adding the series resistance, R_F, in the conduction path, as shown in Figure 2.3(C). In Figure 2.3(D), a leakage conductance is added in parallel with the model of C to model reverse diode leakage.

The ideal diode and its variations are useful for pencil-and-paper circuit analysis. Detailed simulation of electronic circuits containing diodes is done with electronic circuit analysis programs (ECAPs) such as PSPICE and Micro-Cap, which handle the nonlinearity algebraically as well as compute the diode's voltage-dependent shunt capacitance.

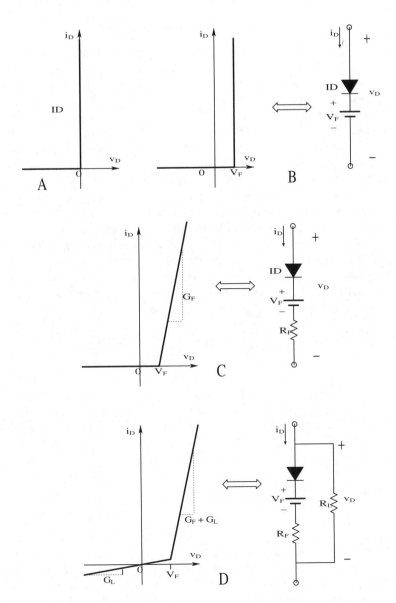

FIGURE 2.3
Various I–V models for junction diodes, excluding avalanche behavior. (A) Ideal diode. (B) Ideal diode in series with fixed forward voltage drop. (C) Ideal diode in series with fixed forward voltage drop and forward resistance. (D) Ideal diode in series with fixed forward voltage drop and forward resistance, and reverse leakage resistance.

2.2.3   High-Frequency Behavior of Diodes

A fundamental limitation to the high-frequency performance of *pn* semiconductor diodes is their voltage-dependent, small-signal junction capacitance.
The junction capacitance mechanism is different for forward conduction
($v_D > 0$) and reverse bias conditions ($v_D < 0$).

As demonstrated earlier, when a diode is dc reverse-biased, a very small
(nA) reverse leakage current flows, part of which is due to the thermal
(random) generation of hole–electron pairs in the depletion region of the
device. The depletion region is a volume around the junction in the p- and
n-doped semiconductor sides that is free of mobile carriers (holes and electrons, respectively). The electric field from the negative v_D causes the carriers
to move away from the junction, creating what is essentially a layer of charge-
free intrinsic semiconductor around the junction. The more negative v_D is,
the stronger the electric field and the larger the depletion region. The charge-
free depletion region behaves like a leaky dielectric in a parallel-plate capacitor. The capacitor's "plates" are the dense conductive semicon region where
majority carriers still exist and conductivity is high. Recall that the capacitance of a simple parallel-plate capacitor is given by:

$$C = \frac{A\kappa\varepsilon_o}{d} \text{ farads} \tag{2.6}$$

where κ is the dielectric constant of silicon; A is the area of the diode junction
in m²; and d is the effective "plate" separation in m. Note that the effective
d increases as v_D goes more negative and the electric field increases at the
junction. Thus C_d decreases as v_D goes more negative and is maximum at
$v_D = 0$. Diode depletion capacitance can be modeled by the function:

$$C_d(v_D) = \frac{C_d(0)}{\left(1 - v_D/\psi_o\right)^n} \text{ farads, for } v_D < 0 \tag{2.7}$$

where $C_d(0)$ is the value of the depletion capacitance at $v_D = 0$ and ψ_o is the
contact potential of the *pn* junction determined by the carrier doping densi-
ties at the junction and their gradients. ψ_o ranges from 0.2 to 0.9 V, and is in
the neighborhood of 0.75 V at room temperature for a typical silicon small-
signal diode. The exponent, n, ranges from 0.33 to 3, depending on the
doping profile near the *pn* junction; $n = 0.5$ for an abrupt (symmetrical step)
junction. For depletion, $v_D < 0$ in Equation 2.7. Note that, as v_D goes positive
and approaches ψ_o, C_d approaches ∞. Clearly, Equation 2.7 is intended to
model diode capacitance for $-V_Z < v_D < 0$. Typical values for $C_d(0)$ are in the
range of tens of picofarads. A typical reverse-biased, *pn* diode's junction
capacitance vs. v_D is shown in Figure 2.4. A detailed analysis of *pn* junction
behavior can be found in Millman (1979), Yang (1988), or Gray and Meyer
(1984).

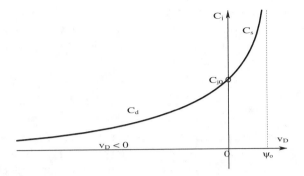

FIGURE 2.4
How the equivalent junction capacitance of a pn diode varies with v_D. C_d is mostly depletion capacitance (see text) and C_s is due to stored minority carriers associated with forward conduction.

A forward-biased diode's pn junction is characterized by a large, current-dependent diffusion or charge storage capacitance, which involves an entirely different mechanism from depletion capacitance. Under forward bias conditions, minority carriers are injected across the junction, where they quickly recombine. That is, electrons are injected into the p-side from the n-side and holes are injected into the n-side from the p-side. The mean lifetime of electrons in the p-side is τ_n and of holes in the n-side, τ_p. These injected minority carriers represent a stored charge, Q_s, around the junction. By definition, the small-signal diffusion capacitance can be written for a symmetrical junction where $\tau = \tau_p = \tau_n$:

$$C_D = \frac{dQ_s}{dv_D} = \frac{\tau di_D}{dv_D} = \tau g_d = \frac{\tau i_{DQ}}{\eta V_T} = \frac{\tau I_{rs}\exp\!\left(v_{DQ}/V_T\right)}{\eta V_T} \text{ farads for } v_D > 0 \; CD \quad (2.8)$$

where g_d is the small-signal conductance of the forward-biased diode at its dc operating (Q) point; $g_d \equiv \partial i_D/\partial v_D$ at Q. i.e., $g_d = d[I_{rs}\exp(v_D/\eta V_T)]/dv_D|_Q = I_{rs}\exp(v_{DQ}/\eta V_T)/(\eta V_T) = i_{DQ}/\eta V_T$ siemens. If the diode junction doping is asymmetrical, it can be shown (Nanavati, 1975) that the diffusion capacitance is given by:

$$C_D = \frac{1}{\eta V_T}\left(I_{DnQ}\tau_n + I_{DpQ}\tau_p\right) \text{ farads} \quad (2.9)$$

The diode forward current is broken into the electron and hole injection currents. For example, calculate the diffusion capacitance of a silicon diode with a symmetrically doped step junction at 300 K, forward-biased with $i_{DQ} = 10$ mA. Take $\tau = 1$ μs, $\eta = 2$.

$$C_D = \frac{1\,\text{E-6} \times 1\,\text{E-2}}{2 \times 0.026} = 0.192 \; \mu\text{F} \quad (2.10)$$

This is a relatively enormous small-signal capacitance that appears in parallel with the diode model. The capacitance, C_D, affects the speed at which the diode can turn off. However, the forward-biased diode has the time constant:

$$\tau_d = C_D/g_d = 1.92 \text{ E-7}/\left(1 \text{ E-2}/(2 \times 0.026)\right) \cong 1 \text{ μs} \qquad (2.11)$$

which is basically the mean minority carrier lifetime, τ. Thus, C_D has little effect on mid-frequency, small-signal performance, but the stored charge does affect the time to stop conducting when v_D goes step negative.

Figure 2.5 illustrates the current, voltage, and excess minority charge waveforms in the n-material for a *pn* junction diode in which a step of forward voltage is followed by a step of reverse voltage. Note that V_D remains at the forward value following switching to V_R until all the excess minority carriers have been discharged from C_D. Then $V_D \rightarrow -V_R$ and depletion capacitance dominates the junction behavior. The storage time is on the order of nano-seconds for most small-signal Si, *pn* diodes.

2.2.4   Schottky Diodes

The Schottky barrier diode (SBD), also called a *hot carrier diode*, consists of a rectifying, metal insulator–semiconductor (MIS) junction. SBDs actually pre-date *pn* junction diodes by about 50 years. The first detectors in early crystal set radios were "cat's whisker" diodes, in which a fine lead wire made contact with a metallic mineral crystal, such as galena, silicon, or germanium. Such cat's whisker detectors were, in fact, primitive SBDs. Because their rectifier characteristics were not reproducible, cat's whisker SBDs were only suited for early radio experimenters and were replaced by *pn* junction diodes in the 1950s.

The presence of a very thin, insulating interfacial oxide layer from 0.5 to 1.5 nm thick between the metal and the semicon makes a modern SBD different from an ordinary ohmic, metal–semiconductor connection. Figure 2.6 shows the static I–V characteristics of a *pn* diode and an SBD. Note that the SBD has a lower cut-in voltage (approximately 0.3 V) than the *pn* diode (approximately 0.55 V) as well as about 1000 times the reverse leakage current (0.1 μA vs. 1 nA), which does not saturate. A schematic cross section of an SBD (after Boylstead and Nashelsky, 1987) is shown on the figure.

The SBD is a majority carrier device; a *pn*D is a minority carrier device. In order for a *pn*D to block reverse current, the stored minority carriers must be swept out of the junction by the reverse electric field. This discharging limits the turn-off time to microseconds. On the other hand, the SBD has no minority carrier storage and can switch off in tens of nanoseconds, meaning the SBD can rectify currents in the hundreds of megahertz. Figure 2.7 shows a high-frequency SSM for the SBD when conducting. Note that the SS forward

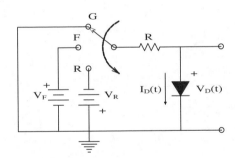

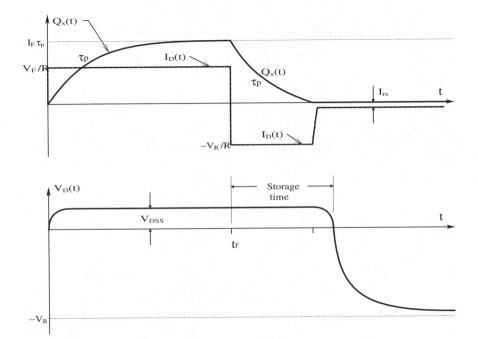

FIGURE 2.5

Schematic showing the effect of switching a diode from $v_D = 0$, $i_D = 0$, to forward conduction. With V_F applied, v_D quickly rises to the steady-state forward drop, $v_{DSS} \cong 0.7$ V, and the XS minority carriers build up to a charge, Q_x. When the applied voltage is switched to $-V_R$, a finite time is required for Q_x to be dissipated before the diode can block current. During this storage time, v_D remains at v_{DSS}.

resistance, r_d, and the junction capacitance, C_J, are dependent on i_D and v_D, respectively. Hewlett–Packard hot carrier diodes of the 5082-2300 series have reverse currents of approximately 50 to 100 nA at $v_D = -10$ V, and $C_J = 0.3$ pF at $v_D = -10$ V.

Besides high-frequency rectification and detection, SBDs can be used to speed up transistor switching in logic gates. Figure 2.8 illustrates a SBD placed in parallel with the *pn* base-to-collector diode in an npn BJT. In normal

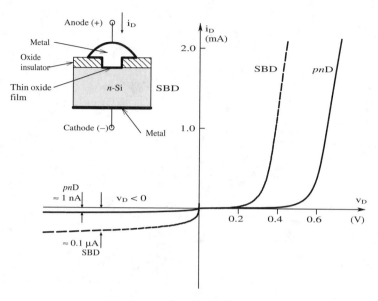

FIGURE 2.6
The static I–V curves of a Schottky barrier diode and a *pn* junction diode.

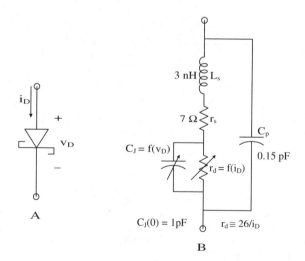

FIGURE 2.7
(A) Symbol for SDB (not to be confused with that for the zener diode). (B) High-frequency equivalent circuit for a SBD.

linear operation, the C–B junction is reverse-biased. When the transistor is saturated, the B–E and the C–B junctions are forward-biased. Without the SBD, there is large minority charge storage in the C–B junction. With the SBD, much of the excess base current will flow through the SBD, preventing large excess charge storage in the C–B junction and allowing the BJT to turn

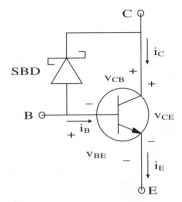

FIGURE 2.8
Use of an SBD to make a Schottky transistor. The SBD prevents XS stored charge in the BJT's
C–B junction.

off much more quickly (Yang, 1988). SBD thin film technology is also used
in the fabrication of certain MOS transistors (Nanavati, 1975).

2.3   Mid-Frequency Models for BJT Behavior

2.3.1   Introduction

Most BJTs found on ICs are silicon *pnp* or *npn*. (Other fabrication materials,
such as gallium arsenide, exist but will not be treated here.) A heuristic view
of BJTs is shown by the "layer cake" models shown in Figure 2.9(B). BJTs
are generally viewed as current-controlled current sources in their "linear"
operating regions. As in the case of *pn* diodes, the large-signal, dc behavior
of these three terminal devices will first be examined. Figure 2.9(C) illustrates
typical volt–ampere curves for a small-signal (as opposed to power) *npn* BJT.

For purposes of dc biasing and crude circuit calculations on paper, an *npn*
BJT in its active region can be represented by the simple circuit shown in
Figure 2.10(A). The voltage drop of the forward-biased B–E junction is represented by V_{BEQ} on the order of 0.6 V. The dc collector current is approximated by the current-controlled current source (CCCS) with gain β_o. β_o is the
transistor's nominal (forward) dc current gain. Figure 2.10(B) illustrates the
dc model for the transistor when it is saturated. Saturation occurs for $i_B >
i_C/\beta_o$, i.e., for high base currents. In saturation, the B–E and C–B junctions
are forward-biased, producing a V_{CEsat} that can range from approximately
0.2 to 0.8 V for high collector currents. The collector-emitter saturation curve
can be approximated by the simple Thevenin circuit shown: $r_{csat} = \partial v_{CE}/\partial i_C$
at the operating point on the saturation curve; V_{CEsat} is used to make the
model fit the published curves.

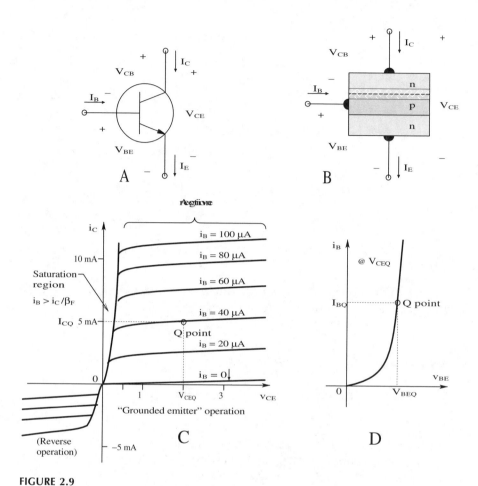

FIGURE 2.9

(A) Symbol for an *npn* BJT. (B) "Layer cake" cross section of a forward-biased *npn* BJT. The cross-hatched layer represents the depletion region of the normally reverse-biased *C–B* junction. (C) Collector–base I–V curves as a function of i_B for the *npn* BJT. (D) Base–emitter I–V curve at constant V_{CEQ}. The *B–E* junction is normally forward biased.

When a *pnp* BJT's large-signal behavior is considered, the actual dc currents *leave* the base and collector nodes and *enter* the emitter node. Consequently, in the $i_C = f(v_{CE}, i_B)$ and $i_B = g(v_{BE}, v_{CE})$ curves shown in Figure 2.11, all currents and voltages are taken as *negative* (with respect to the directions and signs of the *npn* BJT). Figure 2.10(C) and Figure 2.10(D) illustrate the dc biasing models for a *pnp* BJT. Note that the sign of the CCCS is not changed; a negative I_B times a positive β yields a negative I_C, as intended.

Figure 2.12 illustrates how the dc biasing model of Figure 2.10(A) is used to set an *npn* transistor's operating point in its active region. As an example, the required base-biasing resistor, R_B, given the transistor's $β_o$, and the desired Q-point (I_{CQ}, V_{CEQ}) for the device will be found, as well as the necessary R_C and R_E. V_{CC} and the requirement that $V_{CEQ} = V_{CC}/2$ and $V_E =$

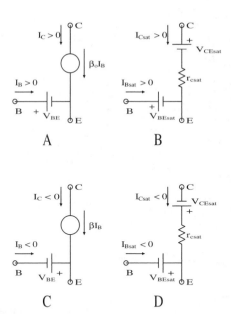

FIGURE 2.10
(A) Simple dc biasing model for an *npn* BJT in its forward linear operating region (see text for examples). (B) dc biasing model for an *npn* BJT in forward saturation. (C) Simple dc biasing model for a *pnp* BJT in its forward linear operating region. (D) dc biasing model for a *pnp* BJT in forward saturation.

0.5 V are given. Pick numbers: $V_{CC} \equiv 12$ V at the Q-point, $V_{CEQ} \equiv 6$ V, and the desired $I_{CQ} \equiv 1$ mA. $\beta_o \equiv 80$ and $V_{BEQ} \equiv 0.5$ V. It is known that $V_C = V_E + V_{CEQ} = 6.5$ V; thus the voltage across R_C is 5.5 V. From Ohm's law, $R_C = 5.5/0.001 = 5.5$ kΩ. Furthermore, $I_{BQ} = I_{CQ}/\beta_o = 0.001/80 = 12.5$ μA and $V_B = V_{BEQ} + V_E = 1$ V, so $R_B = (12 - 1)/12.5 = 880$ kΩ. Note that the emitter current is $I_E = (\beta + 1)I_B = I_C(1 + 1/\beta)$. Thus, $R_E = 0.5/(1 + 1/80) = 494$ Ω.

2.3.2 Mid-Frequency Small-Signal Models for BJTs

To find the voltage amplification factor or gain of a simple *npn* BJT amplifier, we use what is called a *two-port, mid-frequency, small-signal model* (MFSSM) for the transistor. The MFSSM also allows calculation of the amplifier's input and output resistances. The most common MFSSM for BJTs is the common-emitter h-parameter model shown in Figure 2.13. The two-input *h*-parameters define a Thevenin input circuit between the base and emitter, and the output *h*-parameter pair defines a Norton equivalent circuit between the collector and emitter. The input resistance, h_{ie}, is derived operationally from the slope of the nonlinear $I_B = f(V_{BE}, V_{CE})$ curves at the Q-point, as shown in Figure 2.11. That is:

$$h_{ie} = \frac{\Delta v_{BE}}{\Delta i_B}\bigg|_{Q, V_{ce}=\text{const.}} \quad \text{Ohms} \tag{2.12}$$

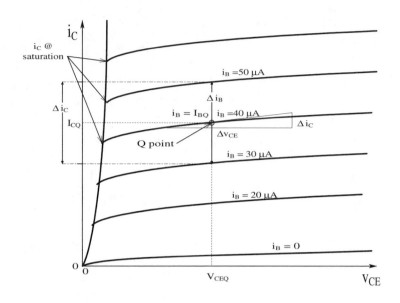

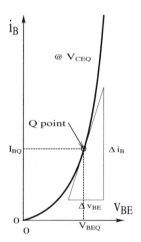

FIGURE 2.11

Top: a large-scale plot of a typical BJT's i_C vs. v_{CE} curves. The Q point is the transistor's quiescent operating point. The small-signal conductance looking into the collector–emitter nodes is approximated by $g_o = \Delta i_C / \Delta v_{CE}$ siemens. The small-signal collector current gain is $\beta = \Delta i_C / \Delta i_B$. Bottom: the i_B vs. v_{BE} curve at the Q point. The small-signal resistance looking into the BJT's base is $r_b = \Delta v_{BE} / \Delta i_B$ ohms.

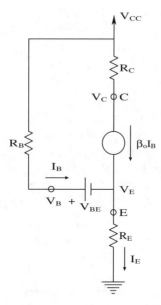

FIGURE 2.12
Model for dc biasing of an *npn* BJT with collector, base, and emitter resistors. See text for analysis.

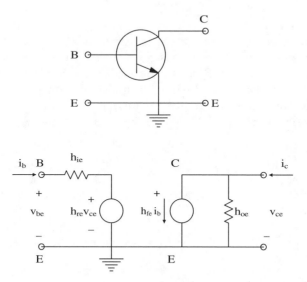

FIGURE 2.13
Top: an *npn* BJT viewed as a two-port circuit. Bottom: the linear, common-emitter, two-port, small-signal, *h*-parameter model for the BJT operating around some Q in its linear region. Note that the input circuit is a Thevenin model and the output is a Norton model.

h_{re} is the gain of a voltage-controlled voltage source (VCVS), which models how the base voltage is modulated by changes in v_{CE}. In other terms, h_{re} is the open-circuit reverse transfer voltage gain.

$$h_{re} = \frac{\Delta v_{BE}}{\Delta v_{CE}}\bigg|_{Q, i_B = \text{const.}} \tag{2.13}$$

For most pencil-and-paper transistor gain calculations using the C–E SMF-SSM, h_{re} is set to zero because it (1) has a second-order contribution to calculations and (2) simplifies calculations. For the collector–base Norton model, h_{oe} is the output conductance that results from the $i_C = f(v_{CE}, i_B)$ curves having a finite upward slope. Figure 2.11 shows that h_{oe} is given by:

$$h_{oe} = \frac{\Delta i_C}{\Delta v_{CE}}\bigg|_{Q, i_B = \text{const.}} \quad \text{siemens} \tag{2.14}$$

Finally, the forward, current-controlled current source gain, h_{fe}, is found:

$$h_{fe} = \frac{\Delta i_C}{\Delta i_B}\bigg|_{Q, V_{ce} = \text{const.}} \tag{2.15}$$

h_{fe} is also called the transistor's β.

One question that invariably arises concerns the MFSSM to be used when a grounded emitter *pnp* transistor is considered. The answer is simple: the same model as for an *npn* BJT. Whether a BJT is *npn* or *pnp* affects the dc biasing of the transistors, not their gains and small-signal input and output impedances. The quiescent operating point of *pnp* and *npn* transistors affects the numerical values of the C–E h-parameters. For example, h_{re} can be approximated by:

$$h_{re} = r_x + r_\pi \text{ ohms} \tag{2.16}$$

where r_x = the base spreading resistance, a fixed resistor with a range of 15 to 150 Ω, and r_π = the dynamic, SS resistance of the forward-biased base–emitter junction.

The value of r_π can be estimated from the basic diode equation for the B–E junction:

$$I_B = I_{bs} \exp(V_{BEQ}/\eta V_T) \text{ amps} \tag{2.17}$$

The resistance, r_π, is given by:

$$r_\pi = \frac{1}{g_\pi} = \frac{1}{\partial i_B/\partial v_{BE}} = \frac{\eta V_T}{I_{BQ}} = \frac{\eta V_T h_{fe}}{I_{CQ}} \text{ ohms} \tag{2.18}$$

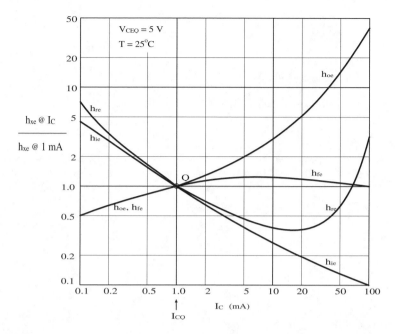

FIGURE 2.14

A normalized plot of how the four common-emitter, small-signal *h*-parameters vary with collector current at constant V_{CEQ}. Note that the output conductance, h_{oe}, increases markedly with increasing collector current, while the input resistance, h_{ie}, decreases linearly. (Note that the same sort of plot can be made of normalized, *C–E h*-parameters vs. at constant I_{CQ}.)

For a silicon BJT with $I_{BQ} = 5 \times 10^{-5}$ A, $r_\pi = 1.04$ kΩ.

Figure 2.14 illustrates how the four *C–E h*-parameters vary with I_C/I_{CQ} at constant V_{CEQ}. Note that the forward current gain, h_{fe}, is the most constant with I_C/I_{CQ}. The collector–emitter Norton conductance, h_{oe}, increases monotonically with I_C/I_{CQ} because, as I_C increases, the $I_C = f(V_{CE}, I_B)$ curves tip upward. h_{ie} decreases monotonically with increasing I_C, as predicted by Equation 2.18. All four h_{xe} parameters increase with temperature.

Another MFSSM used to analyze transistor amplifier behavior on paper is the grounded-base, *h*-parameter model, shown in Figure 2.15. Clearly, this MFSSM is useful in analyzing grounded-base BJT amplifiers; however, the same results can be obtained using the more common grounded-emitter, *h*-parameter MFSSM. The GB *h*-parameters are found experimentally from:

$$h_{ib} = \frac{\Delta v_{EB}}{\Delta i_E}\bigg|_{Q, v_{CB}=\text{const.}} \qquad \text{ohms} \qquad (2.19A)$$

$$h_{rb} = \frac{\Delta v_{EB}}{\Delta i_{CB}}\bigg|_{Q, i_e=\text{const.}} \qquad (2.19B)$$

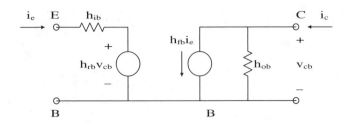

FIGURE 2.15
The common-base *h*-parameter SSM for *npn* and *pnp* BJTs. Using linear algebra, it is possible to express any set of four linear, two-port parameters in terms of any others. (Northrop, R.B., 1990, *Analog Electronic Circuits: Analysis and Applications*, Addison–Wesley, Reading, MA.)

$$h_{fb} = \frac{\Delta i_C}{\Delta i_E}\bigg|_{Q,v_{CB}=\text{const.}} \tag{2.19C}$$

$$h_{ob} = \frac{\Delta i_C}{\Delta v_{CB}}\bigg|_{Q,i_E=\text{const.}} \quad \text{siemens} \tag{2.19D}$$

Most manufacturers of discrete BJTs do not give GB *h*-parameters in their specification data sheets.

2.3.3 Amplifiers Using One BJT

Three basic amplifier configurations can be made with one BJT: (1) the grounded-emitter; (2) the emitter-follower (grounded collector); and (3) the grounded-base amplifier. These three configurations are described and analyzed next.

The first example illustrates how to use the *C–E h*-parameter MFSSM to find expressions for the voltage gain, K_V, and the input and output resistance of a grounded emitter amplifier, shown in Figure 2.16(A). This figure illustrates a basic grounded emitter amplifier driven by a small ac signal, v_s, through a coupling capacitor, C_c. In the MFSSM amplifier model, only small-signal variations around the BJT's operating (Q) point are considered; thus all dc voltage sources are set to zero and replaced with short circuits to ground. Figure 2.16(B) illustrates the complete amplifier model ($h_{re} = 0$ for simplicity). The SS output voltage is, by inspection:

$$v_o = \frac{-h_{fe}i_b}{G_c + h_{oe}} \tag{2.20}$$

The base current is given by Ohm's law, assuming negligible SS current flows in R_B ($R_B \gg h_{ie}$).

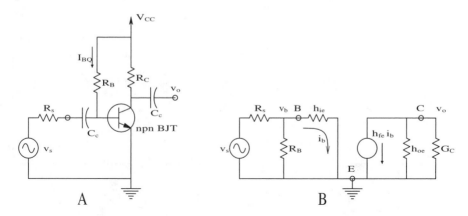

FIGURE 2.16
(A) Schematic of a simple, capacitively coupled, grounded-emitter BJT amplifier. (B) Linear, mid-frequency, small-signal model (MFSSM) of the grounded-emitter amplifier. Note that, at mid-frequencies, capacitors are treated as short circuits and DC source voltages are small-signal grounds. The mid-frequency gain, v_o/v_s, can be found from the model; see text.

$$i_b \cong \frac{v_s}{R_s + h_{ie}} \tag{2.21}$$

Thus, the amplifier's SS voltage gain is found by substituting Equation 2.21 into Equation 2.20:

$$\frac{v_o}{v_s} = \frac{-h_{fe}R_C}{(h_{oe}R_C + 1)(R_s + h_{ie})} = K_V \tag{2.22}$$

By inspection, its SS input resistance is $R_{in} \cong R_s + h_{ie}$ and its (Thevenin) output resistance is $R_{out} = 1/(h_{oe} + G_C)$.

In a second example, a BJT emitter-follower amplifier is shown in Figure 2.17. Figure 2.17(B) illustrates the MFSSM for the emitter follower. To find an expression for the EF gain, write the node equations for the v_b and v_o nodes:

$$v_b [G_s + G_B + g_{ie}] - v_o [g_{ie}] = v_s G_s \tag{2.23A}$$

$$-v_b g_{ie} + v_o [G_E + h_{oe} + g_{ie}] - h_{fe} i_b = 0 \tag{2.23B}$$

where $g_{ie} = 1/h_{ie}$ and $i_b = (v_b - v_o)g_{ie}$. When the expression for i_b is substituted into Equation 2.23B,

$$-v_b \left[g_{ie}(1 + h_{fe}) \right] + v_o \left[G_E + h_{oe} + g_{ie}(1 + h_{fe}) \right] = 0 \tag{2.24}$$

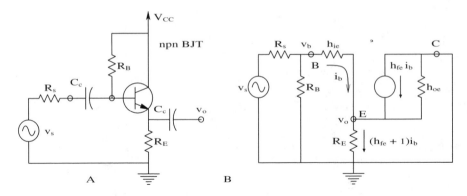

FIGURE 2.17
(A) Schematic of a simple, capacitively coupled, emitter-follower amplifier. (B) MFSSM of the
EF amplifier.

Now Equation 2.23A and Equation 2.24 are solved using Cramer's rule, yielding the voltage gain:

$$\frac{v_o}{v_s} = \frac{G_s g_{ie}\left(1+h_{fe}\right)}{\left(G_s+G_B\right)\left[G_E+h_{oe}+g_{ie}\left(1+h_{fe}\right)\right]+g_{ie}\left(G_E+h_{oe}\right)} = K_V \qquad (2.25)$$

This rather unwieldy expression can be simplified using the *a priori* knowledge that, usually, $G_E \gg h_{oe}$ and $G_s \gg G_B$. Equation 2.25 is multiplied top and bottom by $h_{ie}\, R_E\, R_s$. After some algebra, the simplified EF gain is found to be:

$$K_V \cong \frac{R_E\left(1+h_{fe}\right)}{R_E\left(1+h_{fe}\right)+h_{ie}+R_s} \qquad (2.26)$$

Note that K_v for the EF is positive (noninverting) and slightly less than 1. What then is the point of an amplifier with no gain? The answer lies in the EF's high input impedance and low output impedance. The EF is used to buffer sources and drive coaxial cables and transmission lines with low characteristic impedances. It is easy to show that the EF's input impedance at the v_b node is simply R_B in parallel with $[h_{ie} + R_E (1 + h_{fe})]$ (h_{oe} is neglected). The Thevenin output impedance can be found for the linear MFSSM by taking the ratio of the open circuit voltage (OCV) to its short-circuit current (SCC). The OCV is simply $v_s K_V$:

$$V_{OC} \cong \frac{v_s R_E\left(1+h_{fe}\right)}{R_E\left(1+h_{fe}\right)+h_{ie}+R_s} \qquad (2.27)$$

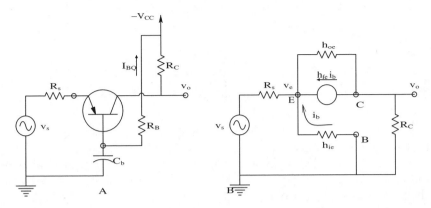

FIGURE 2.18
(A) Schematic of a simple, capacitively coupled, grounded-base amplifier. (B) MFSSM of the
GB amplifier.

The SCC is simply $i_{bsc}(1 + h_{fe})$. When the output is short-circuited, $v_o = 0$
and $i_{bsc} = v_s/(R_s + h_{ie})$. Thus, R_{out} is:

$$R_{out} = \frac{\dfrac{v_s R_E \left(1+h_{fe}\right)}{R_E \left(1+h_{fe}\right)+h_{ie}+R_s}}{\dfrac{v_s \left(1+h_{fe}\right)}{\left(R_s+h_{ie}\right)}} = \frac{R_E \dfrac{\left(R_s+h_{ie}\right)}{\left(1+h_{fe}\right)}}{\dfrac{\left(R_s+h_{ie}\right)}{\left(1+h_{fe}\right)}+R_E} \quad (2.28)$$

Equation 2.28 shows that R_{out} is basically R_E in parallel with $(R_s + h_{ie})/(1 + h_{fe})$.
In general, R_{out} will be on the order of 10 to 30 Ω.

The third single BJT circuit of interest is the grounded-base amplifier,
shown in Figure 2.18. Again, to find the GB amp's gain, the node equations
are written on the v_e and v_o nodes:

$$v_e \left[G_s + g_{ie} + h_{oe}\right] - v_o h_{oe} - h_{fe} i_b = v_s G_s \quad (2.29A)$$

$$-v_e h_{oe} + v_o \left[h_{oe} + G_C\right] + h_{fe} i_b = 0 \quad (2.29B)$$

Now $i_b = -v_e g_{ie}$ is substituted into the preceding equations to get the final
form for the node equations:

$$v_e \left[G_s + h_{oe} + g_{ie}(1+h_{fe})\right] - v_o \left[h_{oe}\right] = v_s G_s \quad (2.30A)$$

$$-v_e \left[h_{oe} + h_{fe} g_{ie}\right] + v_o \left[h_{oe} + G_C\right] = 0 \quad (2.30B)$$

These equations are solved using Cramer's rule. After some algebra, the GB amplifier gain is obtained:

$$K_v = \frac{R_C\left[h_{fe} + h_{oe}h_{ie}\right]}{R_C\left[h_{oe}\left(h_{ie} + R_s\right)\right] + R_s\left[1 + h_{fe} + h_{oe}h_{ie}\right] + h_{ie}} \tag{2.31}$$

It is instructive to substitute typical numerical values into Equation 2.31 and evaluate the gain. Let $R_C = 5$ k; $h_{ie} = 1$ k; $h_{fe} = 100$; $R_s = 100$; and $h_{oe} = 10^{-5}$ S. $K_v = 44.8$. Note that the gain is noninverting. From the numerical evaluation, certain terms in Equation 2.31 are found to be small compared with others (i.e., $h_{oe} \rightarrow 0$), which leads to the approximation:

$$K_v \cong \frac{R_C h_{fe}}{R_s\left(1 + h_{fe}\right) + h_{ie}} \tag{2.32}$$

Next an expression will be found for and R_{in} and R_{out} evaluated for the GB amplifier. R_{in} is the resistance the Thevenin source (v_s, R_s) "sees" looking into the emitter of the GB amplifier. Assume $h_{oe} \rightarrow 0$. The resistance looking into the emitter is approximately:

$$R_{inem} \cong \frac{v_e}{i_e} - \frac{v_e}{-i_b\left(h_{fe} + 1\right)} = \frac{v_e}{-\left(-v_e/h_{ie}\right)\left(h_{fe} + 1\right)} = \frac{h_{ie}}{\left(h_{fe} + 1\right)} \tag{2.33}$$

To get a feeling for the size of R_{in}, substitute realistic circuit parameter values. Let $R_C = 5000$ Ω; $R_s = 100$ Ω; $h_{fe} = 100$; $h_{oe} = 10^{-5}$ S; and $h_{ie} = 1000$ Ω. Thus, $R_{inem} = 9.9$ Ω. The output resistance is the Thevenin resistance seen looking into the collector node with R_C attached. If $h_{oe} \rightarrow 0$ is set again, $R_{out} \cong R_C$, by inspection.

2.3.4 Simple Amplifiers Using Two Transistors at Mid-Frequencies

Figure 2.19 illustrates four common two-BJT amplifier architectures. An *npn* Darlington pair is shown in Figure 2.19(A). Darlington pairs can also use *pnp* BJTs. These pairs are often used as power amplifiers in the emitter-follower architecture or as grounded-base amplifiers. Figure 2.19(B) is called a *feedback pair*; it *is not* a Darlington. It, too, is often used as a power amplifier in the EF or GE modes and will be analyzed later. Figure 2.19(C) is an EF–GB pair, used for small-signal, high-frequency amplification. Figure 2.19(D) is called a *cascode pair*; it is also used as a small-signal, high-frequency amplifier.

In the first example, an expression for the mid-frequency, small-signal voltage gain, as well as input and output resistances for a grounded-emitter Darlington amplifier, are found. The amplifier circuit and its MFSS CE

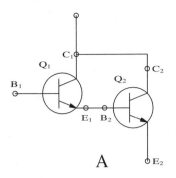

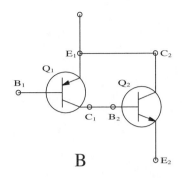

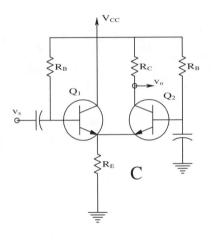

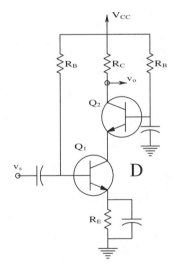

FIGURE 2.19
Four common two-BJT amplifier configurations: (A) The Darlington pair. Note that Q_1's emitter is connected directly to Q_2's base. (B) The feedback pair. The collector of the *pnp* Q_1 is coupled directly to the *npn* Q_2's base. (C) The emitter-follower–grounded-base (EF–GB) BJT pair. (D) The cascode pair.

h-parameter model are shown in Figure 2.20. To simplify analysis, assume $R_B \to \infty$, $h_{oe1} \to 0$, and $h_{oe2} \to 0$. From Ohm's law, $i_{b1} = (v_s - v_{b2})/(R_s + h_{ie1})$, $i_{b2} = v_{b2}/h_{ie2}$.

Now write node equations for the v_{b2} and the v_o nodes:

$$v_{b2}\left[1/h_{ie2} + 1/(R_s + h_{ie1})\right] - h_{fe1}i_{b1} = v_s/(R_s + h_{ie1}) \qquad (2.34A)$$

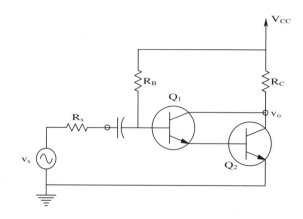

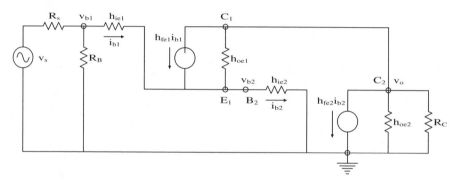

FIGURE 2.20
Top: a common-emitter Darlington amplifier. Bottom: C–E h-parameter MFSSM of the Darlington amplifier. Analysis is in the text.

$$v_o [G_C] + h_{fe1}i_{b1} + h_{fe2}i_{b2} = 0 \tag{2.34B}$$

and then substitute the relations for i_{b1} and i_{b2} and find:

$$v_o[0] + v_{b2}\left[1/h_{ie2} + (1+h_{fe1})/(R_s + h_{ie1})\right] = v_s\left[(1+h_{fe1})/(R_s + h_{ie1})\right] \tag{2.35A}$$

$$v_o[G_C] + v_{b2}\left[h_{fe2}/h_{ie2} - h_{fe1}/(R_s + h_{ie1})\right] = -v_s h_{fe1}/(R_s + h_{ie1}) \tag{2.35B}$$

Using Cramer's rule, find the GE Darlington amplifier's voltage gain:

$$\frac{v_o}{v_s} \cong -\frac{R_C\left(1+h_{fe1} + h_{fe1}h_{fe2}\right)}{\left(R_s + h_{ie1}\right) + h_{ie2}\left(1+h_{fe1}\right)} = K_v \tag{2.36}$$

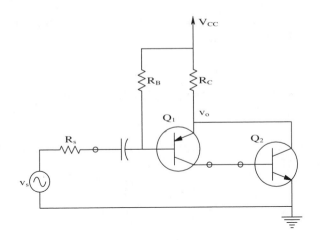

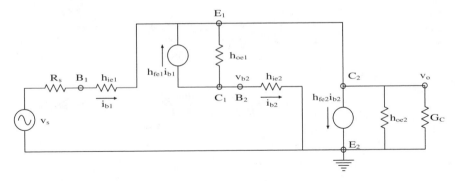

FIGURE 2.21
Top: feedback pair amplifier with load resistor, R_C, attached to common Q_1 emitter + Q_2 collector. Bottom: MFSSM of the feedback pair amplifier above. Analysis in text shows this circuit behaves like a super emitter follower.

By inspection, the Thevenin $R_{out} \cong R_C$ and $R_{in} \cong h_{ie1} + (1 + h_{fe1})h_{ie2}$. As the section on BJT amplifier frequency response demonstrates, the GE Darlington has relatively poor high-frequency response, trading off gain for bandwidth.

This example considers the feedback pair amplifier shown in Figure 2.19(B) and Figure 2.21. Note that in this amplifier, it is the collector of the *pnp* Q_1 that drives the base of the *npn* Q_2, and Q_2's collector is tied to Q_1's emitter. The auxiliary equations are:

$$i_{b1} = (v_s - v_o)/(R_s + h_{ie1}) \tag{2.37A}$$

$$i_{b2} = v_{b2}/h_{ie2} \tag{2.37B}$$

Again, for mathematical convenience, use the approximations $h_{oe1} \to 0$ and $h_{oe2} \to 0$, and write the node equations for v_o and v_{b2}:

$$v_o\left[G_C + 1/\left(R_s + h_{ie1}\right)\right] + h_{fe2}i_{b2} - h_{fe1}i_{b1} = v_s/\left(R_s + h_{ie1}\right) \qquad (2.38A)$$

$$v_{b2}\left[1/h_{ie1}\right] + h_{fe1}i_{b1} = 0 \qquad (2.38B)$$

Now substitute the auxiliary relations for i_{b1} and i_{b2} into Equations 2.38A and Equation 2.38B:

$$v_o\left[G_C + \frac{1+h_{fe1}}{R_s + h_{ie1}}\right] + v_{b2}\left[h_{fe2}/h_{ie2}\right] = v_s\frac{1+h_{fe1}}{R_s + h_{ie1}} \qquad (2.39A)$$

$$-v_o\frac{h_{fe1}}{R_s + h_{ie1}} + v_{b2}\left[1/h_{ie2}\right] = -\frac{v_s}{R_s + h_{ie1}} \qquad (2.39B)$$

The two preceding equations are solved by Cramer's rule to find K_v.

$$\Delta = \left(1/h_{ie1}\right)\left[G_C + \frac{1+h_{fe1}}{R_s + h_{ie1}}\right] + \frac{h_{fe1}h_{fe2}}{h_{ie2}\left(R_s + h_{ie1}\right)} \qquad (2.40)$$

$$\Delta v_o = \frac{\left(1+h_{fe1}\right)h_{ie2} + h_{fe2}h_{ie1}}{h_{ie1}h_{ie2}\left(R_s + h_{ie1}\right)} \qquad (2.41)$$

Thus, the voltage gain is:

$$\frac{v_o}{v_s} \cong \frac{R_C\left[\left(1+h_{fe1}+h_{fe2}h_{fe1}\right)\right]}{R_C\left[\left(1+h_{fe1}+h_{fe1}h_{fe2}\right)\right] + \left(R_s + h_{ie1}\right)} = K_v \qquad (2.42)$$

Taking "typical" numerical values, $R_s + h_{ie1} = 1050 \ \Omega$; $h_{fe1} = 100$; $h_{fe2} = 20$; and $R_C = 5000 \ \Omega$, then $K_v = 0.999895$. It appears that the feedback pair amplifier of Figure 2.21 behaves like a super emitter follower with (almost) unity gain.

Next, examine R_{in} and R_{out} of the FBP amplifier. To find R_{out}, use the open-circuit voltage/short-circuit current method. The OCV approximated by $v_s \cong v_{oc}$ because of the near unity gain of the amplifier. The short-circuit current at the C_2–E_1 node is:

$$i_{sc} = (1 + h_{fe1})\, i_{b1} - h_{fe2}\, i_{b2} \qquad (2.43)$$

With the output short-circuited, $v_o = 0$ and $i_{b1} = v_s/(R_s + h_{ie1})$. Neglecting h_{oe1}, it is possible to write:

$$i_{b2} = -h_{fe1} \, i_{b1} = -h_{fe1} \, v_s / (R_s + h_{ie1}) \tag{2.44}$$

Thus:

$$i_{sc} = (1 + h_{fe1}) v_s / (R_s + h_{ie1}) + h_{fe2} \, h_{fe1} \, v_s / (R_s + h_{ie1}) \tag{2.45}$$

Clearly, $R_{out} = v_{oc} / i_{sc}$, yielding:

$$R_{out} \cong \frac{R_s + h_{ie1}}{1 + h_{fe1} + h_{fe1} h_{fe2}} \tag{2.46}$$

If the numbers used previously are substituted, $R_{out} = 0.5 \, \Omega$ — significantly smaller than a single BJT's emitter follower. R_{in} looking into the B_1 node is just v_s / i_{b1}. That is:

$$R_{in} = v_s h_{ie1} / (v_s - v_o) = h_{ie1} / (1 - v_o / v_s) = \cfrac{h_{ie1}}{1 - \cfrac{R_C [1 + h_{fe1} + h_{fe1} h_{fe2}]}{R_C [1 + h_{fe1} + h_{fe1} h_{fe2}] + h_{ie1}}}$$

$$\downarrow \tag{2.47}$$

$$R_{in} = R_C [1 + h_{fe1} + h_{fe1} h_{fe2}] + h_{ie1}$$

$R_{in} \cong 10.51 \, \text{M}\Omega$, using the previous parameters.

Next, examine the behavior of the feedback pair when the load resistor is connected to E_2 and C_2–E_1 is connected to V_{cc}. The circuit is shown in Figure 2.22. It is not necessary to solve two simultaneous node equations to find K_v; by Ohm's law, $i_{b1} = v_s / (R_s + h_{ie1})$ and $i_{b2} = -i_{b1} h_{fe1}$. Now it is clear that:

$$v_o = i_{b2} (1 + h_{fe2}) R_E = -i_{b1} h_{fe1} (1 + h_{fe2}) R_E = \frac{-v_s h_{fe1} (1 + h_{fe2}) R_E}{R_s + h_{ie1}} = v_{oOC} \tag{2.48}$$

Thus,

$$K_v = -\frac{R_E h_{fe1} (1 + h_{fe2})}{(R_s + h_{ie1})} \tag{2.49}$$

R_{in} for this amplifier is found by inspection; $R_{in} = h_{ie1}$. R_{out} is found by v_{oOC} / i_{oSC}:

$$R_{out} = \frac{\dfrac{-v_s h_{fe1} (1 + h_{fe2}) R_E}{(R_s + h_{ie1})}}{\dfrac{-v_s h_{fe1} (1 + h_{fe2})}{(R_s + h_{ie1})}} = R_E \tag{2.50}$$

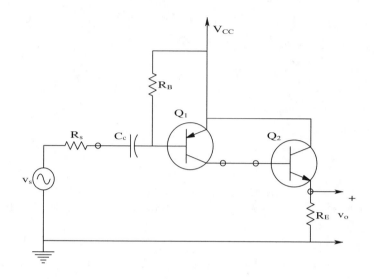

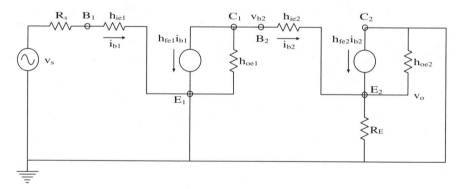

FIGURE 2.22

Top: feedback pair amplifier with load resistor in Q_2's emitter. Bottom: MFSSM of the amplifier shown above. Analysis in text shows this amplifier has a high inverting mid-frequency gain; it does not emulate an emitter follower.

Next, examine the gain, R_{in} and R_{out}, of the emitter-follower-grounded base amplifier shown in Figure 2.19(C). Figure 2.23 illustrates the MFSSM for this amplifier. Again, for algebraic simplicity, assume that h_{oe1} and h_{oe2} are negligible; also, $R_1 = R_s + h_{ie1}$, all capacitors behave as short circuits at mid-frequencies, and $R_B \rightarrow \infty$. Two node equations can be written for the MFSSM:

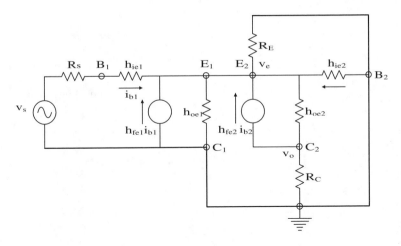

FIGURE 2.23
MFSSM for the EF–GB amplifier of Figure 2.19(C). See text for analysis.

$$v_o \, [G_C] + h_{fe2} \, i_{b2} = 0 \tag{2.51A}$$

$$v_e \, [G_E + 1/h_{ie2} + G_1] - h_{fe2} \, i_{b2} - h_{fe1} i_{b1} = v_s \, G_1 \tag{2.51B}$$

where:

$$i_{b2} = -v_e/h_{ie2} \tag{2.51C}$$

$$i_{b1} = (v_s - v_e)G_1 \tag{2.51D}$$

Substituting Equation 2.51C and Equation 2.51D into the node equations yields:

$$v_o \, [G_C] - v_e \, [h_{fe2}/h_{ie2}] = 0 \tag{2.52A}$$

$$v_o[0] + v_e\left[G_E + \left(1 + h_{fe2}\right)\big/h_{ie2} + G_1\left(1 + h_{fe1}\right)\right] = v_s \, G_1\left(1 + h_{fe1}\right) \tag{2.52B}$$

From Equation 2.52A and Equation 2.52B,

$$v_o = v_e \, R_C \, [h_{fe2}/h_{ie2}] \tag{2.53}$$

can be written and

$$v_e = \frac{v_s G_1\left(1 + h_{fe1}\right)}{\left[G_E + \left(1 + h_{fe2}\right)\big/h_{ie2} + G_1\left(1 + h_{fe1}\right)\right]} \tag{2.54}$$

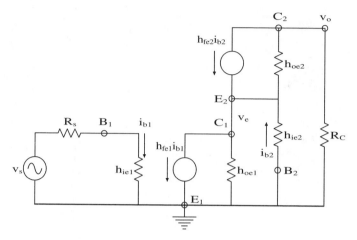

FIGURE 2.24
MFSSM for the cascode amplifier of Figure 2.19(D). See text for analysis.

Now Equation 2.54 is substituted into Equation 2.53 to find K_v:

$$K_v = \frac{v_o}{v_s} = \frac{R_C h_{fe2}\left(1+h_{fe1}\right)}{h_{ie2}\left(R_1/R_E\right)+R_1\left(1+h_{fe2}\right)+h_{ie2}\left(1+h_{fe1}\right)} \tag{2.55}$$

Substitute typical values $R_C = 5000\ \Omega$; $R_1 = 1050\ \Omega$; $h_{fe1} = h_{fe2} = 100$; and $h_{ie2} = 1000\ \Omega$, and find $K_v = +244$, i.e., the EF–GB amplifier is noninverting. The EF–GB amplifier will be shown to have excellent high-frequency response. It is left as an exercise for the reader to find expressions for the mid-frequency R_{in} and R_{out} for this amplifier.

The final two-BJT amplifier stage to be analyzed using the CE MFSSM is the cascode amplifier, shown in Figure 2.19(D). The MFSSM for this amplifier is shown in Figure 2.24. Again, assume capacitors behave as short circuits at mid-frequencies, $h_{oe1} = h_{oe2} = 0$, and $R_B \to \infty$. Clearly, $v_o = -h_{fe2}\, i_{b2}\, R_C$ and $i_{b2} = -v_e/h_{ie2}$, so $v_o = v_e\, h_{fe2}\, R_C/h_{ie2}$ and $i_{b1} = v_s/R_1$. To find v_e, write the node equation:

$$v_e\left[1/h_{ie2}\right] + h_{fe1}i_{b1} - h_{fe2}\,i_{b2} = 0 \tag{2.56}$$

Substituting for i_{b1} and i_{b2} into Equation 2.56 yields:

$$v_e = \frac{-v_s h_{fe1} h_{ie2} G_1}{1+h_{fe2}} \tag{2.57}$$

Equation 2.57 is substituted into the preceding equation for v_o to find K_v:

$$K_v = \frac{v_o}{v_s} = \frac{-h_{fe1}R_C h_{fe2}}{R_1\left(1+h_{fe2}\right)} \approx \frac{-h_{fe1}R_C}{R_1} \tag{2.58}$$

By inspection, $R_{in} = R_1$, $R_{out} \cong R_C$. Like the EF–GB amplifier, the cascode amplifier has a high-frequency bandwidth. It also can be described as a GE–GB amplifier.

2.3.5 The Use of Transistor Dynamic Loads To Improve Amplifier Performance

In many analog IC designs, including those with differential amplifiers, transistors and small transistor circuits are used to create small-signal, dynamic high impedances that, when used in amplifiers to replace conventional resistors, increase amplifier gain or differential amplifier common-mode rejection ratio. Figure 2.25 illustrates four BJT circuits that act as dc current sources or sinks with high, small-signal, Norton resistances. For example, if 2 mA dc flows through a potential difference of 5 V in an electronic circuit, a 2.5-k resistor is needed. If a dynamic current source is used, the equivalent small-signal (Norton) resistance can range from 100 k to 10 M, depending on the circuit. A good way to view such dynamic resistances is to treat the circuit as a dc current source in parallel with a Norton resistance of 100 k to 10 M.

The most basic dynamic resistance is realized by looking into the collector of a BJT with an emitter resistance that is not bypassed, as shown in Figure 2.25(A). Figure 2.26 illustrates how the MFSSM is used to find the resistance looking into the collector. Note that the base is bypassed to ground at signal frequencies. Clearly, from Ohm's law, $R_{incol} = v_t/i_t$. (v_t is a small-signal test source.)

Begin analysis by finding an expression for $v_e = f(v_t)$. Writing the node equation:

$$v_e\left[\left(1/h_{ie}\right) + G_E + h_{oe}\right] - \beta i_b = v_t h_{oe} \tag{2.59A}$$

$$i_b = -v_e/h_{ie} \tag{2.59B}$$

$$\downarrow$$

$$v_e\left[\left(1/h_{ie}\right)(1+\beta) + G_e + h_{oe}\right] = v_t h_{oe} \tag{2.59C}$$

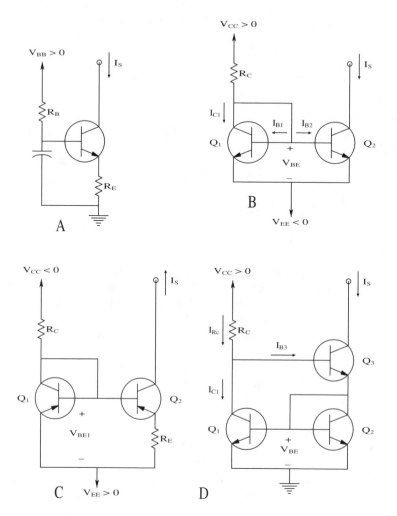

FIGURE 2.25
Four BJT circuits used for high-impedance current sources and sinks in the design of differential amplifiers and other analog ICs. They can serve as high-impedance active loads. (A) Collector of simple BJT with unbypassed emitter resistance. (B) Basic two-BJT current sink. (C) Widlar current source (*pnp* BJTs are used). (D) Wilson current sink.

Thus, v_e is:

$$v_e = \frac{v_t h_{oe}}{(1/h_{ie})(1+\beta) + G_E + h_{oe}} \tag{2.60}$$

and the test current is:

$$i_t = v_e \left[(1/h_{ie}) + G_E \right] \tag{2.61}$$

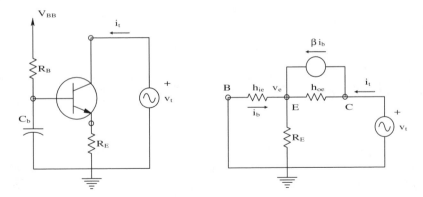

FIGURE 2.26
Left: test circuit for calculating small-signal resistance looking into BJT's collector. An ac test source, v_t, is used; i_t is measured. Right: MFSSM of the test circuit used to calculate the expression for the small-signal resistance looking into collector.

When Equation 2.60 is substituted into Equation 2.61, it is possible to solve for R_{incol}:

$$R_{incol} = \frac{v_t}{i_t} = \frac{1 + \dfrac{\beta R_E + h_{oe} h_{ie} R_E}{R_E + h_{ie}}}{h_{oe}} \qquad (2.62)$$

Looking into the collector of a BJT with no R_E, $R_{incol} \cong h_{oe}^{-1}$ Ω can be seen. To see how much R_E increases R_{incol}, substitute some typical parameter values into Equation 2.62: $R_E = 5k$; $h_{ie} = 1k$; $\beta = 100$; and $h_{oe} = 10^{-5}$ S. Crunching the numbers, $R_{incol} = 8.4$ MΩ. Note that the BJT's base was bypassed to ground in the preceding development. If the base *is not* bypassed, $h_{ie} \to h_{ie} + R_B$ in Equation 2.62, where R_B is the Thevenin resistance that the base "sees." The unbypassed base causes R_{incol} to decrease markedly, but it still remains above $1/h_{oe}$.

More sophisticated, high dynamic resistance dc current sources are shown in Figure 2.25(B) and Figure 2.25(C). Figure 2.25(B) is the basic, two-BJT current sink; its dynamic input resistance is about $1/h_{oe}$ Ω. Figure 2.25(C) is the Widlar current source (note *pnp* BJTs are used). Figure 2.25(D) is a Wilson current sink. Note that a collector–base junction in all three current source/active load circuits is short-circuited (Q_1 in Figure 2.25(B) and Figure 2.25(C), Q_2 in Figure 2.25(D)). The transistor with the shorted collector–base junction then behaves as a forward-biased, base–emitter diode junction.

Analysis of the basic two-BJT current sink (Figure 2.25(B)) is made easy when it is assumed that Q_1 and Q_2 have identical parameters. Because both transistors have the same V_{BE}, their collector currents are equal, i.e., $I_{C1} = I_{C2}$. Summing currents at Q_1's collector,

$$I_{Rc} - I_{C1} = 2I_{C1}/\beta \qquad (2.63)$$

and thus:

$$I_{C1} = \frac{I_{Rc}}{1 + 2/\beta} = I_{C2} \tag{2.64}$$

If β is large (≥ 100), I_{C2} is nearly equal to the reference current:

$$I_{C2} \cong I_{Rc} = (V_{CC} - V_{BE})/R_C \tag{2.65}$$

Thus R_C can be manipulated to obtain the desired quiescent dc current, I_{C2}.

If V_{CE2} varies, there will be a small variation in the dc I_{CE2}. I_{CE2} can be expressed in terms of V_{BE2} and Q_2's *Early voltage* ($|V_x|$), which is used to model the upward tilt of the $I_{C2} = f(V_{BE2}, V_{CE2})$ curves. Gray and Meyer (1984) model I_{C2} by:

$$I_{C2} = I_{CS}\left[\exp\left(V_{BE2}/V_T\right)\right]\left(1 + V_{CE2}/|V_x|\right) \tag{2.66}$$

Now,

$$\frac{\partial I_{C2}}{\partial V_{CE2}} = I_{CS}\left[\exp\left(V_{BE2}/V_T\right)\right]\left(1/|V_x|\right) \tag{2.67}$$

so the variation in I_{C2} is:

$$\Delta I_{C2} = I_{CS}\left[\exp\left(V_{BE2}/V_T\right)\right]\left(1/|V_x|\right)\Delta V_{CE2} \tag{2.68}$$

A very detailed treatment of the transistor current sources and active loads used in IC design beyond the scope of this text can be found in Chapter 4 of Gray and Meyer (1984). These authors show how certain active load designs can be used to reduce the overall dc temperature coefficient (tempco) of certain amplifier stages, as well as to increase gain and CMRR.

2.4   Mid-Frequency Models for Field-Effect Transistors

2.4.1   Introduction

The two basic types of field-effect transistor are the junction field-effect transistor (JFET), which can be further characterized as n-channel or p-channel, and the metal-oxide semiconductor FET (MOSFET), which can also be sub-divided into p- and n-channel devices and is further distinguished by whether it operates by enhancement or depletion of charge carriers in the channel. Surprisingly, one mid-frequency small-signal model describes the behavior of *all* types of FETs, although the dc biasing varies. MFSSMs for FETs use a voltage-controlled current source (transconductance) model in parallel with an output conductance to model the drain-to-source behavior. The following sections examine the behavior of JFETs and how they work as amplifiers.

2.4.2 JFETs at Mid-Frequencies

Figure 2.27 illustrates the symbols for n- and p-channel JFETs and the volt–ampere curves for an n-channel JFET. Note that the gate-to-channel *pn* junction is normally reverse-biased in a JFET; thus, the gate current is the reverse saturation current of this diode (I_{rs}), which is on the order of nA. In the n-channel JFET, all the currents and voltages are positive as written, with v_{GS} being negative. In the p-channel JFET, all the signs are reversed: i_D and v_{DS} are negative and v_{GS} is positive. The operating region of the JFET's (i_D, v_{DS}) curves is ohmic to the *left* of the I_{DB} line and saturated to the *right* of the I_{DB} line.

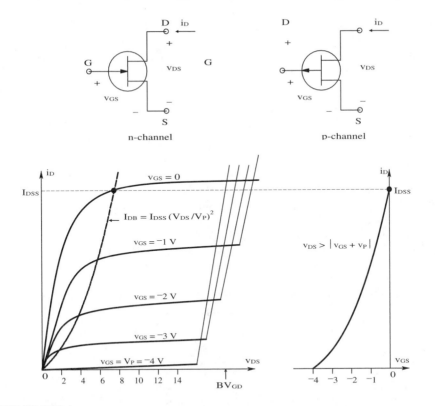

FIGURE 2.27
Top: symbols for n- and p-channel JFETs. Bottom left: i_D vs. v_{DS} curves for an n-channel JFET. Area to left of I_{DB} parabola has ohmic FET operation; area to right of I_{DB} line has saturated (channel) operation. Bottom right: the i_D vs. v_{GS} curve for saturated operation [$v_{DS} > |v_{GS} + V_P|$]. The pinch-off voltage $V_P = -4$ V in this example.

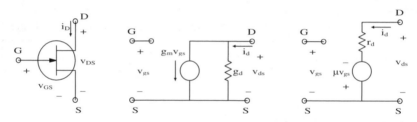

FIGURE 2.28
Left: symbol for n-channel JFET. Center: Norton MFSSM for p- and n-channel JFETs. Right:
Thevenin MFSSM for JFETs.

Just as there is a mathematical model for *pn* junction diode current, there
is also a mathematical approximation to JFET behavior in the saturation
region. This is:

$$I_D = I_{DSS}(1 - V_{GS}/V_P)^2 \text{ for } V_{DS} > |V_{GS} + V_p| \text{ and } |V_{GS}| < |V_P| \qquad (2.69)$$

In the ohmic region, I_D is modeled by:

$$I_D = I_{DSS}\left[2(1 + V_{GS}/V_P)(V_{DS}/V_P) - (V_{DS}/V_P)^2\right] \text{ for } 0 < V_{DS} < |V_{GS} + V_p| \quad (2.70)$$

For $V_{GS} \ll V_P$,

$$I_D = I_{DSS}\left[2(1 + V_{GS}/V_P)(V_{DS}/V_P)\right] \qquad (2.71)$$

where I_{DSS} is the drain current defined for $V_{GS} = 0$ and $V_{DS} > |V_{GS} + V_P|$. V_P
is the pinch-off voltage, i.e., $V_P = V_{GS}$ where $I_D \to 0$, given $V_{DS} > |V_{GS} + V_P|$.
In the ohmic region, the JFET behaves like a voltage-controlled conductance:

$$g_d = \left.\frac{\partial i_D}{\partial v_{DS}}\right|V_{GS} = I_{DSS}\left[2(1 + (V_{GS}/V_P))/V_P\right] \qquad (2.72)$$

In the saturation region, n- and p-channel JFETs have the same MFSSM,
shown in Figure 2.28. The transconductance of the VCCS is defined by:

$$g_m = \left.\frac{\partial i_D}{\partial v_{DS}}\right|Q, V_{GS} = \text{const.} \qquad (2.73)$$

By differentiating Equation 2.69, an algebraic expression is found for g_m:

$$g_m = \frac{2I_{DSS}}{|V_P|}(1 - V_{GS}/V_P) \qquad (2.74)$$

Note from Equation 2.69 that $\sqrt{I_D}$ can be written as:

$$\sqrt{I_D} = \sqrt{I_{DSS}}\left(1 - V_{GS}/V_P\right) \tag{2.75}$$

Now Equation 2.75 can be substituted into Equation 2.74 to find:

$$g_m = \frac{2I_{DSS}}{|V_P|}\sqrt{\frac{I_{DQ}}{I_{DSS}}} = g_{mo}\sqrt{\frac{I_{DQ}}{I_{DSS}}} \quad \text{for } V_{DS} > |V_{GS} + V_P| \tag{2.76}$$

Equation 2.76 gives an algebraic means of estimating a JFET's g_m in terms of its quiescent drain current (I_{DQ}) and the manufacturer-specified parameters, I_{DSS} and V_P. g_{mo} is the JFET's (maximum) transconductance at $V_{GS} = 0$ and $V_{DS} > |V_{GS} + V_P|$.

The MFSSM for a saturated-channel JFET is also characterized by an output conductance in parallel with the VCCS. This small-signal conductance is due in part to the upward slope of the $i_D = f(v_{GS}, v_{DS})$ curve family :

$$g_d = \left.\frac{\partial i_D}{\partial v_{DS}}\right|_{V_{GS}} = \left.\frac{\Delta I_D}{\Delta V_{DS}}\right|_{Q, V_{GS}=\text{const.}} \quad \text{Siemens} \tag{2.77}$$

To model the upward slope of the $i_D = f(v_{GS}, v_{DS})$ curve family, we choose a voltage V_x such that:

$$I_D \cong I_{DSS}\left(1 - V_{GS}/V_P\right)^2\left(1 - V_{DS}/V_x\right) \quad \text{for } V_{DS} > |V_{GS} + V_P| \text{ and } |V_{GS}| < |V_P| \tag{2.78}$$

Note that the intercept voltage, V_x, is typically 25 to 50 V in magnitude. V_x is negative and V_{DS} is positive for n-channel JFETs and V_x is positive and V_{DS} is negative for p-channel JFETs. An algebraic expression for g_d can be found by differentiating Equation 2.78.

$$g_d = \left.\frac{\partial I_D}{\partial V_{DS}}\right|_Q = I_{DSS}\left(1 - V_{GS}/V_P\right)^2\left(-1/V_x\right) = -\left(I_{DQ}/V_x\right) > 0 \tag{2.79}$$

An estimate of V_x can be found by extrapolating the $i_D = f(v_{GS}, v_{DS})$ curves in the saturation region back to the negative V_{SD} axis, as shown in Figure 2.29.

The Norton drain–source model shown in Figure 2.28 can be made into a Thevenin model in which the series Thevenin resistance is just $r_d = 1/g_d$ and the open-circuit voltage is given by a VCVS, μv_{GS}. (Note the sign of the VCVS; *it is the same for n- and p-channel JFETs.*

The voltage gain, μ, is easily seen to be given by:

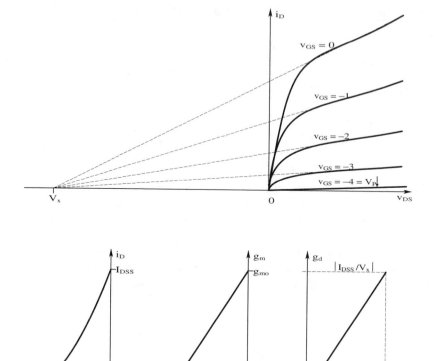

FIGURE 2.29
Top: large-signal i_D vs. v_{DS} curves for an n-channel JFET showing the geometry of the FET equivalent of the BJT Early voltage, V_x. Bottom, left to right: small-signal i_D vs. v_{GS} for a saturated channel. Small-signal g_m vs. v_{GS} for a saturated channel. Small-signal Norton drain conductance, g_d vs. i_D for a saturated channel.

$$\mu = g_m/g_d = g_{mo}\sqrt{\left(I_{DQ}/I_{DSS}\right)}\left(\left|V_x/I_{DQ}\right|\right) = \frac{g_{mo}\left|V_x\right|}{\sqrt{I_{DQ}I_{DSS}}} \qquad (2.80)$$

In the saturation region of operation, μ varies inversely with I_{DQ}. Either the Norton or Thevenin model is valid. Most engineers use the Norton model because manufacturers generally provide V_P, I_{DSS}, and g_{mo} for a given JFET.

2.4.3 MOSFET Behavior at Mid-Frequencies

MOSFETS are also known as insulated gate field-effect transistors (IgFETS). The gate electrode is insulated from the channel, thus gate leakage current is on the order of picoamperes or less. Symbols for n-channel, p-channel, and the $i_D = f(v_{GS}, v_{DS})$ curves for an n-channel depletion MOSFET are shown

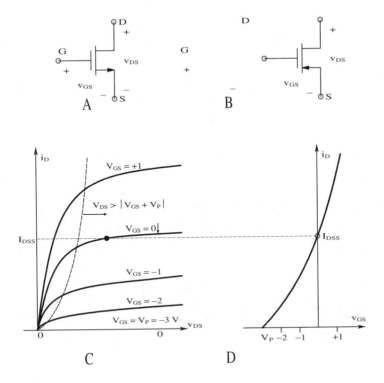

FIGURE 2.30
(A) Symbol for an n-channel MOSFET. (B) Symbol for a p-channel MOSFET. (C) The $i_D = f(v_{GS},$ $v_{DS})$ curves for an n-channel depletion MOSFET. (D) The $i_D = f(v_{GS})$ curve for a saturated-channel, n-channel depletion MOSFET.

in Figure 2.30. In the depletion device, a lightly doped p-substrate underlies a lightly doped n-channel connecting two heavily doped n-regions for the source and drain. This device has a negative pinch-off voltage (V_P); however, $I_D = I_{DSS}$ when $V_{GS} = 0$ and the saturated channel conducts heavily for $V_{GS} > 0$.

Similar to the n-channel JFET, it is possible to model the $i_D = f(v_{GS}, v_{DS})$ curves of the depletion n-channel MOSFET in the saturation region by:

$$i_D = I_{DSS}\left[1 - \left(v_{GS}/V_P\right)\right]^2 \text{ for } v_{DS} > |v_{GS} + V_P| > 0 \qquad (2.81)$$

and in the ohmic region:

$$i_D = I_{DSS}\left[2\left(1 + v_{GS}/V_P\right)\left(v_{DS}/V_P\right) - \left(v_{DS}/V_P\right)^2\right] \text{ for } 0 < v_{DS} < |v_{GS} + V_P| \quad (2.82)$$

When the $i_D = f(v_{GS}, v_{DS})$ curves of the enhancement n-channel MOSFET shown in Figure 2.31 are considered, it can be seen that there is no I_{DSS} for this family of device. Channel cut-off occurs at a threshold voltage, $v_{GS} = V_T$,

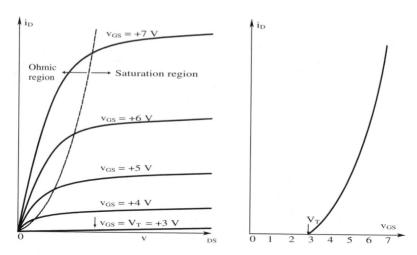

FIGURE 2.31

Left: the $i_D = f(v_{GS}, v_{DS})$ curves for an n-channel enhancement MOSFET. Right: the $i_D = f(v_{GS})$ curve for a saturated-channel, n-channel enhancement MOSFET.

where i_D reaches some defined low value, e.g., 10 μA. The mathematical model for n-channel enhancement MOSFET $i_D = f(v_{GS}, v_{DS})$ in the saturation region is:

$$i_D = K(v_{GS} - V_T)^2 = K\,V_T^2\left(1 - v_{GS}/V_T\right)^2 \quad \text{for } 0 < |v_{GS} - V_T| < |v_{DS}| \quad (2.83)$$

In the ohmic channel operating region:

$$i_D = K\left[2(v_{GS} - V_T)v_{DS} - v_{DS}^2\right] \quad \text{for } 0 < |v_{DS}| < |v_{GS} - V_T| \quad (2.84)$$

The line separating the saturated- and ohmic-channel regions is

$$I_{DB} = K\,V_{DS}^2 \quad (2.85)$$

p-channel MOSFETs have $i_D = f(v_{GS}, v_{DS})$ curves with the signs opposite those for n-channel devices. It is easy to see from Equation 2.73, which defines the small-signal transconductance, and Equation 2.72, which defines the small-signal drain conductance, that all FETs (JFETs, MOSFETs, n-channel, p-channel, enhancement, depletion) have the same parsimonious MFSSM — a case of electronic serendipity.

2.4.4   Basic Mid-Frequency Single FET Amplifiers

Just as in the case of BJTs, there are so-called grounded-source amplifiers, grounded-gate amplifiers, and source followers. In order to find the small-

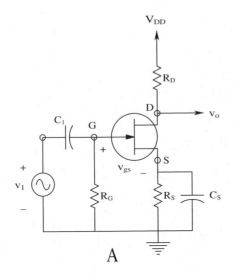

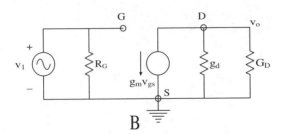

FIGURE 2.32
(A) An n-channel JFET "grounded-source" amplifier. C_S bypasses small ac signals at the JFET's source to ground, making $v_s = 0$. (B) MFSSM of the amplifier. The same MFSSM would obtain if a p-channel JFET were used.

signal voltage gain of each if these amplifiers, as well as their input and output resistances, first examine a JFET grounded-source amplifier, shown in Figure 2.32. At mid-frequencies, the external coupling and bypass capacitors are treated as short circuits. Thus, the source is at small-signal ground, so $v_s = 0$. The amplifier's mid-frequency gain is found from the node equation:

$$v_o [G_D + g_d] = -g_m v_{gs} = -g_m v_1 \tag{2.86}$$

$$\downarrow$$

$$K_v = \frac{v_o}{v_1} = \frac{-g_m r_d R_D}{R_D + r_d} \tag{2.87}$$

From inspection of the MFSSM of the circuit, $R_{in} \to \infty$ and $R_{out} = R_D r_d / (R_D + r_d)$.

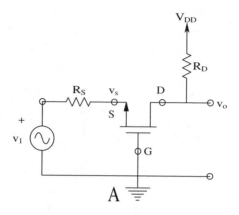

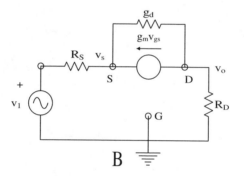

FIGURE 2.33
(A) An n-channel MOSFET grounded-gate amplifier. (B) MFSSM of the MOSFET G-G amplifier.
See text for analysis.

Next, consider an n-channel MOSFET grounded-gate amplifier at mid-frequencies. The electrical circuit and its MFSSM are shown in Figure 2.33. Write two node equations, one for the v_s node and the other for the drain (output) node.

$$v_s [G_S + g_d + g_m] - v_o [g_d] = v_1 G_S \tag{2.88A}$$

$$-v_s [g_d + g_m] + v_o [g_d + G_D] = 0 \tag{2.88B}$$

Using Cramer's rule:

$$\Delta = G_S g_d + G_D [G_S + g_d + g_m] \tag{2.89}$$

$$\frac{v_s}{v_1} = \frac{R_D + r_d}{R_D + r_d + R_S(1 + g_m r_d)} \tag{2.90}$$

$$\frac{v_o}{v_1} = \frac{R_D(1 + g_m r_d)}{R_D + r_d + R_S(1 + g_m r_d)} = K_v \tag{2.91}$$

The input resistance, R_{in}, of the MOSFET GG amplifier is found from:

$$R_{in} = \frac{v_1}{i_s} = \frac{v_1 R_S}{v_1(1 - v_s/v_1)} = \frac{R_S}{1 - \dfrac{R_D + r_d}{R_D + r_d + R_S(1 + g_m r_d)}} = R_S + \frac{R_D + r_d}{(1 + g_m r_d)} \tag{2.92}$$

R_{out} is approximately R_D for the GG amplifier.

Finally, examine the MOSFET source-follower amplifier at mid-frequencies. The circuit and its MFSSM are shown in Figure 2.34. This an easy circuit to analyze because the drain is at SS ground. The output node equation is:

$$v_o [G_C + g_d + g_m] = g_m v_1 \tag{2.93}$$

Equation 2.93 leads to the SF amplifier's gain:

$$K_v = \frac{v_o}{v_1} = \frac{R_D g_m r_d}{r_d + R_D(1 + g_m r_d)} < 1 \tag{2.94}$$

By inspection, $R_{in} \to \infty$; R_{out} can be found by v_{oc}/i_{sc}.

$$R_{out} = \frac{v_{oc}}{i_{sc}} = \frac{\dfrac{v_1 R_D g_m r_d}{r_d + R_D(1 + g_m r_d)}}{g_m v_1} = \frac{R_D r_d/(1 + g_m r_d)}{R_D + r_d/(1 + g_m r_d)} \tag{2.95}$$

Single FET amplifiers generally have higher R_{in}, about the same R_{out}, less gain, and more even harmonic distortion than equivalent BJT amplifiers.

2.4.5 Simple Amplifiers Using Two FETs at Mid-Frequencies

As in the case of BJTs, certain basic building blocks for analog ICs can be made from two transistors. Figure 2.35 illustrates four such circuits using field-effect transistors. Notably absent is the difference amplifier; because of its great importance in analog electronic circuits, the DA is treated separately in Chapter 3 of this text. Figure 2.35(A) illustrates a Darlington amplifier in which the input transistor is an n-channel MOSFET acting as a voltage control-led current source driving the base of a power *npn* BJT. Figure 2.35(B) shows the FET–BJT equivalent for the "feedback pair" power amplifier. In Figure 2.35(C), a source-follower/grounded-gate high-frequency amplifier can be seen and an FET–FET cascode amplifier is shown in Figure 2.35(D).

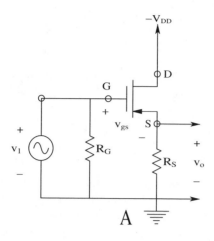

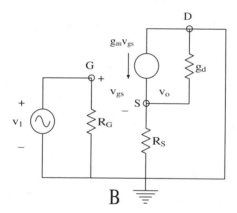

FIGURE 2.34
(A) A p-channel MOSFET source follower. (B) MFSSM for the MOSFET S-F.

It is necessary first to examine the gain of the FET–BJT Darlington connected as an emitter follower. This circuit and its MFSSM are shown in Figure 2.36. Analysis begins by writing the node equations for the v_s and v_o nodes; note that $i_b = g_{ie} (v_s - v_o)$; $v_{gs} = v_1 - v_s$; $\mu = g_m r_d$; and $g_{ie} = 1/h_{ie}$.

$$v_s [g_d + g_{ie} + g_m] - v_o g_{ie} = v_1 g_m \qquad (2.96A)$$

$$-v_s [g_{ie} (1 + h_{fe})] + v_o [g_{ie} (1 + h_{fe}) + G_E] = 0 \qquad (2.96B)$$

Using Cramer's rule,

$$\Delta = (g_d + g_m)g_{ie} (1 + h_{fe}) + G_E (g_d + g_{ie} + g_m) \qquad (2.97)$$

$$\Delta v_o = v_1 g_m g_{ie} (1 + h_{fe}) \qquad (2.98)$$

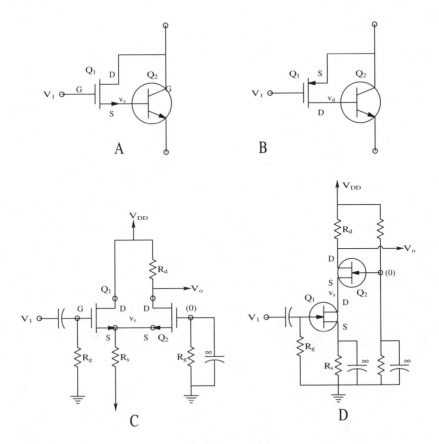

FIGURE 2.35
(A) An n-channel MOSFET/*npn* BJT Darlington configuration. (B) A p-channel MOSFET/*npn* BJT feedback pair configuration. (C) An n-channel MOSFET source-follower–grounded-gate amplifier. (D) An n-channel JFET cascode amplifier.

Solving for v_o/v_1 yields:

$$\frac{v_o}{v_1} = \frac{R_E\left(1+h_{fe}\right)\mu}{R_E\left(1+h_{fe}\right)\left(1+\mu\right)+h_{ie}\left(1+\mu\right)+r_d} \tag{2.99}$$

As expected, this voltage gain is <1. The amplifier's input resistance is extremely high and the output resistance can be found by the open-circuit output voltage, given by Equation 2.99, divided by the short-circuit output current, which is simply $i_b(1 + h_{fe})$ for $v_o = 0$, (R_{out} = OCV/SCC). R_{out} is on the order of single ohms.

Next, find the gain for the FET–BJT feedback pair amplifier shown in Figure 2.35(B). The node equations are:

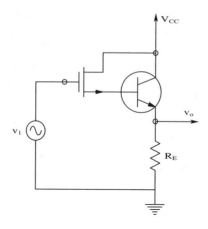

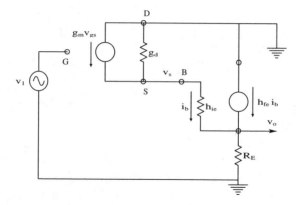

FIGURE 2.36
Top: A MOSFET/BJT Darlington connected as an emitter-follower. Bottom: MFSSM of the Darlington EF. See analysis in text.

$$v_d [g_d + g_{ie}] - v_o [g_{ie}] = - v_1 g_m \qquad (2.100A)$$

$$-v_d [g_{ie} (1 + h_{fe})] + v_o [G_E + g_{ie} (1 + h_{fe})] = 0 \qquad (2.100B)$$

Using Cramer's rule,

$$\Delta = g_d [G_E + g_{ie} (1 + h_{fe})] + g_{ie} G_E \qquad (2.101)$$

$$\Delta v_o = - v_1 g_m g_{ie} (1 + h_{fe}) \qquad (2.102)$$

from which the mid-frequency voltage gain is found:

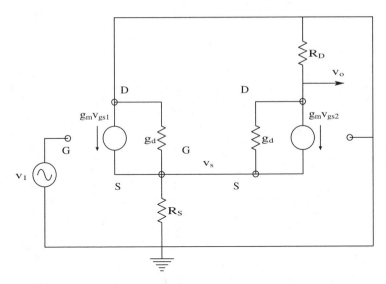

FIGURE 2.37
MFSSM for the two-MOSFET SF/GG amplifier. See text for analysis.

$$\frac{v_o}{v_1} = \frac{-R_E\mu\left(1+h_{fe}\right)}{R_E\left(1+h_{fe}\right)+h_{ie}+r_d} = \frac{-\mu R_E}{R_E+\left(h_{ie}+r_d\right)/\left(1+h_{fe}\right)} = K_v \qquad (2.103)$$

Again, R_{in} is very high because of the MOSFET and R_{out} can be found from $R_{out} = OCV/SCC$. It can be shown that R_{out} is R_E in parallel with $(h_{ie}+r_d)/(1+h_{fe})$ ohms.

The MFSSM of the FET–FET SF-GG amplifier of Figure 2.35(C) is shown in Figure 2.37. Proceeding as before, write the node equations for v_s and v_o, then use Cramer's rule to find the amplifier's MFSS gain; note that $v_{gs1} = v_1 - v_s$ and $v_{gs2} = -v_s$.

$$v_s\left[2(g_d + g_m) + G_S\right] - v_o\left[g_d\right] = g_m\,v_1 \qquad (2.104A)$$

$$-v_s\left[g_d + g_m\right] + v_o\left[G_D + g_d\right] = 0 \qquad (2.104B)$$

$$\Delta = 2G_D\,(g_d + g_m) + g_d\,(g_m + G_S) + G_S\,G_D \qquad (2.105)$$

$$\Delta v_o = v_1\,g_m\,(g_d + g_m) \qquad (2.106)$$

The voltage gain is found from Equation 2.105 and Equation 2.106:

$$\frac{v_o}{v_1} = \frac{+R_D\mu}{R_D + 2r_d + r_d\left(r_d + R_D\right)/\left[R_S(1+\mu)\right]} = K_v \qquad (2.107)$$

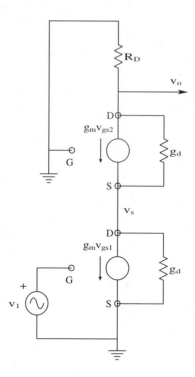

FIGURE 2.38
MFSSM for the two-JFET cascode amplifier. See text for analysis.

Note that the gain is noninverting; R_{in} is on the order of 10^{13} Ω and R_{out} is slightly lower than R_D.

The final two-FET amplifier considered is the cascode amplifier using two JFETs shown in Figure 2.35(D). The MFSSM of the cascode is shown in Figure 2.38. Note that $v_{gs1} = v_1$, $v_{gs2} = -v_s$, the JFETs are matched, and $\mu = g_m r_d$. The node equations are:

$$v_s \left[2g_d + g_m \right] - v_o \, g_d = - g_m v_1 \tag{2.108A}$$

$$-v_s \left[g_d + g_m \right] + v_o \left[G_D + g_d \right] = 0 \tag{2.108B}$$

$$\Delta = 2g_d \, G_D + 2g_d^2 + g_m G_D + g_m \, g_d - g_d^2 - g_m \, g_d = G_D(2g_d + g_m) + g_d^2 \tag{2.109}$$

$$\Delta v_o = - v_1 \, g_m \left[g_d + g_m \right] \tag{2.110}$$

The cascode amplifier's mid-frequency voltage gain is found to be:

$$\frac{v_o}{v_1} = \frac{-R_D \mu (1 + \mu)}{R_D + r_d (1 + \mu)} = K_v \tag{2.111}$$

The JFET cascode amplifier's R_{in} is on the order of gigaohms; its R_{out} is slightly lower than R_D.

Two-transistor amplifiers using FETs generally have very high input resistances, gains that are not as high as equivalent two-BJT amplifiers, and more distortion in the output signal because of the nonlinear $I_D(V_{GS})$ characteristics of all FETs.

2.5 High-Frequency Models for Transistors, and Simple Transistor Amplifiers

2.5.1 Introduction

The limitation of the high-frequency bandwidth of all transistor amplifiers can be modeled by small capacitances that shunt the transistor's small-signal model elements to ground or that connect input to output. High bandwidth is certainly not required for conditioning recorded physiological signals such as the ECG, EMG, EEG, EOG, etc. Such signals require only a low audio bandwidth for faithful reproduction. High bandwidth (into the tens of megahertz) is required for pulsed and CW ultrasound signals.

Pulse signals from sensors in imaging systems in which radioactive emissions are measured (e.g., SPECT, PET, scintimammography, etc.) also require amplifiers with bandwidths in the hundreds of megahertz or higher. Emitted ionizing radiation is detected using scintillation crystal/photomultiplier tube systems or direct semiconductor radiation sensors (Northrop, 2002).

A major goal of electronic amplifier design is to develop amplifier designs that overcome certain basic limitations on high-frequency bandwidth. A major limitation on high-frequency response is called the *Miller effect*. In this effect, a small-signal parasitic capacitor couples the inverting output of an ideal VCVS amplifier to its input. The circuit is shown in Figure 2.39(A); clearly, $V_o = -\mu V_g$ (the amplifier is inverting). Feedback to the input node is through the parasitic capacitance, C_{io} (normally approximately 1 to 3 pF in small-signal transistors). A node equation is written on the V_g node:

$$V_g\left[G_s + j\omega\, C_{io}\right] - V_o\, j\omega\, C_{io} = G_s V_s \qquad (2.112)$$

from which

$$\frac{V_o}{V_s}(j\omega) = \frac{-\mu}{1 + j\omega C_{io}(1+\mu)R_s} \qquad (2.113)$$

is obtained.

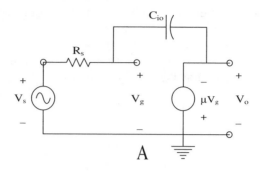

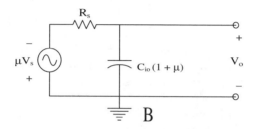

FIGURE 2.39
(A) Simple VCVS with negative feedback through capacitor C_{io} illustrating the cause of the Miller effect. (B) Simple circuit showing the Miller capacitor of the equivalent input low-pass filter. See text for analysis.

Equation 2.113 is the frequency response function of an equivalent simple R–C low-pass filter shown in Figure 2.39(B). Note that the equivalent capacitor shunting the V_g node to ground is (1 minus the voltage gain) times the parasitic feedback capacitor, C_{io}. This high-frequency attenuation of the input signal due to C_{io} is called the Miller effect.

When the ideal inverting VCVS is replaced by a Thevenin equivalent, as shown in Figure 2.40, the effect of C_{io} is more complex. Now it is necessary to write two node equations:

$$V_g [G_s + j\omega C_{io}] - V_o j\omega C_{io} = V_s G_s \tag{2.114A}$$

$$-V_g [j\omega C_{io} - \mu G_o] + V_o [G_o + j\omega C_{io}] = 0 \tag{2.114B}$$

Using Cramer's rule to solve for V_g and V_o:

$$\Delta = \begin{vmatrix} G_s + j\omega C_{io} & -j\omega C_{io} \\ -[j\omega C_{io} - \mu G_o] & [G_o + j\omega C_{io}] \end{vmatrix} = G_s G_o + j\omega C_{io}[G_s + G_o(1 + \mu)] \tag{2.115}$$

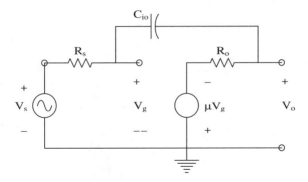

FIGURE 2.40
Another circuit illustrating the Miller effect; the effect of an output resistance is included.

$$\Delta V_o = V_s\, G_s\, [j\omega C_{io} - \mu G_o] \tag{2.116}$$

$$\Delta V_g = V_s\, G_s\, [j\omega C_{io} + G_o] \tag{2.117}$$

Thus:

$$\frac{V_o}{V_s}(j\omega) = \frac{-\mu\big[1 - j\omega C_{io} R_o/\mu\big]}{1 + j\omega C_{io}\big[(1+\mu)R_s + R_o\big]} \tag{2.118}$$

and:

$$\frac{V_g}{V_s}(j\omega) = \frac{1 + j\omega C_{io} R_o}{1 + j\omega C_{io}\big[(1+\mu)R_s + R_o\big]} \tag{2.119}$$

From Equation 2.118, it can be seen that the break frequency of the pole still depends inversely on the Miller capacitance in the input circuit, $C_M = C_{io}(1 + \mu)$. The Thevenin output resistance also contributes to the amplifier's time constant. Note that the larger the gain magnitude, μ, is, the lower the break frequency. This property suggests a trade-off between gain and amplifier high-frequency bandwidth, called the *gain–bandwidth product* (GBWP). More will be said concerning the GBWP in following sections.

BJTs and the various types of FETs have parasitic capacitances between the input and output nodes and ground, and between the input and output nodes (the latter able to form the "evil" Miller capacitance). The following sections examine the high-frequency SSMs for BJTs and FETs, as well as the behavior of the three major single-BJT amplifiers (grounded emitter, grounded base, and emitter follower). The three major single-FET amplifiers (the grounded source, the grounded gate and source follower) will also be discussed.

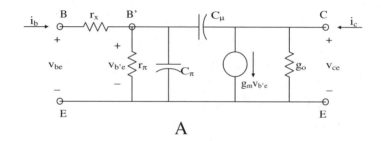

A

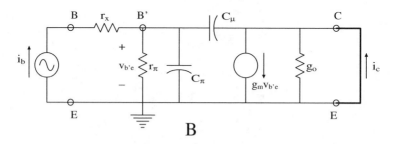

B

FIGURE 2.41

(A) The hybrid pi, high-frequency SSM for a BJT. A common-emitter configuration is assumed. (B) A hy-pi HFSSM circuit used to calculate a BJT's complex short-circuit output current gain, $h_{fe}(j\omega)$, and f_T, where $\left| h_{fe}(j2\pi f_T) \right| = 1$.

2.5.2 High-Frequency SSMs for BJTs and FETs

The simplified, hybrid-pi (hy-pi) high-frequency, small-signal model (HFSSM) is widely used to model and predict the high-frequency behavior of *npn* and *pnp* BJTs. The hy-pi model is illustrated in Figure 2.41(A). The capacitance, C_μ, is largely due to the depletion capacitance of the normally reverse-biased, collector–base junction and thus is voltage dependent. The capacitance, C_π, is the capacitance of the forward-biased, base–emitter junction and its value can be considered to be dependent on the total emitter current. Note that the hy-pi SSM uses a Norton model for the BJT's collector–emitter port. The output conductance, g_o, can be related to the BJT's mid-frequency, *h*-parameter, SSM by $g_o \cong (h_{oe} - g_m\,h_{re})$ (Northrop, 1990). The VCCS has a small-signal transconductance, g_m, given by:

$$g_m = \left. \frac{\partial i_c}{\partial v_{b'e}} \right|_{v_{Ce}=0} \cong \frac{h_{fe}}{r_\pi} = \frac{\left| I_{CQ} \right|}{V_T} \tag{2.120}$$

The g_m of BJTs is large compared with FETs and depends on the dc operating point of the device; for example, if $I_{CQ} = 1$ mA, $g_m \cong 0.04$ S. g_m is measured under small-signal, short-circuit collector–emitter conditions.

An important BJT parameter is its f_T, the frequency at which $|h_{fe}| = 1$. Recall that:

$$h_{fe} = \frac{\partial i_c}{\partial i_b}\bigg|_{v_{ce}=0} \qquad (2.121)$$

When i_b and i_c are sine waves, h_{fe} can be written as a complex (vector) function of frequency:

$$h_{fe}(j\omega) = \frac{I_c}{I_b}(j\omega)\bigg|_{V_{ce}=0} \qquad (2.122)$$

Thus, by definition of f_T,

$$\left|h_{fe}(j2\pi f_T)\right| \equiv 1 \qquad (2.123)$$

To develop an expression for f_T in terms of the hy-pi SSM parameters, consider the model shown in Figure 2.41(B). Because of the small-signal short-circuit conditions on the model, the collector current is:

$$I_c(j\omega) = g_m V_{b'e} - j\omega C_\mu V_{b'e} \qquad (2.124)$$

$V_{b'e}$ is found by writing a node equation on the B' node:

$$V_{b'e} = \frac{I_b}{g_\pi + j\omega(C_\pi + C_\mu)} \qquad (2.125)$$

Substituting Equation 2.125 into Equation 2.124 yields the final result for $h_{fe}(j\omega)$:

$$h_{fe}(j\omega) = \frac{I_c}{I_b}(j\omega)\bigg|_{V_{ce}=0} = \frac{h_{fe}(0)}{1 + j\omega r_\pi(C_\pi + C_\mu)} \qquad (2.126)$$

$h_{fe}(0)$ is the low- and mid-frequency, common-emitter, h-parameter current gain, also known as the BJT's beta. Set the magnitude of the expression of Equation 2.126 equal to unity and solve for f_T:

$$f_T = \frac{g_m}{2\pi(C_\pi + C_\mu)} = \frac{h_{fe}(0)}{2\pi(C_\pi + C_\mu)r_\pi} = \frac{|I_{CQ}|}{2\pi(C_\pi + C_\mu)V_T} \text{Hz} \qquad (2.127)$$

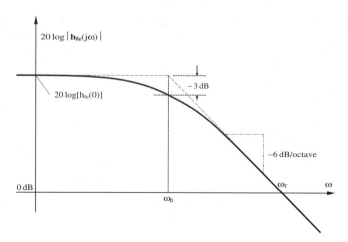

FIGURE 2.42
Bode frequency response magnitude of $|h_{fe}(j\omega)|$.

Thus, the f_T frequency for unity current gain magnitude is seen to be a function of C_π and C_μ, as well as the BJT's Q-point.

A Bode magnitude plot of $h_{fe}(j\omega)$ vs. ω is shown in Figure 2.42. Note that $h_{fe}(j\omega)$ has a (current) gain-bandwidth product. This is easily written from Equation 2.126:

$$\text{GBWP} = \frac{h_{fe}(0)}{2\pi r_\pi \left(C_\pi + C_\mu\right)} \text{ Hz} \qquad (2.128)$$

Note that the h_{fe} GBWP = f_T.

It is important to note that the hy-pi HFSSM is generally valid for frequencies below $f_T/3$. To examine high-frequency BJT circuit behavior above $f_T/3$, one must use SPICE or MicroCap™ computer simulations, which use more detailed, nonlinear BJT models that include effects such as carrier transit times, charge storage, how C_π changes with V_{CB}, etc.

A simple, linear fixed-parameter model for FET high-frequency behavior is shown in Figure 2.43. For simple modeling of FET amplifier high-frequency response, the three voltage-dependent capacitances, C_{gs}, C_{gd}, and C_{ds}, are assigned values determined from the FET's quiescent operating point. Manufacturers of discrete FETs generally do not give specific values for C_{gs}, C_{gd}, and C_{ds}; instead they specify C_{iss}, the common-source short-circuit input capacitance measured with $v_{ds} = 0$ (small-signal drain–source voltage = 0). From inspection of the FET HFSSM, it is obvious that $C_{iss} = C_{gd} + C_{gs}$, at some specific Q-point. Also given by manufacturers is C_{rss}, the reverse transfer capacitance measured with $v_{gs} = 0$. From the HFSSM, it is obvious that $C_{rss} = C_{ds} + C_{gd}$. In general, $C_{gd} \gg C_{ds}$, so $C_{rss} \cong C_{gd}$ and $C_{gs} \cong C_{iss} - C_{rss}$.

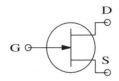

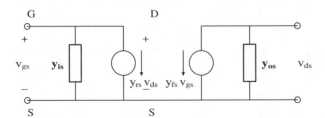

FIGURE 2.43
A simple fixed-parameter HFSSM for all FETs. In JFETs, in particular, C_{gd} and C_{gs} are voltage dependent. Their values at the Q-point must be used.

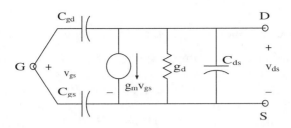

FIGURE 2.44
The more general y-parameter HFSSM for FETs.

At VHF and UHF frequencies, the simple HFSSM of Figure 2.43 is no longer valid, so a two-port, y-parameter model is commonly used for computer modeling in which the four y-parameters are frequency dependent. The y-parameter model is illustrated in Figure 2.44. Note that this is a Norton two-port. In general, $y_{fs}(j\omega) = g_{fs} + jx_{fs}$ and, at mid- and low-frequencies, $y_{fs} = g_{fs} = g_m$; $y_{rs} \rightarrow 0$; $y_{is} \rightarrow 0$; and $y_{os} = g_d$ S.

FETs are characterized by a maximum operating frequency, f_{max}, at which the small-signal current magnitude into the gate node, $I_g(j\omega)$, equals the current magnitude, $|y_{fs} V_{gs}|$, with $v_{ds} = 0$. From the VHFSS y-model of Figure 2.44, it is clear that f_{max} satisfies:

$$V_{gs}|y_{is}(j2\pi f_{max})| = V_{gs}|y_{fs}(j2\pi f_{max})| \qquad (2.129)$$

It is easily seen from the fixed-parameter HFSSM of Figure 2.43 that:

$$f_{max} \cong \frac{g_m}{2\pi C_{iss}} \qquad (2.130)$$

Note that f_{max} is a device figure of merit, not a circuit figure of merit. The unity gain frequency for a grounded-source or grounded-gate FET amplifier is apt to be lower than f_{max} because of the Miller effect and capacitive loading, etc.

2.5.3 Behavior of One-BJT and One-FET Amplifiers at High Frequencies

Figure 2.45(A) illustrates a simple, grounded-emitter (G-E) BJT amplifier. Note that the emitter is not actually grounded, but tied to ground through a parallel R_E, C_E. R_E provides temperature stabilization of the BJT's dc operating point; C_E bypasses the emitter to ground at signal frequencies, putting the emitter at small-signal ground. Figure 2.45(B) illustrates the HFSSM of the circuit. Note that some output capacitance is generally present; it has been omitted in the model for algebraic simplicity. The base spreading resistance, r_x, has also been eliminated so that two, rather than three, node equations govern the amplifier's HF behavior. To analyze the circuit, begin by writing node equations for the V_b and V_o nodes:

$$V_b \left[G_s + g_\pi + j\omega(C_\pi + C_\mu) \right] + V_o \left[j\omega C_\mu \right] = V_s G_s \qquad (2.131A)$$

$$-V_b \left[j\omega C_\mu - g_m \right] + V_o \left[j\omega C_\mu + G_c \right] = 0 \qquad (2.131B)$$

Using Cramer's rule and a good deal of algebra, it is possible to find the mid- and high-frequency response function for the amplifier in time-constant form:

$$\frac{V_o}{V_s}(j\omega) = \frac{-g_m R_C \left[r_\pi / (R_s + r_\pi) \right] \left(1 - j\omega C_\mu / g_m \right)}{\left[1 - \omega^2 C_\mu C_\pi R_C \left(R_s r_\pi / (R_s + r_\pi) \right) \right] +} \qquad (2.132)$$
$$j\omega \left[C_\pi \left(R_s r_\pi / (R_s + r_\pi) \right) + C_\mu R_C + C_\mu \left(1 + g_m R_C \right) \left(R_s r_\pi / (R_s + r_\pi) \right) \right]$$

Note that this quadratic frequency response function has a zero at $\omega = g_m / C_\mu$ r/s, which is well above the BJT's ω_T, where the results predicted by the hy-pi model are no longer valid. It is therefore prudent to neglect the $(1 - j\omega C_\mu / g_m)$ term. Without this term, the frequency response function is that of a second-order low-pass filter. The Miller capacitance is $C_\mu (1 + g_m R_C)$; its presence provides a significant reduction of the amplifier's high-frequency –3-dB point.

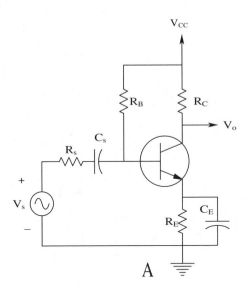

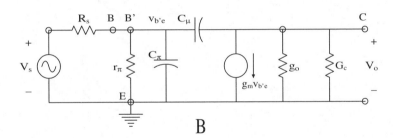

FIGURE 2.45

(A) A basic BJT "grounded-emitter" amplifier; the emitter is assumed to be at small-signal ground at mid- and high-frequencies. (B) Hybrid pi HFSSM for the amplifier. Note that C_μ makes a Miller feedback path between the output node and the $v_{b'e}$ node.

A numerical evaluation of Equation 2.132 for the grounded-emitter BJT amplifier's frequency response is useful to appreciate its practical behavior. Let $g_m = 0.01$ S; $r_\pi = 1.5$ kΩ; $R_C = 10^4$ Ω; $R_s = 1$ kΩ; $C_\pi = 20$ pF; $C_\mu = 2$ pF; $g_o = 0$ S; and $r_x = 0$. The zero is found to be at $\omega_o = g_m/C_\mu = 5 \times 10^9$ r/s, well over the amplifier's ω_T, which is found to be 4.55×10^8 r/s. Thus, the zero is ignored.

The denominator is factored with Matlab™ and is found to have two real poles: one at $\omega_1 = 6.60 \times 10^6$ r/s and the other at $\omega_2 = 6.32 \times 10^8$ r/s. Because ω_2 is also well over $\omega_T/3$, it can be neglected. The mid-frequency gain is $A_{vo} = -60$ and the Miller capacitance is $C_M = C_\mu (1 + g_m R_C) = 202$ pF. Finally, the G-E amplifier's high frequency response function can thus be approximated by the one-pole LPF:

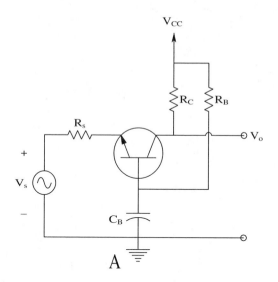

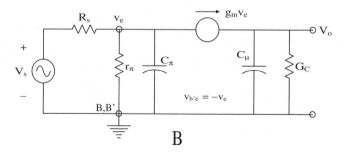

FIGURE 2.46
(A) A BJT grounded-base amplifier. (B) The HFSSM for the amplifier. Note that the model does not have a Miller feedback capacitor.

$$\frac{V_o}{V_s}(j\omega) \cong \frac{-60.0}{\left(1 + j\omega/6.60 \times 10^6\right)} \qquad (2.133)$$

The Hertz to 3-dB break frequency is $f_x = 6.60 \times 10^6/2\pi = 1.05$ MHz, not really very high. Recall that the amplifier's GBWP tends to remain constant; thus, to estimate f_x, one can divide the BJT's f_T by its mid-frequency gain: $\hat{f}_x = 7.24 \times 10^7/60 = 1.21 \times 10^6$ Hz (slightly higher than f_x, but in the range).

The next single-BJT amplifier circuit is the grounded-base amplifier, shown in Figure 2.46(A) and Figure 2.46(B). In the preceding treatment of the BJT G-E amplifier, feedback from the collector to the base coupled through the small-signal, collector-to-base capacitance, $C_{\mu'}$ gave rise to the Miller effect, which caused a lowered high-frequency response. In the grounded-base (G-B) amplifier, no such feedback occurs and no Miller effect is present. Consequently, a G-B amplifier's high-frequency response is generally better than that for a G-E amplifier, other conditions being equal.

To begin analysis of the G-B amplifier, note that the transistor's base is bypassed to ground, causing the small-signal $v_b = 0$. Thus, $V_{b'e} = V_{be} = V_b - V_e = V_e$. Assume that r_x and $g_o = 0$ for algebraic simplicity. Using the hy-pi HFSSM for the BJT, write node equations for the V_e and V_o nodes:

$$V_e \left[G_s + g_\pi + g_m + j\omega C_\pi \right] = V_s\, G_s \tag{2.134A}$$

$$V_o \left[G_C + j\omega C_\mu \right] - V_e\, g_m = 0 \tag{2.134B}$$

Because the two node equations are independent, it is simple to write:

$$V_e = \frac{V_s}{1 + R_s \left(g_\pi + g_m \right) + j\omega C_\pi R_s} \tag{2.135}$$

$$V_o = \frac{V_e g_m R_C}{1 + j\omega C_\mu R_C} \tag{2.136}$$

Substitute Equation 2.135 into Equation 2.136 and find the G-B amplifier's frequency response function:

$$\frac{V_o}{V_s}(j\omega) = \frac{g_m R_C \big/ \left[1 + R_s \left(g_\pi + g_m \right) \right]}{\left(1 + j\omega C_\mu R_C \right) \left\{ 1 + j\omega C_\pi R_s \big/ \left[1 + R_s \left(g_\pi + g_m \right) \right] \right\}} \tag{2.137}$$

Now evaluate the frequency response function's parameters. Let $R_s = 200\ \Omega$; $r_\pi = 2\ \text{k}\Omega$; $g_m = 0.01$; $R_C = 10^4\ \Omega$; $C_\mu = 2\ \text{pF}$; $C_\pi = 20\ \text{pF}$; $r_x = 0$; and $g_o = 0$. From these parameters, find the noninverting, mid-frequency gain, $A_{vo} = +32.26$; $\omega_1 = 1/(R_C C_\mu) = 5 \times 10^7$ r/s; $\omega_2 = [1 + R_s (g_\pi + g_m)]/R_s C_\pi = 7.75 \times 10^8$ r/s; and $\omega_T = 4.55 \times 10^8$ r/s. Disregard ω_2 because it is above ω_T. Thus, the approximate frequency response function for the G-B BJT amplifier is:

$$\frac{V_o}{V_s}(j\omega) \cong \frac{+32.26}{\left(1 + j\omega / 5 \times 10^7 \right)} \tag{2.138}$$

The GBWP for this amplifier is $32.27 \times 5 \times 10^7 = 1.61 \times 10^9$ r/s. Clearly, the G-B amplifier has improved high-frequency response because no Miller effect is present.

The final BJT amplifier to be considered is the emitter-follower (E-F) or grounded-collector amplifier. An E–F amplifier and its HFSSM are shown in

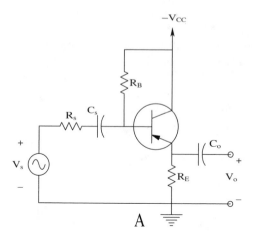

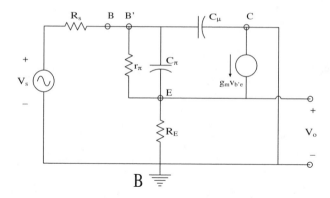

FIGURE 2.47
(A) A BJT emitter-follower. (B) The HFSSM for the amplifier.

Figure 2.47. Node equations are written for the V_b and the $V_o = V_e$ nodes. Assume that $R_b \gg R_s$ and $r_x = g_o = 0$. Also, $V_{b'e} = V_{be} = (V_b - V_o)$.

$$V_b\left[\left(G_s + g_\pi\right) + s\left(C_\mu + C_\pi\right)\right] - V_o\left[g_\pi + sC_\pi\right] = V_s G_s \qquad (2.139\text{A})$$

$$-V_b\left[g_\pi + g_m\right] + sC_\pi + V_o\left[\left(G_E + g_\pi + g_m\right) + sC_\pi\right] = 0 \qquad (2.139\text{B})$$

From Cramer's rule:

$$\Delta V_o = V_s G_s \left[\left(g_\pi + g_m \right) + s C_\pi \right] \tag{2.140}$$

$$\Delta = s^2 C_\pi C_\mu + s \left[C_\pi \left(G_s + G_E \right) + C_\mu \left(G_E + g_m + g_\pi \right) \right] + G_s \left(G_E + g_m + g_\pi \right) + g_\pi G_E \tag{2.141}$$

The emitter follower's frequency response function can then be written, letting $s \rightarrow j\omega$:

$$\frac{V_o}{V_s}(s) = \frac{R_E \left(g_m + g_\pi \right) \left[1 + s C_\pi / \left(g_m + g_\pi \right) \right]}{s^2 C_\pi C_\mu R_E R_s + s \left\{ C_\pi \left(R_E + R_s \right) + C_\mu R_s \left[1 + R_E \left(g_m + g_\pi \right) \right] \right\} + \left\{ 1 + R_E \left(g_m + g_\pi \right) + g_\pi R_s \right\}} \tag{2.142}$$

Note that the preceding frequency response function is *not* in time-constant format; to put in standard TC format, one must divide all terms by $\{[1 + R_E (g_m + g_\pi)] + g_\pi R_s\}$. The mid-frequency gain of the E-F amplifier is simply:

$$A_{vo} = \frac{R_E \left(1 + g_m r_\pi \right)}{R_E \left(1 + g_m r_\pi \right) + R_s + r_\pi} < 1 \tag{2.143}$$

Note that no Miller effect is present in an E-F amplifier, as well as no feedback from output to input; the gain is positive and <1. Let $C_\mu = 2$ pF; $C_\pi = 20$ pF; $g_m = 0.01$ S; $g_\pi = 5 \times 10^{-4}$ S; $R_s = 200\ \Omega$; and $R_E = 10^4\ \Omega$. The frequency of the zero is 5.25×10^8 r/s and it can be neglected. The E-F's poles (break frequencies) are found to be at 2.058×10^9 r/s and 4.102×10^9 r/s. $\omega_T = 4.55 \times 10^8$ r/s. Because the break frequencies are 10 times the transistor's ω_T, the results are not particularly valid. What they do illustrate, however, is that the E-F has amazing bandwidth. Capacitance shunting G_C (output capacitance) will lower the E-F's high frequency response.

It is now appropriate to consider the high-frequency behavior of the three FET amplifiers analogous to the BJT amplifiers described previously: the FET grounded-source (G-S) amplifier; the grounded-gate (G-G) amplifier; and the source follower (S-F). Figure 2.48 illustrates a typical G-S amplifier and its HFSSM. It is clear that there will be a Miller effect for this amplifier because it has an inverting gain with magnitude >1 and a small capacitance C_{gd} coupling the output node to the input. The node equations for the G-S amplifier's HFSSM are:

$$V_g \left[G_1 + s(C_{gs} + C_{gd}) \right] - V_o[sC_{gd}] = V_1 G_1 \tag{2.144A}$$

$$-V_g[-g_m + sC_{gd}] + V_o[G_D' + s(C_{ds} + C_{gd})] = 0 \tag{2.144B}$$

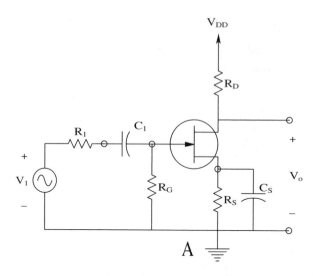

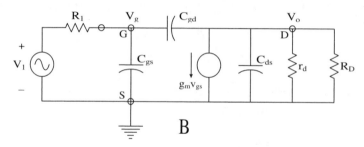

FIGURE 2.48
(A) A JFET grounded-source amplifier. (B) The HFSSM for the amplifier.

where $G_D' = G_D + g_d$. These equations are solved with Cramer's rule:

$$\Delta = G_1 G_D' + s(C_{ds} + C_{gd})G_1 + s(C_{gs} + C_{gd})G_D' + s^2 [(C_{gs} + C_{gd})C_{ds} + C_{gd} C_{gs}] \quad (2.145)$$

$$\Delta V_o = V_1 G_1 [-g_m + sC_{gd}] \quad (2.146)$$

Thus, the detailed frequency response function for the FET G-S amplifier is:

$$\frac{V_o}{V_1}(s) = \frac{-g_m R_D' \left[1 - sC_{gd}/g_m\right]}{s^2 \left[\left(C_{gs} + C_{gd}\right)C_{ds} + C_{gd}C_{gs}\right]R_1 R_D' +} \quad (2.147)$$

$$s\left[R_1 C_{gd}\left(1 + g_m R_D'\right) + R_D'\left(C_{gd} + C_{ds}\right) + R_1 C_{gs}\right] + 1$$

Pick some reasonable parameters for the JFET: $g_d = 2 \times 10^{-5}$ S; $I_{DSS} = 10$ mA; $I_{DQ} = 5$ mA; $g_{mo} = 7 \times 10^{-3}$ S; $C_{gs} = C_{gd} = 2.5$ pF; $C_{ds} = 0.5$ pF; $R_1 = 600$ Ω; and $R_D = 3$ kΩ. Thus, $G_D' = 3.533 \times 10^{-4}$ S and $g_m = g_{mo}\sqrt{(I_{DQ}/I_{DSS})} = 4.243 \times 10^{-3}$ S.

Now the zero is at $g_m/C_{gd} = 1.70 \times 10^9$ r/s, which is ridiculously high, so neglect it. The mid-frequency gain is simply $A_{vo} = g_m R_D' = -12.0$. To find the G-S amplifier's two break frequencies (poles), it is necessary to factor the denominator of Equation 2.147. The two break frequencies are found to be $\omega_1 = 3.451 \times 10^7$ r/s, or 5.492×10^6 Hz, and $\omega_2 = 1.950 \times 10^9$ r/s. The first, lower-frequency pole is dominant and the second pole is neglected, giving the approximate frequency response for the G-S amplifier:

$$\frac{V_o}{V_1}(j\omega) \cong \frac{-12}{\left[1 + j\omega/(3.451 \times 10^7)\right]} \tag{2.148}$$

The FET analog to the BJT grounded-base circuit is the FET grounded-gate amplifier, shown in Figure 2.49(A). Assume that the dc I_{DQ} flows through R_s and V_1, self-biasing the Q point of the JFET so that V_{GSQ} is appropriately negative. Figure 2.49(B) shows the HFSSM of the G-G amplifier. Write node equations at V_s and V_o:

$$V_s\left[G_s + g_d + g_m + s(C_{gs} + C_{ds})\right] - V_o\left[g_d + sC_{ds}\right] = V_1 G_s \tag{2.149A}$$

$$-V_s\left[g_m + g_d + sC_{ds}\right] + V_o\left[G_D + g_d + s(C_{dg} + C_{ds})\right] = 0 \tag{2.149B}$$

Using Cramer's rule:

$$\Delta = s^2\left[C_{ds}(C_{dg} + C_{gs}) + C_{gs}C_{dg}\right]$$
$$+ s\left[G_s(C_{dg} + C_{ds}) + g_d(C_{ds} + C_{gs})G_D(C_{ds} + C_{gs}) + g_m C_{dg}\right] \tag{2.150}$$
$$+ \left[G_s(G_D + g_d) + G_D(g_d + g_m)\right]$$

$$\Delta V_o = V_1 G_s\left[g_m + g_d + sC_{ds}\right] \tag{2.151}$$

The frequency response function for the JFET G-G amplifier can finally be written after some algebra:

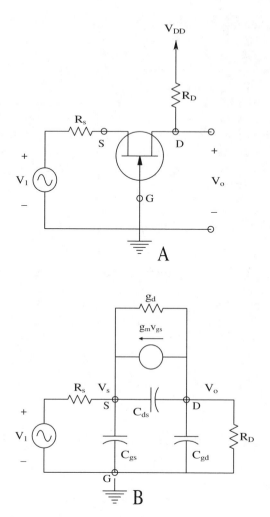

FIGURE 2.49
(A) A JFET grounded-gate amplifier. (B) The HFSSM for the amplifier.

$$\frac{V_o}{V_1}(s) = \frac{+R_D(g_m + g_d)\left[1 + sC_{ds}r_d/(1 + g_m r_d)\right]}{s^2\left[C_{ds}(C_{dg} + C_{gs}) + C_{gs}C_{dg}\right]R_s R_D +} \quad \cdots \quad (2.152)$$

$$s\left[G_s(C_{dg} + C_{ds}) + (G_D + g_d)(C_{ds} + C_{gs}) + g_m C_{dg}\right] +$$

$$\left[1 + g_d R_D + R_s(g_d + g_m)\right]$$

The numerical values of the FET HFSSM parameters are the same as for the G-S amplifier: $g_d = 2 \times 10^{-5}$ S; $I_{DSS} = 10$ mA; $I_{DQ} = 5$ mA; $g_{mo} = 7 \times 10^{-3}$ S;

$C_{gs} = C_{gd} = 2.5$ pF; $C_{ds} = 0.5$ pF; $R_s = 600$ Ω; and $R_D = 3$ kΩ; and $g_m = g_{mo}$ $\sqrt{(I_{DQ}/I_{DSS})} = 4.243 \times 10^{-3}$ S. The G-G amplifier's mid-band gain is:

$$A_{vo} = \frac{R_D(g_m r_d + 1)}{R_s(g_m r_d + 1) + R_D + r_d} = 3.535 \qquad (2.153)$$

The frequency of the zero is sufficiently high, so it can be neglected:

$$\omega_o = \frac{(g_m r_d + 1)}{C_{ds} r_d} = 8.526 \times 10^9 \text{ r/s} \qquad (2.154)$$

Using numerical values, the quadratic denominator is factored to find the break frequencies, which are $\omega_1 = 1.29 \times 10^8$ and $\omega_2 = 1.78 \times 10^9$ r/s. Now the approximate low-pass transfer function of the G-G JFET amplifier can be written:

$$\frac{V_o}{V_1}(j\omega) \cong \frac{3.535}{\left[1 + j\omega/(1.29 \times 10^8)\right]} \qquad (2.155)$$

Note the GBWP for the G-G amplifier is 4.57×10^8 r/s and the GBWP for the JFET G-S amplifier with the same parameters is found to be 4.14×10^8 r/s, illustrating that gain-bandwidth product is substantially independent of amplifier gain and design for a given device.

As a final example in this one-transistor amplifier section, consider the FET source follower (S-F), shown in Figure 2.50(A). From the HFSSM, the node equations can be written:

$$V_g\left[G_1 + s(C_{gd} + C_{gs})\right] - V_o\left[sC_{gs}\right] = V_1 G_1 \qquad (2.156A)$$

$$-V_g\left[g_m + sC_{gs}\right] + V_o\left[g_m + G_s + g_d + s(C_{gs} + C_{ds})\right] = 0 \qquad (2.156B)$$

Cramer's rule yields:

$$\Delta = s^2\left[C_{gd}(C_{gs} + C_{ds}) + C_{gs}C_{ds}\right] + s\left[(C_{gs} + C_{ds})G_1 + C_{gd}(g_m + g_d + G_s) + C_{gs}(G_s + g_d)\right] +$$
$$\left[G_1(g_m + g_d + G_s)\right] \qquad (2.157)$$

$$\Delta V_o = V_1 G_1[g_m + sC_{gs}] \qquad (2.158)$$

After some algebra, the frequency response function can be written:

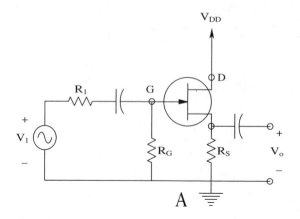

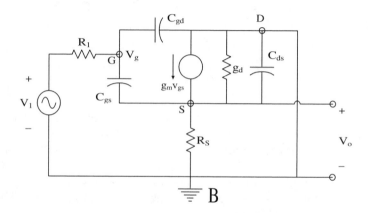

FIGURE 2.50
(A) A JFET source-follower amplifier. (B) The HFSSM for the amplifier.

$$\frac{V_o}{V_1}(s) = \frac{R_S g_m \left[1 + s C_{gs}/g_m\right]}{s^2 \left[C_{gd}\left(C_{gs} + C_{ds}\right) + C_{gs}C_{ds}\right]R_1 R_S +} \qquad \ldots \; (2.159)$$

$$s\left\{R_S\left(C_{gs} + C_{ds}\right) + R_1 C_{gd}\left[1 + R_S\left(g_m + g_d\right)\right] + R_1 C_{gs}\left[1 + g_d R_s\right]\right\} +$$

$$\left[R_S\left(g_m + g_d + G_s\right)\right]$$

From Equation 2.159, the mid-frequency gain is:

$$A_{vo} = \frac{R_S\left(g_m r_d\right)}{R_S\left(g_m r_d + 1\right) + r_d} = 0.923 \qquad (2.160)$$

using the parameters of the preceding FET amplifiers. The zero is at $\omega_o = g_m/C_{gs} = 1.70 \times 10^9$ r/s.

The two poles found by factoring the quadratic denominator in numerical form are $\omega_1 = 1.26 \times 10^9$ and $\omega_2 = 5.96 \times 10^8$ r/s. Thus, the approximate mid- and high-frequency response of the JFET S-F is:

$$\frac{V_o}{V_1}(j\omega) \cong \frac{+0.923}{\left[1+ j\omega/\left(5.96 \times 10^8\right)\right]} \tag{2.161}$$

This section has shown how the Miller effect reduces high-frequency response in conventional grounded-emitter BJT amplifiers and grounded-source FET amplifiers. It has also shown that G-B, G-G, E-F, and S-F amplifiers do not suffer from the Miller effect and generally have their first high-frequency break frequency well above that for the same transistors used in G-E and G-S amplifiers. The following section shows that good high-frequency amplifiers essentially free of Miller effect can be made using two transistors.

2.5.4 High-Frequency Behavior of Two-Transistor Amplifiers

The loss of high-frequency amplification from the Miller effect comes from the negative feedback from output to input nodes supplied through the small drain-to-gate capacitance in FETs or through the collector-to-base capacitance in BJTs, configured as G-S and G-E amplifiers, respectively. Clearly, a good high-frequency amplifier design must avoid the Miller effect at all costs.

The first broadband amplifier configuration can be realized with two BJTs, two FETs, or an FET and a BJT. It is called the *emitter-follower/grounded-base* (EF–GB) configuration when made from BJTs. Figure 2.51 illustrates the circuit and its HFSSM. As in the previous examples of single-transistor, high-frequency amplifier analysis, write the *three* node equations for the HFSSM of the amplifier:

$$V_o\left[G_C + sC_{\mu 2}\right] - g_{m2}V_e = 0 \tag{2.162A}$$

$$V_b\left[G_s + g_{\pi 1} + s\left(C_{\mu 1} + C_{\pi 1}\right)\right] - V_e\left[g_{\pi 1} + sC_{\pi}\right] = V_sG_s \tag{2.162B}$$

$$-V_b\left[g_{m1} + g_{\pi 1} + sC_{\pi 1}\right] + V_e\left[\left(g_{\pi 1} + g_{\pi 2} + g_{m1} + g_{m2}\right) + G_E + s\left(C_{\pi 1} + C_{\pi 2}\right)\right] = 0 \tag{2.162C}$$

Note that the V_o node equation is depends only on V_e; thus:

$$\frac{V_o}{V_e}(s) = \frac{g_{m2}R_C}{1+ sC_{\mu 2}R_C} \tag{2.163}$$

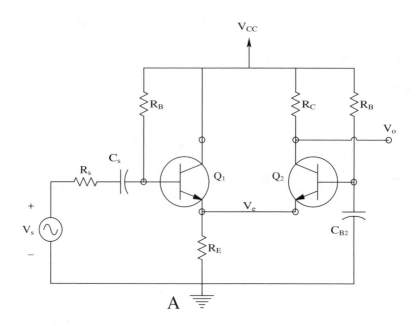

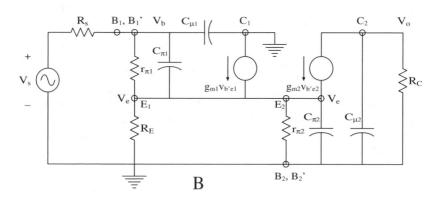

FIGURE 2.51
(A) A BJT emitter-follower–grounded-base amplifier. (B) The HFSSM for the amplifier.

To simplify the algebra, assume the transistors are identical and have the same I_{CQ}. Thus,

$$C_{\pi 1} = C_{\pi 2} = C_{\pi}, \; g_{m1} = g_{m2} = g_m, \; r_{\pi 1} = r_{\pi 2} = r_{\pi}, \; C_{\mu 1} = C_{\mu 2} = C_{\mu},$$

$$r_{x1} = r_{x2} = 0, \text{ and } g_{o1} = g_{o2} = 0 \qquad (2.164)$$

and, using Cramer's rule and a plethora of algebra, the frequency response for V_e can be found (let $s = j\omega$):

$$\frac{V_e}{V_s}(s) = \frac{(1+g_m r_\pi)[1+sC_\pi r_\pi/(1+g_m r_\pi)]}{s^2[2C_\pi C_\mu + C_\pi^2]R_s r_\pi +} \tag{2.165}$$

$$s\{C_\pi[2r_\pi + R_s(g_m r_\pi + 2 + G_E r_\pi)] + C_\mu R_s[2(1+g_m r_\pi) + G_E r_\pi]\} +$$

$$[2(1+g_m r_\pi) + G_E r_\pi + R_s(g_m + G_E)]$$

The mid-frequency gain of the amplifier is found by substituting Equation 2.165 into Equation 2.163 and letting $s = j\omega = 0$:

$$A_{vo} = \frac{V_o}{V_s} = \frac{g_m R_C}{2 + [r_\pi + R_s(1+g_m R_E)]/[R_E(1+g_m r_\pi)]} \tag{2.166}$$

Note that the small-signal term, $g_m r_\pi$, is equal to the BJT's beta or h_{fe}. Define reasonable numerical values for the EF–GB circuit's parameters: $I_{CQ} = 1$ mA; $g_m = 0.0384615$ S; $r_\pi = 2.6 \times 10^3$ Ω; $R_s = 300$ Ω; $R_C = 6$ kΩ; $RE = 3$ kΩ; $C_\mu = 2$ pF; and $C_\pi = 200$ pF.

Substituting these parameters in the preceding expressions yields $A_{vo} = +108.66$. The frequency of the zero is $\omega_o = (1 + g_m r_\pi)/C_\pi r_\pi = 1.942 \times 10^8$ r/s. The collector break frequency is at $\omega_3 = 1/C_\mu R_C = 8.333 \times 10^7$ r/s. The other two break frequencies are found from finding the roots of the denominator of Equation 2.165; they are $\omega_1 = 1.961 \times 10^8$ and $\omega_2 = 3.438 \times 10^7$ r/s. Thus the overall frequency response function for the EF–GB amplifier is:

$$\frac{V_o}{V_s}(j\omega) = \frac{+108.66[1+j\omega/(1.942 \times 10^8)]}{[1+j\omega/(3.438 \times 10^7)][1+j\omega/(8.333 \times 10^7)][1+j\omega/(1.961 \times 10^8)]} \tag{2.167}$$

Note that the HF pole nearly cancels the HF zero, so the final (approximate) frequency response is

$$\frac{V_o}{V_s}(j\omega) \cong \frac{V_o + 108.66}{V_s[1+j\omega/(3.438 \times 10^7)][1+j\omega/(8.333 \times 10^7)]} \tag{2.168}$$

Note from the HFSSM of the EF–GB amplifier that it has no Miller capacitance coupling the output to the input and the gain is noninverting. By way of comparison, substitute the hy-pi transistor model parameters used previously into the frequency response expression for a conventional single G-E amplifier, given by Equation 2.132 in the previous section. The mid-frequency gain for this amplifier is found to be -230.8 and the dominant break frequency is at $\omega_1 = 5.348 \times 10^6$ r/s, considerably lower that that for the EF–GB amplifier.

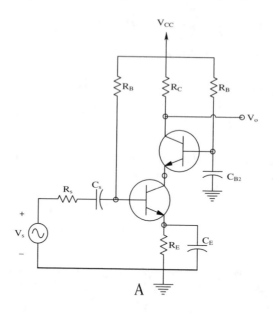

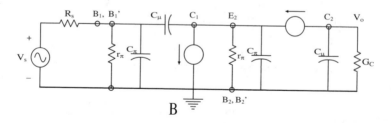

FIGURE 2.52
(A) A BJT cascode amplifier. (B) The HFSSM for the amplifier.

A second two-transistor amplifier that substantially avoids the Miller effect is the well-known cascode amplifier, shown in Figure 2.52(A). The two-BJT cascode amp is illustrated, but it is possible to use an FET for the lower transistor and a BJT for the top, or to use two FETs. As in the preceding example, assume that $C_{\pi 1} = C_{\pi 2} = C_{\pi}$, $g_{m1} = g_{m2} = g_m$, $r_{\pi 1} = r_{\pi 2} = r_{\pi}$, $C_{\mu 1} = C_{\mu 2} = C_{\mu}$, $r_{x1} = r_{x2} = 0$, and $g_{o1} = g_{o2} = 0$. The node equations for the HFSSM of Figure 2.52(B) are

$$V_b \left[(G_s + g_{\pi}) + s(C_{\pi} + C_{\mu}) \right] - V_e \left[sC_{\mu} \right] = V_s\, G_s \qquad (2.169A)$$

$$- V_b \left[-g_m + sC_{\mu} \right] + V_e \left[(g_{\pi} + g_m) + s(C_{\pi} + C_{\mu}) \right] = 0 \qquad (2.169B)$$

$$V_o \left[G_C + sC_{\mu} \right] - V_e\, g_m = 0 \qquad (2.169C)$$

From Equation 2.169 can easily be written:

$$\frac{V_o}{V_e}(s) = \frac{g_m R_C}{1 + sR_C C_\mu} \tag{2.170}$$

Using Cramer's rule on Equation 2.169A and Equation 2.169B:

$$\Delta = s^2 \left[2C_\mu C_\pi + C_\pi^2\right] + s\left[g_\pi\left(C_\pi + C_\mu\right) + g_m\left(C_\pi + 2C_\mu\right)\right] + \tag{2.171}$$
$$\left[G_s\left(g_\pi + g_m\right) + g_\pi\left(g_\pi + g_m\right)\right]$$

$$\Delta V_e = -V_s G_s g_m \left[1 - sC_\mu/g_m\right] \tag{2.172}$$

The frequency response function for V_e can be written from the two preceding equations:

$$\frac{V_e}{V_s}(s) = \frac{-g_m r_\pi \left[1 - sC_\mu/g_m\right]}{s^2\left[2C_\mu C_\pi + C_\pi^2\right] + sR_s\left[C_\pi\left(1 + g_m r_\pi\right) + C_\mu\left(1 + 2g_m r_\pi\right)\right] +} \tag{2.173}$$
$$\left[\left(1 + g_m r_\pi\right) + R_s\left(g_\pi + g_m\right)\right]$$

From Equation 2.173 and Equation 2.169C, the cascode amplifier's mid-frequency gain, A_{vo}, can be found:

$$A_{vo} = \frac{V_o}{V_s} = \frac{-g_m R_C\left[g_m r_\pi/\left(1 + g_m r_\pi\right)\right]}{\left(1 + R_s/r_\pi\right)} \tag{2.174}$$

Now, using the hy-pi HFSSM parameters used in the EF–GB HF amplifier, evaluate the zero, poles, and gain, A_{vo}, for the cascode amplifier, $A_{vo} = -204.9$. The zero is at $\omega_o = 1.923 \times 10^{10}$ r/s (the zero is negligible). The collector pole for the upper BJT is $\omega_3 = 1/(R_C C_\mu) = 8.333 \times 10^7$ r/s. The two poles for the V_e frequency response function, Equation 2.173, are found to be $\omega_1 = 1.739 \times 10^8$ and $\omega_2 = 2.036 \times 10^7$ r/s. Note that ω_2 is the dominant, lowest break frequency. The simplified frequency response function is thus:

$$\frac{V_o}{V_s}(j\omega) = \frac{-204.9}{\left[1 + j\omega/\left(2036 \times 10^7\right)\right]} \tag{2.175}$$

The high break frequency for the BJT cascode amplifier compares favorably with that for the EF–GB amplifier analyzed previously. There is no Miller effect for the upper (G-B) BJT and the Miller effect for the lower (G-E) BJT is very small because the V_e/V_s voltage gain magnitude is <1. Namely,

$$\frac{V_e}{V_s}(0) = \frac{-g_m r_\pi \big/ \left(1 + g_m r_\pi\right)}{1 + R_s/s_\pi} = -0.8877 \tag{2.176}$$

In summary, certain one- and two-transistor amplifier designs are inherently broadband because they avoid the Miller effect. These designs include the emitter-follower; grounded-base; source-follower; grounded-gate; EF–GB pair; and cascode amplifiers. The next section examines some other schemes for increasing high-frequency response, also known as broadbanding. One way is to trade-off mid-band gain for high-frequency bandwidth by using negative feedback. Another is to use a high-pass zero to cancel a low-pass pole, effectively extending high-frequency bandwidth. Still another is to ensure that the Thevenin source resistance of the first stage's output is very low compared to the input resistance of the second stage; an emitter follower is often used to realize low R_{s1}.

2.5.5   Broadbanding Strategies

In op amps, instrumentation amplifiers, and other IC amplifiers, multiple transistor stages are used to achieve the requisite gain. The gain stages are generally direct coupled (DC), i.e., there is a dc pathway from the output of one stage to the input of the next gain stage. Thus DC amplifiers can amplify dc signals. To match appropriate dc bias voltages between the output of one stage and the input of the following stage, often a resistive voltage divider is used. Another strategy to match dc levels is to alternate *pnp* and *npn* BJTs in the stages (or p-channel and n-channel FETs). An advantage of the voltage divider is that it allows one to use shunt capacitive frequency compensation.

Figure 2.53 illustrates two stages of a DC amplifier in general format; the first stage is represented by a frequency-independent Thevenin model, coupled to the input of the second stage through a voltage divider, (R_1, R_2). The input resistance and capacitance of the second stage are R_i, C_i, respectively. V_2 drives the second stage. The shunt capacitor, C_1, can be used to cancel the low-pass effect of the input capacitance. To illustrate this effect, find the transfer function, V_2/V_1, using the simple voltage-divider relation:

$$\frac{V_2}{V_1}(s) = \frac{\dfrac{1}{G_{in} + sC_i}}{\dfrac{1}{G_{in} + sC_i} + R_{s1} + \dfrac{1}{G_1 + sC_1}} \tag{2.177}$$

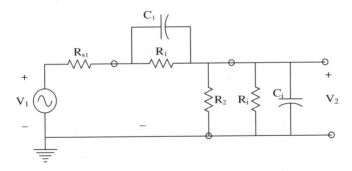

FIGURE 2.53
An *R–C* voltage divider model for direct coupling between amplifier stages. It is shown that a
nearly flat frequency response occurs when $R_1C_1 = C_i (R_i \| R_2)$.

where:

$$R_{in} = \frac{1}{G_2 + G_i} = 1/G_m \qquad (2.178)$$

Adjust C_1 so that $C_1R_1 = C_iR_{in}$ and do algebra to find:

$$\frac{V_2}{V_1}(s) = \frac{\dfrac{R_{in}}{R_{in} + R_1 + R_{s1}}}{1 + \dfrac{sC_iR_{s1}R_{in}}{R_{in} + R_1 + R_{s1}}} \qquad (2.179)$$

Note that, if $R_{s1} \to 0$, $V_2/V_1 \to R_{in}/(R_{in} + R_1)$ (V_2/V_1 is independent of
frequency); otherwise the break frequency is quite high.

Another general principle of extending the high-frequency bandwidth of
a multistage, inverting-gain amplifier is to trade-off mid-band gain for bandwidth through the use of negative feedback. The classic illustration of the
gain-bandwidth constancy is done with op amps in Section 6.3 in Chapter 6.
A similar example will be examined here; see Figure 2.54 for the circuit.
Without feedback ($R_F = \infty$), an inspection shows that the amplifier's frequency response is:

$$\frac{V_o}{V_s}(j\omega) = \frac{-\mu}{1 + j\omega\tau_a} \qquad (2.180)$$

The gain-bandwidth product of this amplifier without feedback is:

$$\text{GBWP}_o = \mu/\tau_a \text{ r/s} \qquad (2.181)$$

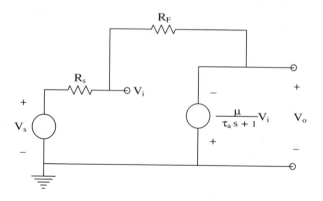

FIGURE 2.54
Circuit illustrating the trade-off of gain for bandwidth using negative feedback. See text for analysis.

With feedback, V_i is given by the node equation:

$$V_i[G_s + G_F] - V_o G_F = V_s G_s \tag{2.182A}$$

$$\downarrow$$

$$\frac{-(s\tau_a + 1)V_o}{\mu}[G_s + G_F] - V_o G_F = V_s G_s \tag{2.182B}$$

$$\downarrow$$

$$\frac{V_o}{V_s}(s) = \frac{-R_F \mu / \left[R_F + R_s(1+\mu)\right]}{\dfrac{s\tau_a(R_F + R_s)}{\left[R_F + R_s(1+\mu)\right]}} \tag{2.182C}$$

The gain-bandwidth product with feedback is:

$$GBWP_f = \mu / \left[\tau_a\left(1 + R_s/R_F\right)\right] \tag{2.183}$$

Assuming that $\mu \gg 1$ and $\mu R_s \gg R_F$ yields the approximate frequency response function:

$$\frac{V_o}{V_s}(j\omega) \cong \frac{-R_F/R_s}{\dfrac{j\omega\tau_a}{\mu R_s/(R_s + R_F)} + 1} \tag{2.184}$$

Note the trade-off between closed-loop gain and bandwidth; the lower the mid-band gain magnitude is, $-R_F/R_s$, the higher the break frequency,

$$\omega_b = \frac{\mu R_s/(R_s + R_F)}{\tau_a} \, r/s$$

The choice of transistor for a high-frequency amplifier design is paramount. BJTs must be chosen to have high f_Ts, and FETs to have high f_{max}. Although it may never be necessary to design a discrete or an IC multistage amplifier, the factors described earlier that go into the design of broadband amplifiers should appreciated.

2.6   Photons, Photodiodes, Photoconductors, LEDs, and Laser Diodes

2.6.1   Introduction

This section examines the properties of semiconductor devices that sense photon energy and others that emit photon energy. Photons are an alternate way to describe electromagnetic (EM) radiation generally having wavelengths from 1×10^{-4} m to less than 3×10^{-12} m. These wavelengths include infrared (IR); visible light; ultraviolet (UV); x-rays; and gamma rays. The photon is a quantum EM "particle" used to describe physical interactions of low-power EMR with molecules, atoms, and subatomic particles, such as atomic shell electrons. The electromagnetic wave characterization of EM energy is used throughout the EM spectrum and finds application in describing the operation of antennas, transmission lines, fiber optic cables, and optical elements such as lenses, prisms, and mirrors used in IR, visible, and UV wavelengths. Maxwell's equations for EM wave propagation are also useful in describing such phenomena as diffraction, refraction, and polarization of light (Balanis, 1989; Hecht, 1987).

A photon has essentially zero mass; it moves at the speed of light in a medium and has an individual energy of $\varepsilon = hc/\lambda = h\nu$ joules, where h is Planck's constant (6.6253×10^{-34} joule-second); c is the speed of light in the supporting medium ($c = 2.998 \times 10^8$ m/sec *in vacuo*); λ is the wavelength of the EM radiation in meters; and ν is the Hertz frequency of the EMR (ν of visible light is approximately 10^{14} Hz). Photon energy is also given in electronvolts (eV). To obtain the energy of a photon in eV, divide its energy in joules by 1.602×10^{-19}. (1.602×10^{-19} is the magnitude of the charge on an electron.) For example, a photon of blue light with a wavelength of $\lambda = 450$ nm has an energy of $e = (6.626 \times 10^{-34}$ J s$)(3 \times 10^8$ m/s$)/(450 \times 10^{-9}$ m$) = 4.41 \times 10^{-19}$ J or 2.76 eV. Similarly, a photon of $\lambda = 700$ nm (red light) has an energy of 2.84×10^{-19} J or 1.77 eV. Figure 2.55 illustrates the EM spectrum.

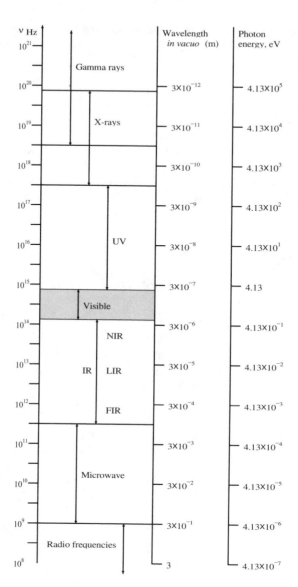

FIGURE 2.55

The electromagnetic spectrum.

Many sensors are used to measure EM energy in biomedical applications. These include, but are not limited to, photodiodes; phototransistors; photoconductors; pyroelectric IR sensors; photomultiplier tubes (PMTs); scintillation crystals + PMTs; etc. (Northrop, 2002).

Next, *pn* junction photon sensors, photoconductors and certain solid-state photon sources will be considered. It will be demonstrated that the interaction of photons in a certain energy range with a semiconductor *pn* junction can cause the generation of a photovoltaic EMF; this EMF is the basis for photodiode behavior and the solar cell as an energy transducer (photons to electrical current flow) capable of doing work. Photodiodes and solar cells can be used to measure incident EM radiation intensity. Also treated in the following sections are the generation of photon energy by special semiconductor diode structures, the light-emitting diode (LED) and the laser diode. Both types of photon-emissive devices have found wide application in biomedical instrumentation (Northrop, 2002).

2.6.2 PIN Photodiodes

Photodiodes are used as sensors for EMR ranging from near infrared (NIR) to near ultraviolet (UVA). Even a standard small-signal silicon *pn* junction diode with a transparent glass envelope will respond to incident EMR of appropriate wavelength, as will a reverse-biased LED. However, photodiodes used for photonic measurements have specialized junction structures that maximize the area over which incident photons are absorbed. Photodiodes are used in a broad range of biomedical instruments, including blood pulse oximeters; finger-tip heart-rate sensors; single-drop blood glucose meters; fiber-optic-based spectrophotometers (used to sense analytes in blood, urine, etc.); spectrophotometric detection of tumors using endoscopes; etc.

Photodiodes fall into two broad categories: (1) three-layer, PIN diodes ("I" stands for intrinsic semiconductor) and (2) avalanche photodiodes (APDs), which are basically four-layer structures (P+IPN). Figure 2.56 illustrates schematic cross sections through two types of PIN devices. Note that to improve the efficiency of photon capture, a thin, $\lambda/4$ layer of antireflective (AR) coating is used on the surface of the PD, similar to the AR coatings commonly used on binocular and camera lenses. Assume an incident photon with the appropriate energy passes through the AR coating, enters the P+ diffusion layer, and interacts (collides) with a valence-band electron. If the electron gains energy greater than the band-gap energy, E_g, it is pulled up into the conduction band, leaving a hole in the valence band.

These electron–hole pairs are formed throughout the P+ layer, the depletion layer, and the N-layer materials. In the depletion layer, the E-field accelerates these photoelectrons toward the N-layer and the holes toward the P-layer. Electrons from the electron–hole pairs generated by photons in the N-layer, along with electrons that have arrived from the P-layer, are left in the N-layer conduction band. Meanwhile the holes diffuse through the N-layer up to the depletion layer while being accelerated and are collected in the P-layer valence band. By these mechanisms, electron–hole pairs, which are generated in proportion to the amount of incident light, are collected in the N- and P-layers of the PD. This results in a positive charge in the P-layer and a negative charge in the N-layer.

When an external circuit is connected between the P- and N-layers, photocurrent electrons will flow away from the N-layer and holes will flow away from the P-layer, toward the opposite electrode. The PIN PD and the external

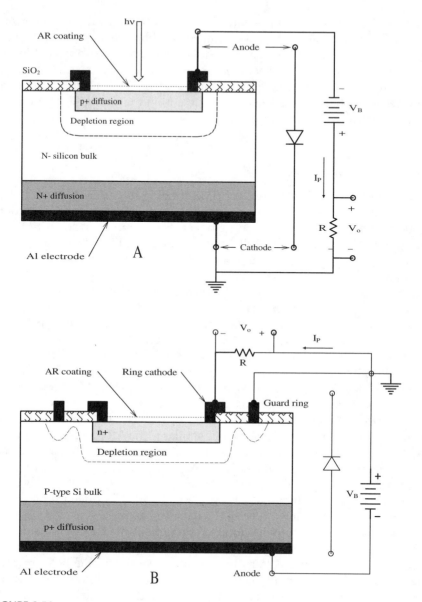

FIGURE 2.56

(A) Layer cake schematic of a three-layer PIN Si photodiode. (B) Layer cake schematic of a three layer, NIP Si photodiode. The AR coating minimizes reflection (and thus maximizes photon absorption) in the range of wavelengths in which the PD is designed to work. The guard ring minimizes dark current.

circuit are shown in Figure 2.56(A). Note that in normal operation of the PD, it is reverse-biased, so the photocurrent is a reverse current flowing in the same direction as the thermally generated leakage current that flows in a reverse-biased *pn* diode.

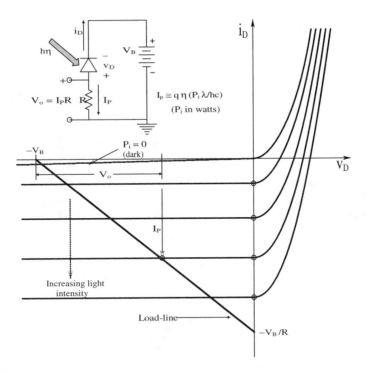

FIGURE 2.57

Top: simple series circuit for PIN PD. Bottom: i_D vs. v_D curves as a function of absorbed photon power, P_i. The load line is determined by the Thevenin equivalent circuit that the PD "sees." Note that the PD's photocurrent, I_P, flows in the reverse direction. V_o across the load resistor can be determined graphically by the intersection of the $i_D = f(P_i)$ line with the load line.

Figure 2.57 illustrates typical PIN PD volt–ampere curves. The load line represents a graphical solution of the PD's (nonlinear) volt–ampere curves with the (linear) Thevenin circuit "seen" by the PD. The zero-current intercept of the load line on the V_D axis is at –Thevenin open-circuit voltage; the zero-voltage intercept is –Thevenin short-circuit current. The load line permits a graphical solution of:

$$i_D(v_D) = \frac{V_B - v_D}{R} \qquad (2.185A)$$

or

$$v_D = V_B - i_D R, \ (V_B < 0 \text{ in reverse-biased diode.}) \qquad (2.185B)$$

The slope of the load line is easily seen to be $-1/R$ and depends only on the Thevenin model parameters. Most PDs are operated in the third quadrant, either with a reverse-bias OCV or under short-circuit conditions ($v_D = 0$). PD signal-conditioning circuits will be described later.

The total PD current can be modeled by:

$$i_D = I_{rs}\left[\exp\left(v_D/V_T\right)-1\right]-I_p \qquad (2.186)$$

where the photocurrent, I_p, flows in the reverse direction and is given by:

$$I_p = \frac{\eta q P_i \lambda}{hc} \text{ amperes} \qquad (2.187)$$

where P_i is the total photon power incident on the PD active surface in watts; $V_T = kT/q$, η is the capture efficiency (approximately 0.8); and I_{rs} is the reverse saturation current. I_{rs} is very temperature dependent; it can be approximated by (Navon, 1975; Millman, 1979):

$$I_{rs}(T) = I_{rs}(T_o)2^{(T-T_o)/10}$$

or

$$\Delta I_{rs}/I_{rs} = \frac{1}{2}\left[3/T + \phi/\left(kT^2\right)\right] \cong 0.08/°\text{K} \qquad (2.188B)$$

where T is the Kelvin temperature; T_o is the Kelvin reference temperature; ϕ is the silicon energy gap (1.15 eV); and k is Boltzmann's constant (1.380 × 10^{-23} J/K). The simple PD model given by Equation 2.186 does not include the ohmic leakage of the reverse-biased PD. Such leakage can be an appreciable portion of the reverse dark i_D for large reverse v_D.

If the PIN PD is operated at zero i_D, photon power produces an open-circuit voltage given by:

$$v_{Doc} = \left(kT/q\right)\ln\left[1+\frac{q\eta\lambda P_i}{hcI_{rs}}\right] \text{ open-circuit volts} \qquad (2.189)$$

Silicon PIN PDs are useful over a wavelength band covering approximately 200 to 1100 nm; their spectral sensitivity rises slowly to a peak at approximately 800 nm, then falls off rapidly. Sensitivity is given by the PD's responsivity in amps per watt; $R(\lambda) = i_D(0)/P_i$. $R(\lambda)$ peaks at approximately 0.55 A/W at approximately 850 nm. Figure 2.58 shows a "typical" Si PIN PD responsivity plot. PDs can also be fabricated using germanium (Ge) and InGaAs. The former material responds from approximately 300 to 1600 nm and the latter composition has a spectral responsivity range from approximately 800 to 2600 nm. Depending on operating conditions, PIN PDs are useful over a range of picowatts to milliwatts of optical power.

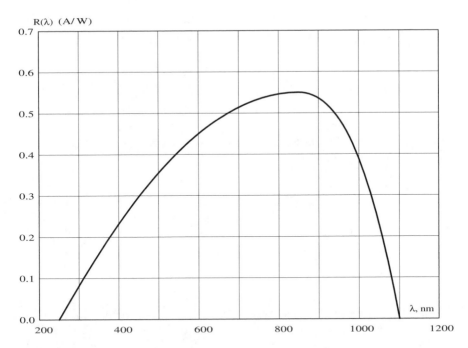

R(λ) (A/W)

λ, nm

FIGURE 2.58
A typical responsivity plot for a Si PIN PD. See text for discussion.

Figures of merit for PDs include the responsivity $R(\lambda)$, described previously; the noise-equivalent (optical) power (NEP); and the detectivity (D*). The NEP is the incident P_i at λ required to generate a short-circuit response current, I_p, equal to the RMS noise current of the detector system (unity output signal-to-noise ratio.) NEP is a measure of the minimum detectable noise power at a given wavelength and bandwidth. In other words,

$$\text{NEP}(\lambda) = \frac{\text{rms noise current}}{\text{responsivity @ } \lambda} \text{ Watts} \qquad (2.190)$$

The noise generated by a PD operating under reverse bias is due to shot noise generated in the dark leakage current and Johnson (thermal) noise generated in the equivalent shunt resistance of the PD. Shot and thermal noises are broadband and considered to have flat white power density spectra (See Chapter 9). The mean-squared shot noise can be shown to be given by:

$$\overline{i_{sn}^2} = 2q I_{DL} B \text{ msA} \qquad (2.191)$$

where q is the magnitude of the electron charge; I_{DL} is the dark leakage current in amperes (I_{DL} is zero for a zero-biased PD); and B is the equivalent

Hertz noise bandwidth over which the noise current is measured. The mean-squared thermal noise can be shown to be given by:

$$\overline{i_{tn}^2} = 4kTGB \quad \text{msA} \tag{2.192}$$

where k = Boltzmann's constant (1.38×10^{-38} J/K); T = Kelvin temperature of PD; B = equivalent Hertz noise bandwidth; and G = net thermal noise producing resistance. The total MS diode noise current is found by adding the two MS current noises:

$$\overline{i_n^2} = \overline{i_{sn}^2} + \overline{i_{tn}^2} \quad \text{msA} \tag{2.193}$$

Thus the total RMS diode noise is:

$$i_n = \sqrt{\overline{i_n^2}} = \sqrt{(2qI_{DL} + 4kTG)}\sqrt{B} \quad \text{rmsA} \tag{2.194}$$

Johnson noise dominates as the dark current $\to 0$. Note that NEP depends on λ, I_{DL} (thus the PD operating circuit), the noise bandwidth B, T, and the net (Norton) conductance, G, in parallel with the photocurrent and noise current sources. The NEP for Si PIN PDs ranges from approximately 10^{-14} W/$\sqrt{\text{Hz}}$ for small-area ($A = 1$ mm²) low-noise PDs, to over 2×10^{-13} W/$\sqrt{\text{Hz}}$ for very large area cells ($A = 100$ mm²). Obviously, the NEP is desired to be as small as possible. Note that manufacturers give NEP independent of the noise Hertz bandwidth, B. NEP must be multiplied by the $\sqrt{B}$ to get the actual NEP in watts.

Often the input light power, P_i, is chopped; that is, the beam is periodically interrupted by a chopper wheel, effectively modulating the beam by multiplying it by a 0,1 square wave. The chopping rate is generally at audio frequencies (e.g., 1 kHz) and the bandwidth of the associated band-pass filter used to condition the PD output determines B. Chopping is used to avoid the excess 1/f diode noise present at DC and very low frequencies.

Figure 2.59 illustrates the equivalent model for a reverse-biased Si PIN PD, showing signal, noise, and dark current sources, the diode small-signal capacitance, C_d, which is a depletion capacitance that depends on $-v_{DQ}$, and diode semiconductor doping and geometry. Note that the DC reverse leakage current has two components: a constant small I_{rs} and a voltage-dependent dark current, I_{DL}. $(I_{DL} + I_{rs})$ are used to calculate i_{sn}. Normally, $R_L \gg R$, so the thermal noise current is found using the external load resistor, R ($1/R = G$). The junction depletion capacitance, C_d, decreases as v_{DQ} goes more negative. Large C_d is deleterious to PD high-frequency response because it shunts $I_P(j\omega)$ to ground. Note that C_d increases with illumination and is smallest in the dark (using the circuit of Figure 2.57). C_d is on the order of picofarads. For example, one Si PIN PD with 1 mm² active area and a $v_{DQ} = -10$ V has a $C_d \cong 4$ pF.

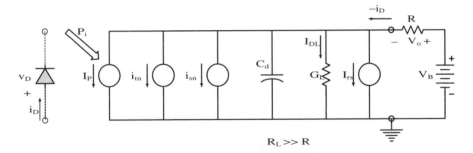

FIGURE 2.59

Model for a reverse-biased Si PIN photodiode. i_{sn} is the DC current-dependent shot noise root power spectrum; i_{tn} is the thermal noise root power spectrum. V_B and R are components of the DC Thevenin circuit biasing the PD.

D^* is $1/\text{NEP}$ for the detector element only, normalized to a 1 cm² active area. D^* is used only for comparisons between PDs of different active areas. D^* units are $\text{cm}\sqrt{\text{Hz}}/\text{W}$. (A "better" PD has a higher D^*.)

2.6.3 Avalanche Photodiodes

A cross-sectional schematic of an avalanche PD (APD) is shown in Figure 2.60. In an APD, a large reverse-biasing voltage is used, about 100 V or more, depending on diode design. The internal E-field completely depletes the π-region of mobile carriers. The E-field in the π-region causes any injected or thermally generated carriers to attain a saturation velocity, giving them enough kinetic energy so that their impact with valence-band electrons causes ionization — the creation of other electron–hole pairs — that in turn are accelerated by the E-field, causing still more impact ionizations, etc.

Photon-generated electron–hole pairs are separated by the E-field in the p- and π-regions; electrons move into the n+ layer and holes drift into the p+ layer, both of which are boundaries of the APD's space-charge region. These photon-generated carriers are multiplied as they pass through the avalanche region by the impact ionization process. At a given reverse operating voltage, $-v_{DQ} = V_R$, one electron generated by photon collision produces M electrons at the APD's anode. The contribution of electrons to I_p is much greater than that from holes because electrons generated in the p- and π-regions are pulled into the avalanche region, whereas holes are swept back into the p+ region (including the holes generated in the avalanche process).

APD noise is due to shot noise. As in the case of the PIN PD, the shot noise is a broadband (white) Gaussian noise whose mean-squared value is proportional to the net DC component of the APD's anode current, I_{Dtot}. The DC anode current has two components; dark leakage current, I_L, and DC photocurrent, I_p. The mean-squared shot noise current is given by:

$$\overline{i_n^2} = 2qBI_{Dtot} \text{ msV} \tag{2.195}$$

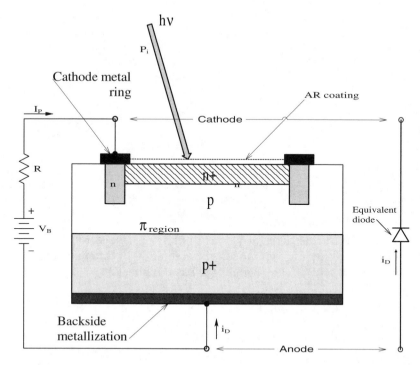

FIGURE 2.60
Cross-sectional layer cake model of an avalanche photodiode.

It is clear that the lowest APD shot noise occurs when the ADP is operated at very low (average) light levels. Figure 2.61 illustrates the peak gain and RMS shot noise current as a function of the DC reverse-bias voltage on a "typical" Si APD. The total leakage current, I_L, can be written as:

$$I_L = I_{LS} + M\,I_{LB} \tag{2.196}$$

where I_{LS} is the surface leakage current (not amplified) and I_{LB} is the bulk leakage current (amplified by the avalanche process). The theoretical MS shot noise current may also be written (Perkin-Elmer, 2003):

$$\overline{i_n^2} = 2qB\Big\{I_{LS} + \big[I_{LB}M^2 + P_i R_1(\lambda)M\big]F\Big\}\ \ \text{msA} \tag{2.197}$$

where q is the electron charge magnitude; I_{LS} is the dark surface leakage current; I_{LB} is the dark bulk leakage current; $I_P = P_i\,R_1(\lambda)\,M$ is the amplified DC photocurrent; and F is the excess noise factor. In general, $F = \rho M + (1 - \rho)$ $(2 - 1/M)$. Because $M \approx 100$, $F \cong 2 + \rho M$. The parameter, ρ, is the ratio of hole to-electron ionization probabilities and is <1. M is the voltage-dependent APD internal gain. It is defined as the ratio of the output current at a given P_i, λ, and DC reverse-bias voltage, V_R, to the output current for the

Gain (M) or Noise Current (pA/√Hz)

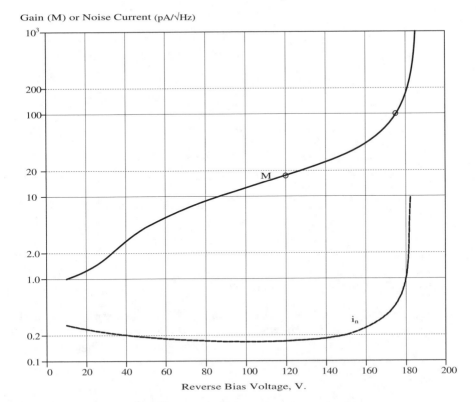

FIGURE 2.61

Plot of peak photonic gain, M, and shot noise root power spectrum, i_n, for a typical avalanche PD.

same input (P_i and λ), but at a low dc reverse-bias voltage, say 10 V. P_i is the incident optical power at wavelength λ, $R(\lambda, V_D)$ is the spectral responsivity in A/W, and B is the Hertz noise bandwidth.

The PE C30902S APD has the following parameters at a reverse voltage of approximately 225 V: $F = 0.02M + 0.98(2 - 1/M)$. $M = 250$ at 830 nm; thus, $F = 6.956$. The responsivity at 830 nm is $R(\lambda) = 128$ A/W. (Dividing the responsivity at 830 nm by M yields $R_1(830) = 0.512$ A/W.) Total dark current is $I_D = 1 \times 10^{-8}$ A. The noise current root spectrum is $i_n = 1.1 \times 10^{-13}$ RMSA/$\sqrt{\text{Hz}}$. The shunt capacitance is $C_d = 1.6$ pF. The rise time and fall time to an 830-nm light pulse with a 50 Ω R_L (10 to 90%) is $t_r = t_f = 0.5$ ns.

The wavelength range of the APD responsivity curve, $R(\lambda)$, depends on APD material; Si APDs are useful between 300 to 1100 nm, Ge APDs between 800 and 1600 nm, and InGaAs devices between 900 to 1700 nm. The peak responsivity depends on the average reverse-bias voltage on the APD. $R_1(\lambda)$ is defined as the APD's responsivity at a low V_R such that $M = 1$. Thus, the APD's (amplified) photocurrent can be written

$$I_P = P_i \, R_1(\lambda) \, M = P_i \, R(\lambda) \text{ amps} \tag{2.198}$$

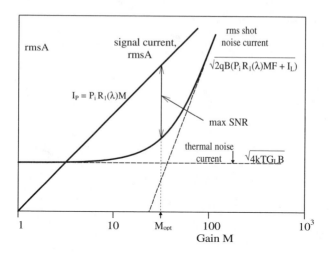

FIGURE 2.62
Plot of signal current and RMS shot noise current for a typical APD vs. gain M, showing the optimum M where the diode's RMS SNR is maximum.

at a given λ and V_R, as shown in Equation 2.195. As noted earlier, the total shot noise from an APD depends not only on dc leakage current, but also on dc photocurrent. There is also a noise current from any Thevenin conductance shunting the APD. Thus, the total diode noise in MSA is given by:

$$\overline{i_n^2} = 2qB\left\{ I_{LS} + \left[I_{LB}M^2 + P_i R_1(\lambda)M \right]F \right\} + 4kTG_L B \text{ msA} \qquad (2.199)$$

The APD's MSSNR can be written, noting that $F \cong 2 + \rho M$:

$$SNR = \frac{P_i^2 R_1^2(\lambda)M^2}{2qB\left\{ I_{LS} + \left[I_{LB}M + P_i R_1(\lambda) \right]MF \right\} + 4kTG_L B}$$

$$= \frac{P_i^2 R_1^2(\lambda)/B}{2q\left\{ I_{LS}/M^2 + \left[I_{LB} + P_i R_1(\lambda)/M \right](2 + \rho M) \right\} + 4kTG_L/M^2} \qquad (2.200)$$

Inspection of the denominator of the right-hand SNR expression shows that it has a minimum at some $M = M_o$, which results in a maximum SNR, other factors remaining constant. This optimum M_o is illustrated in Figure 2.62. Recall that M is set by the DC reverse bias on the APD, V_R, so finding the optimum V_R and M to optimize the APD SNR can be arty.

2.6.4   Signal Conditioning Circuits for Photodiodes

The most basic signal conditioning circuit for a PD is the simple DC Thevenin circuit shown in Figure 2.57. As discussed in the text, the output voltage

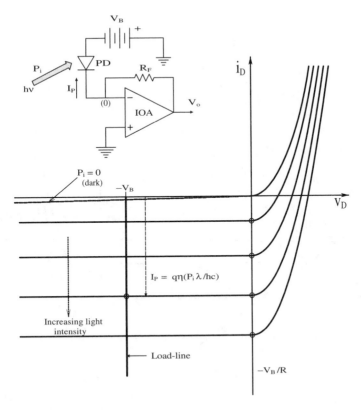

FIGURE 2.63
Top: op amp signal conditioning circuit for a PIN PD operated at constant bias voltage. Bottom:
plot of PD i_D vs. v_D curves showing the constant voltage load line.

from the photocurrent can be found graphically using the load line determined by V_B and R. Neglecting dark current, it is simply:

$$V_o = q\eta(P_i\,\lambda/hc)R \text{ volts} \tag{2.201}$$

An active circuit commonly used to condition PD output is shown in
Figure 2.63. Because the summing junction of the op amp is at virtual ground,
the PD is held at a constant reverse bias, V_B. I_P flows through R_F, so Ohm's
law tells that $V_o = q\eta(P_i\,\lambda/hc)\,R_F$, neglecting leakage (dark) current. By
operating a PIN PD at reverse bias, the junction depletion capacitance, C_d,
is made smaller and the diode's bandwidth is increased. Unfortunately,
reverse bias also increases the leakage current and thus the device's shot
noise. If V_B is made zero, then C_d is maximum and the PD's bandwidth is
lowest. At zero bias, the leakage current $\to 0$ and the diode's shot noise is
minimal, depending only on the photocurrent. As Chapter 9 will show, R_F
and the op amp contribute noise to V_o; this noise will not be discussed here,
however.

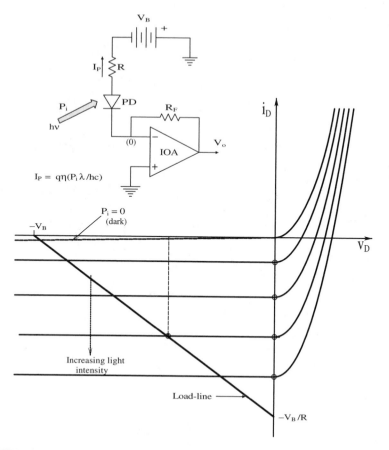

FIGURE 2.64

Top: op amp signal conditioning circuit for a PIN PD biased from a Thevenin dc source. Bottom: plot of PD i_D vs. v_D curves showing the load line.

Sometimes a resistor is added in series with V_B to limit the current through the PD. This circuit is shown in Figure 2.64. Note that the maximum PD current is determined by the load line and is $i_D = -V_B/R$. APDs are run with the same circuit, except V_B is on the order of hundreds of volts and the series R (typically ≥ 1 MΩ) serves to protect the APD from excess reverse current that, for most APDs, is on the order of hundreds of microamperes. Although the series resistor protects the ADP from excess reverse current, it also produces thermal (Johnson) noise over and above the APD's shot noise, as well as the noise produced in the op amp circuit

An op amp circuit can be used to condition the output of a PIN PD to yield a logarithmic output proportional to P_i, as shown in Figure 2.65. The PD is operated in the zero current mode. Solving for v_{Doc}:

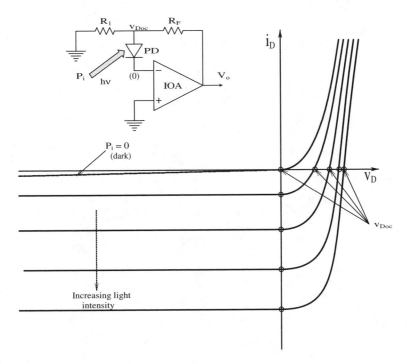

FIGURE 2.65
Top: op amp signal conditioning circuit for a PIN PD operated in the open-circuit photovoltage
mode. Bottom: plot of PD i_D vs. v_D curves showing the operating points.

$$i_D = 0 = I_{rs}\left[\exp\left(v_{Doc}/V_T\right) - 1\right] - q\eta(P_i\lambda/hc) \tag{2.202A}$$

$$\downarrow$$

$$v_{Doc} = V_T \ln\left[1 + \frac{q\eta(P_i\lambda/hc)}{I_{rs}}\right] \tag{2.202B}$$

and, because of the R_1, R_F voltage divider, this yields:

$$V_o = \left(1 + R_F/R_1\right)V_T \ln\left[1 + \frac{q\eta(P_i\lambda/hc)}{I_{rs}}\right] \tag{2.203}$$

At very low light powers, using the relation $\ln(1 + \varepsilon) \cong \varepsilon$, V_o can be
approximated by:

$$V_o \cong \left(1 + R_F/R_1\right)V_T\left(\frac{q\eta(P_i\lambda/hc)}{I_{rs}}\right) \tag{2.204}$$

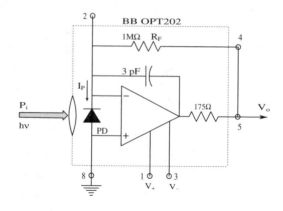

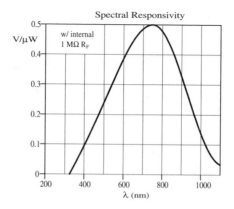

FIGURE 2.66
Top: schematic of the Burr–Brown OPT202 IC photosensor. Bottom: spectral sensitivity of the OPT202 sensor. See text for details.

Typical parameter values are $(1 + R_F/R_1) = 10^3$, $V_T = kT/q = 0.0258$, $q = 1.602 \times 10^{-19}$ Cb, $\eta \cong 0.8$, $\lambda = 512$ nm, $h = 6.625 \times 10^{-34}$ J.sec, $c = 3 \times 10^8$ m/s, $I_{rs} \cong 1$ nA, and NEP $\cong 5 \times 10^{-14}$ W. Neglecting leakage (dark) current, V_o can be calculated for $P_i = 1$ pW at $\lambda = 512$ nm: $\therefore V_o = 8.51$ mV.

Several manufacturers make ICs containing a PIN photodiode with an on-chip amplifier e.g., Burr–Brown makes the OPT202. This photosensor has a 2.29×2.29 mm PD coupled to an op amp with an internal 1-MΩ feedback resistor, as shown in Figure 2.66. This IC works over a wide supply voltage range (± 2.25 to ± 18 V) and has a voltage output responsivity of 0.45 V/μW at $\lambda = 650$ nm with its internal $R_F = 1$ MΩ. It has a -3-dB bandwidth of 50 kHz and a 10 to 90% rise time of 10 μs. To alter system responsivity, the R_F can be made larger or smaller than the internal 1 MΩ R_F. The IC's NEP is 10^{-11} W for $B = 1$ kHz and $\lambda = 650$ nm with $R_F = 1$ MΩ.

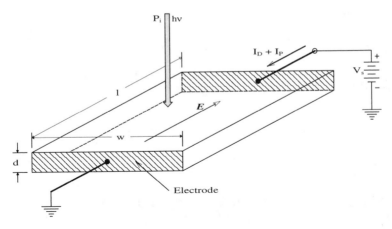

FIGURE 2.67
Geometry of a photoconductor slab.

2.6.5 Photoconductors

Photoconductors (PCs) are transducers that convert photon energy into an increase in electrical conductance; they are also called *light-dependent resistors* or *photoresistors*. Figure 2.67 illustrates the cross-sectional schematic of a typical PC device. PCs can be made from a number of intrinsic and doped semiconductor materials. Each semiconductor has a distinct spectral response to light, ranging from UV to FIR. Table 2.1 lists some of the materials used in PCs, their bandgap energies in electronvolts, and the wavelength of their peak spectral response.

TABLE 2.1

Properties of Some Photoconductors

PC Material	Bandgap Energy, eV	Wavelength of Peak Response, λ_c, μm	Rise Time/ Fall Time
ZnS	3.60	0.345	
CdS	2.40	0.52	30 MS/10 MS
CdSe	1.80	0.69	15 MS/15 MS
CdTe	1.50	0.83	
Si (intrinsic)	1.12	1.10	1 μs/1 μs
Ge (intrinsic)	0.67	1.85	0.1 μs/0.1 μs
PbS	0.37	3.35	
InAs	0.35	3.54	≈ 1 ns
Te	0.33	7.75	
PbTe	0.30	4.13	
PbSe	0.27	4.58	2 μs
HgCdTe (77 K)		5.0	*/5 μs
InSb (77 K)	0.18	6.90	
GeCu (4 K)		25	
GeBe (3 K)		55	

In general, the total current in a PC can be written:

$$I_{PC} = V_s [G_D + G_P] \tag{2.205}$$

where V_s is the bias voltage; G_D is the equivalent dark conductance; and G_P is the photoconductance. G_P can be shown to be given by (Yang, 1988):

$$G_P = \frac{I_P}{V_s} = \frac{q \eta \tau_p (\mu_p + \mu_n)}{l^2} \left[\frac{P_i \lambda}{hc} \right] \text{Siemens} \tag{2.206}$$

where τ_p is the mean lifetime of holes; $\mu_p = |v_p/E|$ = hole mobility in cm²/V.sec; $\mu_n = |v_n/E|$ = electron mobility in cm²/V.sec; v_p and v_n are the mean drift velocities of holes and electrons, respectively; E is the uniform E-field in the semiconductor; and q, η, P_i, λ, h, and c have been defined previously. Note that, in general, $\mu_n > \mu_p$. The expression for G_P is an approximation, valid up to the cut-off wavelength, λ_c. $[P_i \lambda/hc] = \Phi_i$, the incoming number of photons/second on area wl m². The dark conductance of a Si PC can be found simply from the room temperature resistivity of Si, ρ, and the geometry of the PC. For example:

$$G_D = A/\rho l = wd/\rho l = 0.2 \text{ cm} \times 0.001 \text{ cm} \big/ \left(2.3 \times 10^3 \, \Omega \text{ cm} \times 0.02 \text{ cm} \right)$$
$$= 4.348 \times 10^{-6} \text{ S} \tag{2.207}$$

From Equation 2.206, the photoconductance for a Si PC illuminated by 1 µW of 512-nm photons is:

$$G_P = \frac{\overset{Cb}{1.6 \times 10^{-19}} \times \overset{\eta}{0.8 \times 10^{-4}} \overset{\tau_p}{\left(1350 + 450\right)}^{\text{cm}^2/\text{V.sec}}}{\underset{\text{cm}^2}{10^{-4}}} \left[\frac{\overset{W}{10^{-6} \times 512 \times 10^{-9}}^{m}}{\underset{\text{joule.sec}}{6.625 \times 10^{-34} \times 3 \times 10^3}_{\text{m/sec}}} \right] \tag{2.208}$$

$$= 5.935 \times 10^{-4} \text{ Siemens}$$

A great advantage of PCs is their unique ability to respond to MIR and FIR photons at wavelengths not sensed by PIN PDs or APDs. For various materials, as the bandgap energy decreases, λ_c increases and the PC's response time constants decrease.

PCs also are unique in their ability to convert x-ray photons to conductance change. X-ray sensing PCs are made of amorphous selenium (a-Se) (Soltani et al., 1999). An a-Se PC with E 10 V/µm produces approximately 1000 electron–hole pairs per 50-keV x-ray photon. There is a 50% attenuation of a 50-keV electron beam in $d = 365$ µm a-Se. Soltani et al. (1999) describe a charge-coupled x-ray photon-sensing array using a-Se sensors that have superior image resolution to phosphor x-ray sensors.

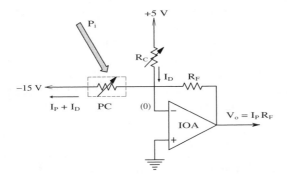

FIGURE 2.68

Op amp circuit for conditioning a photoconductive sensor's output. The current through R_C compensates for the PC's dark current.

Figure 2.68 illustrates a simple op amp circuit that gives $V_o \propto P_i$. Note that R_C is used to cancel the PC's dark current. A Wheatstone bridge can also be used to convert photoconductance to output voltage, albeit nonlinearly. Unlike PDs, PCs make thermal noise; it can be shown that the total MS noise current input to the op amp's summing junction is:

$$\overline{i_{ntot}^2} = \left\{ 4kT\left[G_D + G_P + G_C + G_F \right] + i_{na}^2 \right\} B \text{ msA} \tag{2.209}$$

Note that the MS noise increases with input light power because G_P increases with P_i. In addition to the noise current, the op amp also has an equivalent short-circuit input noise voltage, $e_{na}^2\ B$ MSV. Chapter 9 will consider such noise.

2.6.6 LEDs

Light-emitting diodes are widely used in all electronic applications as pilot lights, status indicators, and warning signals. They are also used in biomedical applications as (approximately) monochromatic light sources for chemical analysis by spectrophotometry. LEDs can be purchased that emit not only near IR, but also visible red, orange, yellow, green, blue, and white light. An important application for LEDs in biomedicine is the two light sources in the pulse oximeter, which is basically a two-wavelength spectrophotometer used to measure blood oxygen saturation (Northrop, 2002). One NIR LED emits at 805 nm, the isobestic wavelength for deoxyhemoglobin (Hb) and oxyhemoglobin (HbO$_2$) absorbance (the wavelength at which Hb and HbO$_2$ absorbances are equal). The other wavelength is at approximately 650 nm (red), where there is a large difference between the absorbances of Hb and HbO$_2$. LEDs are also used as the light sources in the paper strip, blood glucose sensing systems. Again, a two-λ spectrophotometer is used. Even though LEDs are relative broadband emitters, their spectral purity is good enough for simple spectrophotometric measurements.

An LED is a solid-state, *pn* junction device that emits photons upon the application of a forward-biasing current. It converts electric energy directly into photon energy without the intermediate step of thermal conversion. LED p-material is typically doped gallium aluminum arsenide (GaAlAs), while the n-material is doped gallium arsenide (GaAs). Between the *p* and *n* layers is an active layer. When a forward voltage (and current) is applied to the LED, holes from the p-region (GaAlAs) meet electrons from the n-doped GaAs layer in the active layer and recombine, producing photons. Photon wavelength is dependent on the chemical composition and relative energy levels of the two doped semicon layers. It also depends to a small degree on the junction temperature and I_D. Visible-light LEDs typically have plastic dome lenses that serve to expand and diffuse the light from the LED's active layer. The plastic is colored to indicate the color of the emitted light; clear lenses are used for NIR LEDs.

The wavelength of the emitted light can be altered by varying the composition of the doped semicon materials used in the LED. Typical materials used in LED construction include Al, As, Ga, In, P, and N (as nitrides). White light can be made by several mechanisms, but one way is to make a blue LED and use the blue light to excite a mixture of phosphors in the reflector cup that emit at several longer wavelengths; the mixture of wavelengths appears white.

LED forward voltage is on the order of 1.5 V and operating currents range from a few to tens of milliamperes. When a forward current is applied through a *pn* junction, carriers are injected across the junction to establish excess carriers above the thermal equilibrium values. The excess carriers recombine and, in so doing, some energy is released in the form of heat and light (photons). The injected electrons in the *p* side make a downward energy transition from the conduction band to recombine with holes in the valence band. Photons are emitted having energy, E_g, in joules. The emission wavelength is approximately:

$$\lambda = hc/E_g \text{ meters} \tag{2.210}$$

In practice, the emission power spectrum is not a narrow band such as that produced by lasers, but is a curve with a smooth peak and a Q defined by the wavelength of the peak emission power density divided by the $\Delta\lambda$ between the half-power wavelengths on either side of the peak. That is; $Q = \lambda_{pk}/\Delta\lambda$. For example, $Q \cong 16$ for a GaAsP LED with peak emission at 650 nm (Yang, 1988). The Qs for Osram LEDs LS5421, LO5411, LY5421, and LG5411 — emitting power peaks at 635, 610, 586 and 565 nm, respectively — are 14.1, 15.3, 13.0, and 22.6, respectively.

Figure 2.69(A) illustrates the I–V characteristics of a green gallium phosphide (GaP) LED. Compare this curve with the I–V curve for a typical small-signal, Si *pn* junction diode, as shown on Figure 2.69(B). Figure 2.69(C) illustrates the light intensity vs. I_D for the green LED and Figure 2.70 illustrates the relative spectral emission of a GaP green LED. The peak is at approximately

TABLE 2.2

Semiconductor LED Materials and Approximate Emission
Peak Wavelengths[a]

Material	Wavelength (μm)	Photon energy (eV)
GaP (Zn, diffused green)	0.553	2.24
$Ga_{1-x} Al_x As$ (red)	0.688	1.78
GaP (Zn, 0-doped red)	0.698	1.76
GaAs (NIR)	0.84	1.47
InP	0.9	1.37
$Ga(As_x P_{1-x})$	1.41–1.95	
GaSb	1.5	0.82
PbS (MIR)	4.26	0.29
InSb	5.2	0.23
PbTe	6.5	0.19
PbSe	8.5	0.145

[a] Peak emission, λ, depends on temperature and diode current.

561 nm and the half-intensity width is measured at approximately 26 nm,
giving an LED $Q = 21.6$.

Modern LEDs are now available in the near UV, which provides excellent
application in biochemical fluorescence analysis as an inexpensive source of
excitation for DNA microarrays (gene chips) and many other modes of
fluorescent chemical analysis. Their UV can also be used to catalyze the
polymerization of dental fillings and for spot sterilization. For example, the
Nichia NSHU550E UV LED (gallium indium nitride) has a spectral emission
peak centered at 370 nm, quite invisible to the human eye. Nichia also makes
gallium nitride (GaN) single quantum well LEDs that emit blue with a peak
at approximately 470 nm that are intended for excitation in fluorescence
applications, including protein analysis and DNA analysis using SYBR®
green and SYPRO® orange molecular tags.

The following section shows that laser diodes (LADs) have much narrower
spectral emission lines, but also can have under certain operating conditions
many closely spaced emission lines.

2.6.7 Laser Diodes

The basic difference between an LED and an LAD is that the latter has an
optical resonance cavity that promotes lasing. The optical cavity has two end
facet partial mirrors that reflect photons back into the cavity so that a self-
sustaining laser action occurs. The mirrors can be the cleaved surfaces of the
semiconductor crystals or may be optically ground, polished, and coated.
The LAD unit generally contains a photodiode (PD) that is used with an
external circuit to monitor the optical power output, P_o, of the LAD. LADs
are easily damaged by excess I_D causing excess P_o. Often the PD output is
used to provide feedback to limit the optical power output of the LAD so
that the end mirrors are not damaged by heat or XS light. If the end mirrors
are damaged, the LAD becomes an expensive, ineffective LED.

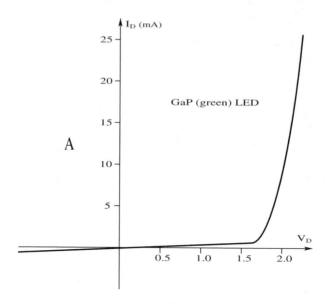

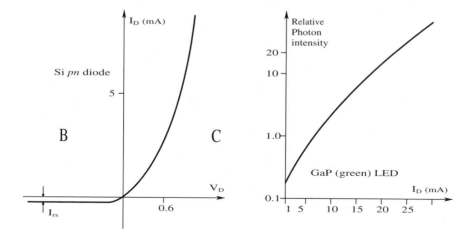

FIGURE 2.69

(A) i_D vs. v_D curve for a GaP (green) LED. Note the high threshold voltage for forward conduction. (B) For comparison, the i_D vs. v_D curve for a typical Si small-signal *pn* diode. (C) Relative light intensity vs. forward current.

Low-power LADs come in a variety of packages; probably the most familiar is the cylindrical can with top (end) window. Such TO-cans are typically 5.6 or 9.0 mm in diameter and have three leads: (1) common, (2) LAD cathode, and (3) PD anode. The PD's cathode and the LAD's anode are connected to the common lead.

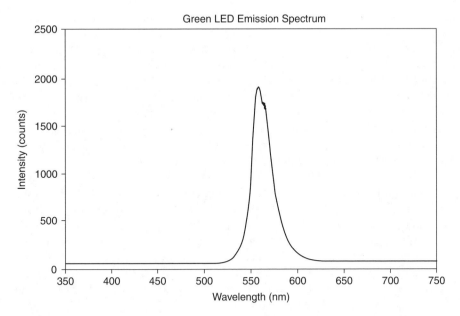

FIGURE 2.70
Spectral emission characteristic of a GaP green LED.

How does diode lasing occur? If some forward current, I_D, generates an electron–hole pair ready to emit a photon of energy $E_g = h\nu_o$ and another photon is present with energy $h\nu_o$, the existing photon stimulates the electron–hole pair to recombine and to emit a photon coherent to the existing one. The probability of stimulated emission is proportional to the density of excess electrons and holes in the active region and to the density of photons. Under low-density conditions, it is negligible. However, if coherent positive feedback is provided by reflecting back some exiting photons with the end mirrors, the stimulated emission can become self-sustaining. This self-sustaining, stimulated emission is the heart of the laser principle.

Several LAD structures are currently used. Early LAD design used homojunction architecture, the boundary between the p- and n-materials serving as the active (laser) region. The length of the active region was much longer (300 to 1000 µm) than its thickness (1 µm) or width (3 µm). The end facets served as the mirrors. A LAD design using alternating layers of p- and n-materials is called a heterojunction structure. For example, if three p-layers are alternated with three n-layers, there are five active regions to lase. When four p-layers are alternated with four n-layers, there are seven active regions, etc. Heterojunction designs have been used to fabricate high-power output LADs. Because of their geometry (long and very thin) homo- and heterojunction LAD output beams tend to be asymmetrical and are often difficult to focus into a small symmetrical (Gaussian) spot.

The new, vertical cavity, surface-emitting laser (VCSEL) diodes consist of a (top) light exit window (it can be round, 5 to 25 μm in diameter), a top-distributed Bragg reflector, a gap to set the emission wave length, two λ-spacers surrounding a GaAs active region, and then a bottom-distributed Bragg reflector sitting on the bottom substrate. VCSEL lasers operate in a single longitudinal mode. They can be designed to have anastigmatic Gaussian beams, which are easy to focus with simple lenses. Because the mirror area is larger, VCSEL lasers are not as prone to overpower damage and optical feedback is not necessary as it is in edge-emitting LADs. They also lase at much lower I_Ds because of their efficient mirrors.

LADs are considered to be current-operated devices; they should be driven from regulated current sources, not voltage sources. Figure 2.71(A) illustrates the optical output power, P_o, from a LAD vs. the forward current, I_D, for a typical heterojunction LAD. I_{Dt} is the threshold current where enough electron–hole pairs are produced to sustain lasing. Note that increasing device temperature moves the $P_o(I_D)$ curve to the right. The steep part of the curve is essentially linear and is characterized by its slope: $\Delta P_o / \Delta I_D = \rho$ watts/amp. In the region of I_D between 0 and I_{Dt}, the LAD is basically a LED. An algebraic model for the $P_o(I_D)$ curve above I_{Dt} is:

$$P_o = \rho I_D - P_x \tag{2.211}$$

where P_x is the intersection of the approximate line with the negative P_o axis. Needless to say, I_{Dt} is much lower for a VCSEL LAD. (An Avalon, AVAP760, VCSEL, 760-nm LAD has $I_{Dt} = 2.0$ mA and $I_{DQ} = 3.0$ mA. I_{DQ} is the operating current for this LAD.)

Although VCSEL LADs have a single mode output (the preceding 760-nm VCSEL has a line Q of 3.95×10^{14} Hz$/100 \times 10^6$ Hz $= 3.95 \times 10^6$), homo- and heterojunction LADs generally emit a multimode "comb" spectral output. The number of spectral lines that appear at the output of a gain-guided LAD depends on the properties of the cavity and mirrors, the operating current, and the temperature. According to the Newport *Photonics Tutorial* (2003):

> The result is that multimode laser diodes exhibit spectral outputs having many peaks around their central wavelength. The optical wave propagating through the laser cavity forms a standing wave between the two mirror facets of the laser. The period of oscillation of this curve is determined by the distance L between the two mirrors. This standing optical wave resonates only when the cavity length L is an integer number m of half wavelengths existing between the two mirrors. In other words, there must exist a node at each end of the cavity. The only way this can take place is for L to be exactly a whole number multiple of half wavelengths λ/2. This means that $L = m(\lambda/2)$, where λ is the wavelength of light in the semiconductor matter and is related to the wavelength of light in free space through the index of refraction n by the relationship $\lambda = \lambda_o/n$. As a result of this situation there can exist many longitudinal modes in the cavity of the laser diode, each resonating at its distinct

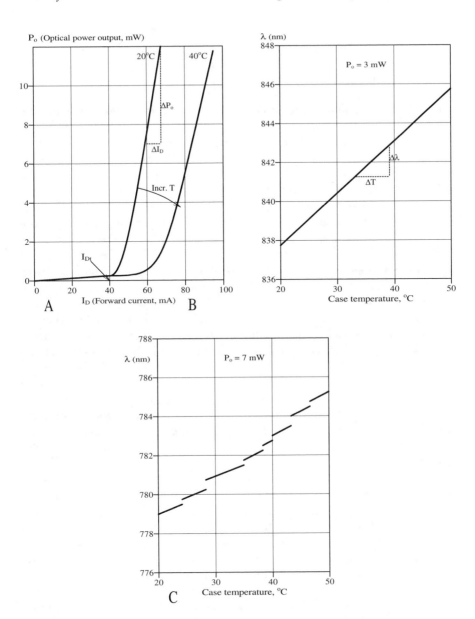

FIGURE 2.71
(A) Optical power output from a laser diode (LAD) vs. forward current. Note that increasing the heterojunction temperature decreases the output power at constant I_D. (B) Increase in output wavelength of an LAD at constant P_o with increasing case temperature. (C) Mode-hopping behavior of LAD output wavelength with increasing case temperature.

wavelength of $\lambda_m = 2L/m$. From this [development] you can note that two adjacent longitudinal laser modes are separated by a wavelength [difference] of $\Delta\lambda = \lambda_o^2/(2nL)$.

> Even single-mode devices [VCSEL LADs] can support multiple [output]
> modes at low output power... As the operating current is increased, one
> mode begins to dominate until, beyond a certain operating power level,
> a single narrow linewidth [output] spectrum appears.

It is also noted that the center λ of an LAD's output increases with operating
temperature. This property is useful in spectroscopy in which the fine structure of a molecular absorbance spectrum is being studied. Newport gives
data for one LAD with a center frequency of 837.6 nm at 20°C. The center
wavelength increases linearly with increasing temperature to 845.5 nm at
50°C. Thus, $\Delta\lambda/\Delta T = 0.263$ nm/°C.

Single-mode LADs can exhibit a phenomenon known as *mode-hopping*.
Here the output λ increases linearly over a short temperature interval, at the
upper end of which it hops discontinuously to a slightly larger λ. The linear
behavior again occurs, followed by another hop, etc. The linear behavior of
$\lambda(T)$ and mode-hopping are shown in Figure 2.71(B) and Figure 2.71(C).
Because of mode-hopping and λ drift with temperature, LADs used for wave
length critical applications are temperature stabilized to approximately 0.1°C
around a desired operating temperature using thermoelectric (Peltier) cooling.

Many circuits have been developed to drive LADs under constant-current
conditions. Some circuits use the signal from the built-in PD to stabilize the
diode's P_o when CW or pulsed output is desired. In communications applications, in which the LAD is driving an optical fiber cable, it is desirable to
on/off modulate P_o at very high rates, up into the gigahertz in some cases.
In biomedical applications, in which the LAD is used as a source for spectrophotometry, the intensity modulation or chopping of the beam is more
conveniently done at audio frequencies to permit the operation of lock-in
amplifiers, etc.

One of the more prosaic applications of LADs is the common (CW) laser
pointer. Some of these devices are operated without any regulation by the
simple expedient of using one current-limiting resistor in series with the two
batteries. The resistor is chosen so that I_D is always less than I_{Dmax} when the
batteries are fresh. Of course the pointer spot gets dimmer as the batteries
become exhausted. Figure 2.72 illustrates this basic series circuit and the
solution of the LAD's $I_D = f(V_D)$ curve with the circuit's load line.

An example of a two-BJT regulator used in laser pointers (Goldwasser,
2001) is shown in Figure 2.73. This is a type 0, negative feedback circuit that
makes P_o relatively independent of ΔV_B and ΔT. Inspection of this circuit
shows that if P_o increases, the PD's I_p increases, decreasing I_{B2}, thus I_{B1} and
I_D, and thus reducing P_o; therefore, negative feedback stabilizes P_o.

When it is desired to modulate an LAD at hundreds of megahertz to
gigahertz for communications applications, very special circuits indeed are
used. LADs can be modulated around some 50% P_o point much faster than
from fully off to fully on. Several semiconductor circuit manufacturers offer
high-frequency single-chip LAD regulator/drivers. For example, the Analog

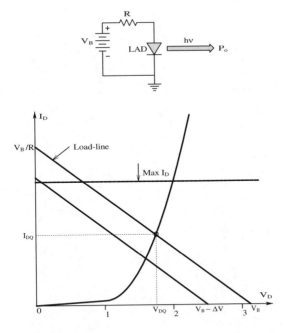

FIGURE 2.72
Top: LAD powered from a simple DC Thevenin circuit. Bottom: an LAD's i_D vs. v_D curve showing max i_D, load lines, and operating point.

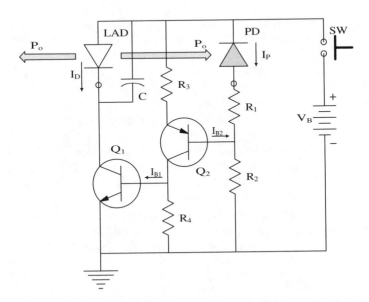

FIGURE 2.73
A simple LAD P_o (thus i_D) regulator circuit. The LAD's built-in PD is used to make a type 0 intensity controller.

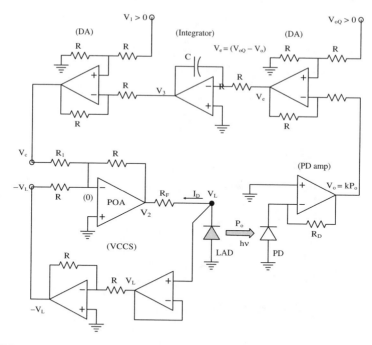

FIGURE 2.74

A type 1 feedback system designed by the author to regulate and modulate LAD P_o. The LAD's built-in PD is used for feedback.

Devices AD9661A driver chip allows LAD on/off switching up to 100 MHz, and has <2 ns rise/fall times. The Maxim MAX3263 is a 155 Mbps LAD driver with <1 ns rise/fall times. Needless to say, getting an LAD to switch at such rates involves the artful use of ferrite beads, as well as consideration of parasitic distributed parameters such as LAD lead inductance and stray capacitances. The MAX3263 chip also has a "slow start" feature to protect the LAD at turn-on. The design of GHz modulation circuits is beyond the scope of this text and will not be treated here.

Figure 2.74 illustrates the architecture of an op amp feedback/modulation circuit designed by the author for spectrophotometric LAD applications. It uses a VCCS to drive the LAD and a feedback loop containing signal conditioning for the on-board PD, a difference amplifier (DA), an integrator, and another DA. The input that sets the LAD's output power is V_{oQ}, which can be an audio-frequency square-wave, a sinewave + DC, or just DC. The VCCS subunit drives the LAD. Its transconductance can be found by KVL, noting:

$$V_2 = -(I_D R_F + V_L) \tag{2.212}$$

The node equation for the power op amp's summing junction can be written:

$$(0)[2G + G_1] - V_c G_1 - V_2 G - V_L G = 0 \tag{2.213}$$

Substituting for V_2:

$$-V_e G_1 - V_L G - G\left[-\left(I_D R_F + V_L\right)\right] = 0 \qquad (2.214A)$$

$$\downarrow$$

$$I_D = \frac{V_c R}{R_1 R_F} = V_c G_M \qquad (2.214B)$$

$$\downarrow$$

$$G_M = R/\left(R_1 R_F\right) \text{ Siemens} \qquad (2.214C)$$

Now refer to the block diagram shown in Figure 2.75, which illustrates the simplified dynamics of the circuit of Figure 2.74. The LAD's $P_o(I_D)$ curve for $I_D > I_{Dt}$ is approximated by the linear relation of Equation 2.211. The output of the PD conditioning amplifier is subtracted from the set-point, V_{oQ}, to create an error voltage, V_e, which is integrated forming V_3. V_3 is then subtracted from $V_1 > 0$, a bias voltage, forming V_c, the input to the VCCS. I_D is the LAD drive current. Application of Mason's rule yields the transfer function:

$$P_o = \frac{V_{oQ}(s)K_i G_M \rho}{s + K_i G_M \rho k} + \frac{V_1(s) s G_M \rho}{s + K_i G_M \rho k} + \frac{-P_x(s) s}{s + K_i G_M \rho k} \qquad (2.215)$$

Note that V_1 and P_x are dc levels. At turn-on, they can be considered to be steps. Using the Laplace initial value theorem:

$$P_o(0+) = s \frac{V_{oQ}}{s} \frac{K_i G_M \rho}{s + K_i G_M \rho k} + s \frac{V_1}{s} \frac{s G_M \rho}{s + K_i G_M \rho k} - s \frac{P_x}{s} \frac{s}{s + K_i G_M \rho k} \qquad (2.216A)$$
$$\lim s \to \infty$$

$$\downarrow$$

$$P_o(0+) = 0 + (V_1 G_M \rho - P_x) \qquad (2.216B)$$

In other words, the *initial* P_o is set by V_1.

Next, use the Laplace final value theorem to find P_{oSS}:

$$P_{oSS} = s \frac{V_{oQ}(s)}{s} \frac{K_i G_M \rho}{s + K_i G_M \rho k} + s \frac{V_1}{s} \frac{s G_M \rho}{s + K_i G_M \rho k} - s \frac{P_x}{s} \frac{s}{s + K_i G_M \rho k} \qquad (2.217A)$$
$$\lim s \to 0$$

$$\downarrow$$

$$P_{oSS} = \frac{V_{oQ} K_i G_M \rho}{K_i G_M \rho k} + 0 + 0 = V_{oQ}/k \qquad (2.217B$$

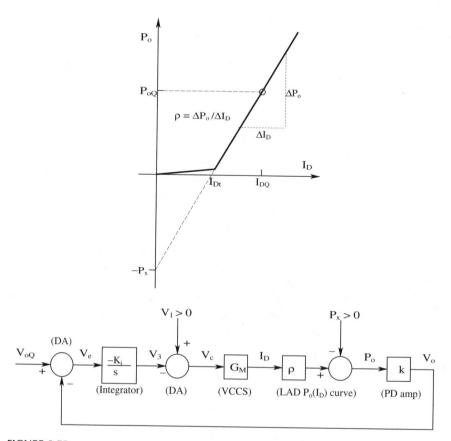

FIGURE 2.75

Top: typical LAD i_D vs. v_D curve, showing desired P_{oQ}. Bottom: simplified block diagram of the regulator/modulator of Figure 2.74. See text for analysis.

Note that the final value of P_o is independent of V_1 and P_x and is set by V_{oQ}.

Driving laser diodes safely is a complex matter; it requires a VCCS and feedback to stabilize P_o against changes in temperature and supply voltage. It also requires a mechanism to protect the LAD against over-current surges at turn-on and when switching I_D. Fortunately, several manufacturers now offer special ICs that stabilize P_o and also permit high-frequency modulation of the laser output intensity.

2.7 Chapter Summary

This chapter introduced models for the basic semiconductor devices used in analog electronic circuits, including *pn* junction diodes; Schottky diodes; bipolar junction transistors (BJTs); field-effect transistors (JFETs, MOSFETs);

and some common solid-state photonic devices widely used in biomedical instrumentation, e.g., PIN photodiodes, avalanche photodiodes, LEDs, and laser diodes.

The circuit element models were seen to be subdivided into DC-to-mid-frequency models and high-frequency models that included small-signal capacitances resulting from charge depletion at reverse-biased *pn* junctions, and from stored charge in forward-conducting junctions. Mid-frequency models were used to examine the basic input resistance, voltage gain, and output resistance of simple, one-transistor BJT and FET amplifiers.

Also examined as analog IC "building blocks" were two-transistor amplifiers. High-frequency behavior of diodes, single-transistor amplifiers, and two-transistor amplifiers was examined. Certain two-transistor amplifier architectures such as the cascode and the emitter (source)-follower–grounded-base (gate) amplifier were shown to give excellent high-frequency performance because they minimized or avoided the Miller effect. Certain other broadbanding strategies were described.

Semiconductor photon sensors were introduced, including pin and avalanche photodiodes, and photoconductors. LEDs and laser diode photon sources were also covered, as well as circuits used in their operation.

Home Problems

2.1 A diode is used as a half-wave rectifier as shown in Figure P2.1A.

    a. Assume the diode is ideal. The voltage source is $v_s(t) = 10 \sin(377t)$ and the load is 10 Ω. Find the average power dissipated in the load, R_L.

    b. Now let the diode be represented by the I–V curve in Figure P2.1B. Find the average power dissipated in the load and also in the diode.

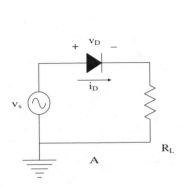
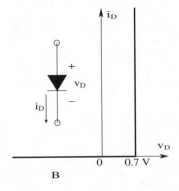

FIGURE P2.1

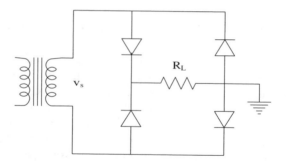

FIGURE P2.2

2.2   A diode bridge rectifier is shown in Figure P2.2. Each diode has the I–V curve of Figure P2.1B. Find the average power in the load, R_L, and also in each diode.

2.3   A zener diode power supply is shown in Figure P2.3. Its purpose is to deliver 5.1 Vdc to an 85-Ω load, in which a 9-V battery is the primary dc source. A 1N751 zener diode is used; its rated voltage is 5.1 V when a 20-mA reverse (zener) current, I_Z, is flowing. Find the required value for R_s. Also find the power dissipation in the diode, R_s and R_L, and the power supplied by the battery.

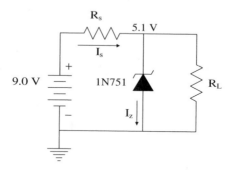

FIGURE P2.3

2.4   Refer to the emitter follower in Figure P2.4. Given: $h_{FE} = 99$, $V_{BEQ} = 0.65$ V.

   a.   Find I_{BQ} and R_B required to make $V_{EQ} = 0$ V.
   b.   Calculate the quiescent power dissipation in the BJT and in R_E.
   c.   Calculate the small-signal h_{ie} for the BJT at its Q-point.

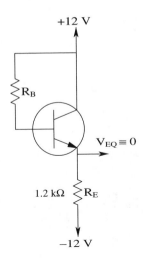

FIGURE P2.4

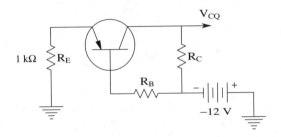

FIGURE P2.5

2.5   A *pnp* BJT grounded-base amplifier is shown in Figure P2.5. Given: h_{FE} = 149, V_{BEQ} = 0.65 V. Find R_B and R_C so that the amplifier's Q-point is at I_{CQ} = −1.0 mA, V_{CEQ} = −5.0 V. Find V_{EQ}.

2.6   The circuit shown in Figure P2.6 is a current mirror. Given: h_{FE} = 100 (all three BJTs), V_{CC} = +6.0 V, R = 12 kΩ, V_{BE1} = 0.65 = V_{BE2}, V_{BE3} = 0.60 V, V_{CE2} ≫ V_{CE2sat}. Find (a) V_{CE1}; (b) I_R; (c) I_{E3}; (d) I_{B3}; and (e) I_{C1} and I_{C2}.

2.7   An *npn* BJT grounded base amplifier is shown in Figure P2.7. Given: V_{BEQ} = 0.65 V, h_{FE} = 119. Find R_B and R_C so the Q-point is at I_{CQ} = 2.5 mA, V_{CEQ} = 7 V.

2.8   A *pnp* BJT emitter follower is shown in Figure P2.8. Given: h_{FE} = 99, V_{BEQ} = −0.65 V.

   a.   Find R_B and I_{BQ} required to make V_{CEQ} = −10 V.
   b.   Find the quiescent power dissipated in the BJT and in R_E.

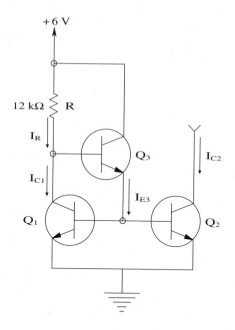

FIGURE P2.6

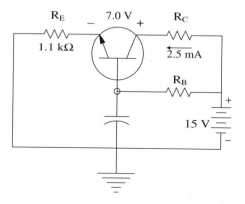

FIGURE P2.7

2.9 Consider the three basic BJT amplifiers shown in Figure P2.9. In each amplifier, find the R_B required to make $I_{CQ} = 1$ mA. Also find V_{CEQ} in each circuit. Given: $h_{FE} = 100$ and $V_{BEQ} = 0.65$ V.

2.10 Three JFET amplifiers are shown in Figure P2.10. A "grounded-source" amplifier is shown in Figure P2.10A. The source resistor, R_S, is bypassed by C_S, making the source node at small-signal ground. R_S is required for self-bias of the JFET. The same JFET is used in all three circuits, in which $I_{DSS} =$

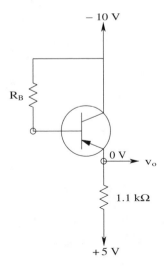

FIGURE P2.8

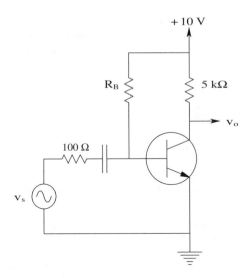

FIGURE P2.9A

6.0 mA; $V_P = -3.0$ V; and $g_{mo} = 4 \times 10^{-3}$ S. In circuits (A) and (B) of Figure P2.10, find g_{mQ}, R_S, and R_D so that $I_{DQ} = 3.0$ mA and $V_{DQ} = 8.0$ V. Give V_{DSQ}. Circuit (C) of Figure P2.10 is a source follower. Find R_1 and R_S required to make $I_{DQ} = 3.0$ mA and $V_{SQ} = 8.0$ V. Neglect gate leakage current.

2.11 The circuit of Figure P2.11 is an emitter-follower–grounded-base amplifier pair, normally used to amplify video frequency signals because it has no Miller effect. Examine its gain at mid-frequencies.

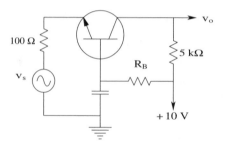

FIGURE P2.9B

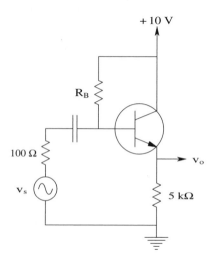

FIGURE P2.9C

a. Draw the mid-frequency SSM for the amplifier. Let $h_{oe} = h_{re} = 0$ for both BJTs.

b. Find an expression for $A_{vo} = v_o/v_1$. Show what happens to A_{vo} when $R_E \rightarrow \infty$ and $\beta_1 = \beta_2 = \beta$.

2.12 A simplified MOSFET feedback pair amplifier is shown in Figure P2.12.

a. Draw the MFSSM for the amplifier. Assume the MOSFETs have different g_ms (g_{m1}, g_{m2}) and $g_{d1} = g_{d2} = 0$ for simplicity.

b. Find an algebraic expression for the amplifier's mid-frequency voltage gain, $A_{vo} = v_o/v_1$.

c. Find an algebraic expression for the amplifier's small-signal, Thevenin output resistance. Use the OCV/SCC method. Note that the OCV is $v_1 A_{vo}$; to find the SCC, replace R_L with a short-circuit to small-signal ground and find the current in it.

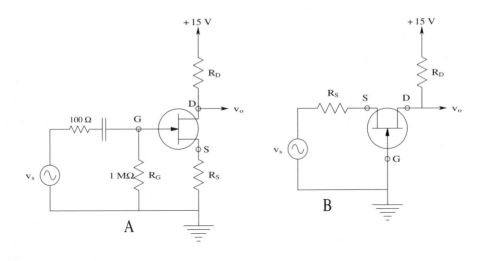

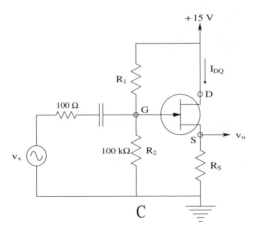

FIGURE P2.10

2.13 See the JFET in Figure P2.13 with drain small-signal short-circuited to ground.

    a. Use the high-frequency SSM for the JFET to derive an expression for the device's complex, short-circuit output transconductance, $G_M(j\omega) = I_d/V_1$, at $V_{ds} \equiv 0$. Assume g_m, g_d, C_{gs}, C_{gd}, $C_{ds} > 0$ in the model.

    b. Neglect the high-frequency zero at g_m/C_{gd} r/s. Find an expression for the Hertz frequency, f_T, such that $r_d |G_M(j2\pi f_T)| = 1$. Express f_T in terms of the quiescent drain current, I_{DQ}. Plot f_T vs. I_{DQ} for $0 \leq I_{DQ} \leq I_{DSS}$.

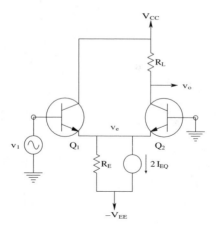

FIGURE P2.11

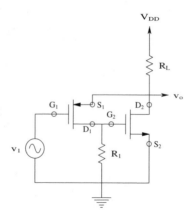

FIGURE P2.12

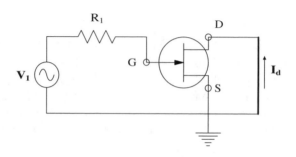

FIGURE P2.13

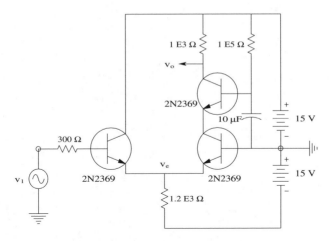

FIGURE P2.14

2.14 An emitter-coupled cascode amplifier uses three 2N2369 BJTs as shown in Figure P2.14.

a. Use an ECAP to do a dc biasing analysis. Plot the dc V_o vs. V_1. Use a 0- to15-V scale for V_o and a ±0.25-V scale for the dc input, V_1. Find the amplifier's maximum dc gain.

b. Make a Bode plot of the amplifier's frequency response, $20 \log |V_o/V_1|$ vs. f for $10^5 \leq f \leq 10^9$ Hz. Give the mid-frequency gain, the –3-dB frequency, and f_T for the amplifier.

c. Now put a 300-Ω resistor in series with V_1. Repeat (b).

2.15 An EF–GB amplifier, shown in Figure P2.15, uses capacitance "neutralization" to effectively cancel its input capacitance and extend its high-frequency, –3-dB bandwidth. Use an ECAP to investigate how C_N affects the amplifier's high-frequency response. First, try $C_N = 0$, then see what happens with C_N values in the tenths of a picofarad. Find C_N that will give the maximum –3-dB frequency with no more than a +3-dB peak to the frequency response Bode plot.

2.16 The MOSFET source follower uses a current mirror to obtain a high equivalent R_S looking into the drain of Q_2. The three MOSFETs have identical MFSSMs (identical g_{mo}, I_{DSS}, and V_P).

a. Draw the MFSSM for the circuit.

b. Find an expression for the mid-frequency gain, $A_{vo} = v_o/v_1$.

c. Find an expression for the Thevenin output resistance presented at the v_o node.

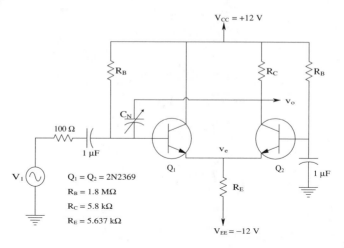

FIGURE P2.15

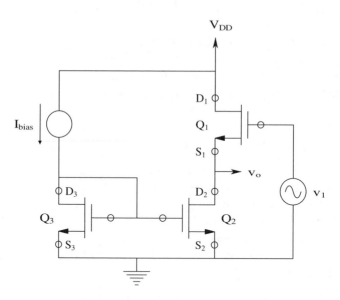

FIGURE P2.16

2.17 A JFET circuit is used as a current sink for a differential amplifier's "long tail."

a. Use the high-frequency SSM for the FET to find an expression for the impedance looking into the FET's drain, $Z_{id}(j\omega)$. (The HiFSSM includes g_m, g_d, C_{ds}, C_{gd}, C_{gs}.)

b. Find the FET's short-circuit, dc drain current, I_{Dsc}. Assume the FET's drain current is given by $I_D = I_{DSS} (1 - V_{GS}/V_P)^2$. Assume saturated drain operation. I_{DSS} and V_P are known.

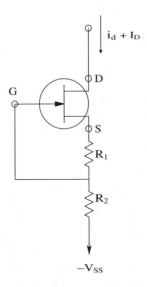

2.18 A Si avalanche photodiode (APD) is connected as shown in Figure P2.18. The total dark current of the APD is $I_D = 10$ nA, its spectral responsivity at $\lambda = 512$ nm is $R(\lambda) = 12$ amps/watt at a reverse $v_D = -150$ V. R_F of the ideal op amp is 1 megohm.

a. Find V_o due to dark current alone.

b. Find the P_i at 512 nm that will give $V_o = 1$ V.

c. The total RMS output noise in the dark in a 1-kHz noise bandwidth is 4.33 μV. Find the P_i at 512 nm that will give a DC $V_o = 13$ μV due to I_p alone (3 × the RMS noise output).

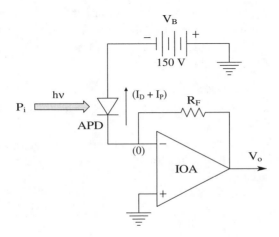

FIGURE P2.18

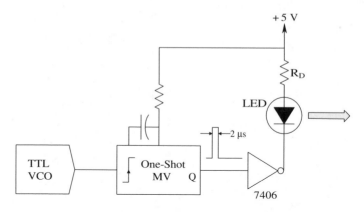

FIGURE P2.19

2.19 A single open-collector, inverting buffer gate (7406) is used to switch a GaP (green) LED on and off in a stroboscope. The ON time is 2 μsec. The flashing rate is variable from 10 flashes/sec to 10^4 flashes/sec. When the LED is ON, the LOW output voltage of the gate is 0.7 V, the LED's forward current is 15 mA, and its forward drop is 2.0 V. The circuit is shown in Figure P2.19.

    a. Find the required value of R_D.

    b. Find the electrical power input to the LED when a dc 15 mA flows.

    c. Find the LED's power input when driven by 2-μsec pulses at 10^4 pps.

2.20 A laser pointer is to be run CW from a 3.1-V (max) alkaline battery. The simple series circuit shown in Figure P2.20A is to be used to save money. Figure P2.20B shows the LAD's $i_D = f(v_D)$ curve and its linear approximation. The maximum (burnout) $i_D = 20$ mA. The desired operating current with the 3.1-V battery is 15 mA. Three load lines are shown: (1) LL_1 gives the desired operating point; (2) LL_2 is always safe because the short-circuit current (SCC) can never exceed 20 mA (with LL_2, the LAD cannot run at the desired 15 mA); and (3) LL_3 is a nonlinear LL that allows 15-mA operation of the LAD, but limits the SCC to 20 mA.

    a. Find the resistance required for LL_1, R_{L1}.

    b. Find the resistance required for LL_2, R_{L2}, and the LAD's operating point at Q_2.

    c. Describe how a simple tungsten lamp or a positive temperature coefficient (PTC) thermistor in series with a fixed resistor can be used to realize LL_3.

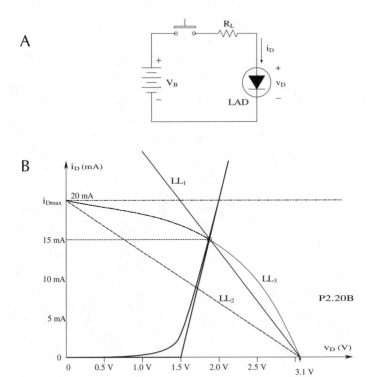

FIGURE P2.20

3

The Differential Amplifier

3.1 Introduction

The differential or difference amplifier (DA) is a cornerstone element in the design of most signal conditioning systems used in biomedical engineering applications, as well as in general instrumentation. All instrumentation and medical isolation amplifiers are DAs as are nearly all operational amplifiers. Why are DAs so ubiquitous? The answer lies in their inherent ability to reject unwanted dc levels, interference, and noise voltages common to both inputs. An ideal DA responds only to the so-called difference-mode signal at its two inputs. Most DAs have a single-ended output voltage, V_o, given by the phasor relation:

$$V_o = A_1 V_1 - A_1' \, V_1' \qquad (3.1)$$

Ideally, the gains A_1 and A_1' should be equal. In practice this does not happen; thus:

$$V_o = A_D \, V_{1d} + A_C \, V_{1c} \qquad (3.2)$$

where:

$$V_{id} \equiv (V_1 - V_1')/2 \text{ (difference-mode input voltage)} \qquad (3.3A)$$

$$V_{1c} \equiv (V_1 + V_1')/2 \text{ (common-mode input voltage)} \qquad (3.3B)$$

and A_D is the complex difference mode gain and A_C is the complex common-mode gain. It can easily be shown by vector summation that:

$$A_D = A_1 + A_1' \qquad (3.4A)$$

$$A_C = A_1 - A_1' \qquad (3.4B)$$

Clearly, if $A_1 = A_1'$, then $A_C \to 0$.

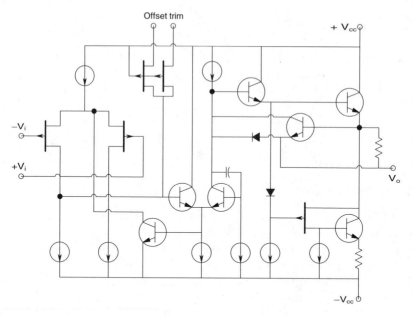

FIGURE 3.1
Simplified schematic of a Burr–Brown OPA606 JFET input DA.

3.2 DA Circuit Architecture

Figure 3.1 illustrates a simplified circuit of the Burr–Brown OPA606 JFET-INPUT op amp. Note that a pair of p-channel JFETS connected as a DA are used as a differential input headstage in the op amp. The single-ended signal output from the left-hand (inverting input) JFET drives the base (input) of a BJT emitter–follower, which drives a second BJT connected as a grounded-base amplifier. Its output, in turn, drives the OA's output stage.

To appreciate how the differential headstage works, consider the simple JFET DA circuit of Figure 3.2. Note that in the op amp schematic, the resistors R_s, R_d, and R_d' are shown as dc current sources and thus can be assumed to have very high Norton resistances on the order of megohms. (See Northrop, 1990, Section 5.2, for a description of active current sources and sinks used in IC DA designs.) Figure 3.3 illustrates the mid-frequency, small-signal model (MFSSM) of the JFET DA. To make the circuit bilaterally symmetric so that the bisection theorem (Northrop, 1990, Chapter 2) can be used in its analysis, two $2R_s$ resistors are put in parallel to replace the one R_s in the actual circuit. Note that all DC voltage sources are represented by small-signal grounds in all SSM$_s$. The scalar A_D and A_C in Equation 3.2 are to be evaluated using the DCSSM. The simplest way to do this is to use the bisection theorem on the DA's MFSSM. First, pure DM excitation is applied

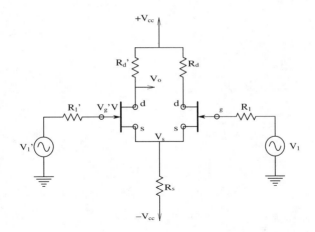

FIGURE 3.2
A JFET differential amplifier. The circuit must be symmetrical to operate well.

where $V_s' = -V_s$. Thus, $V_{sc} = 0$ and the MFSSM can be shown to be redrawn as in Figure 3.3(B). A node equation at the drain (V_{od}) node is written:

$$v_{od} [G_d + g_d] = -g_m v_{sd} \tag{3.5}$$

Thus:

$$A_D = v_{od}/v_{sd} = \frac{-g_m}{G_d + g_d} = \frac{-g_m r_d R_d}{R_d + r_d} \tag{3.6}$$

Now consider pure CM input where $v_s' = v_s$ and $v_{sd} = 0$. The bisection theorem gives the MFSSM shown in Figure 3.3(C). Now two node equations are required for the v_{oc} node:

$$v_{oc} [G_d + g_d] - v_s g_d + g_m (v_{sc} - v_s) = 0 \tag{3.7}$$

and for the v_s node:

$$v_s [G_s/2 + g_d] - v_{oc} g_d - g_m (v_{sc} - v_s) = 0 \tag{3.8}$$

The two node equations are rewritten as simultaneous equations in v_{oc} and v_s:

$$v_{oc} [G_d + g_d] - v_s [g_m + g_d] = -v_{sc} g_m \tag{3.9A}$$

$$-v_{oc} g_d + v_s [G_s/2 + g_d + g_m] = v_{sc} g_m \tag{3.9B}$$

Now Cramer's rule can be used to find v_{oc}:

$$\Delta = G_d G_s/2 + G_d g_d + g_d g_m + g_d G_s/2 \tag{3.10}$$

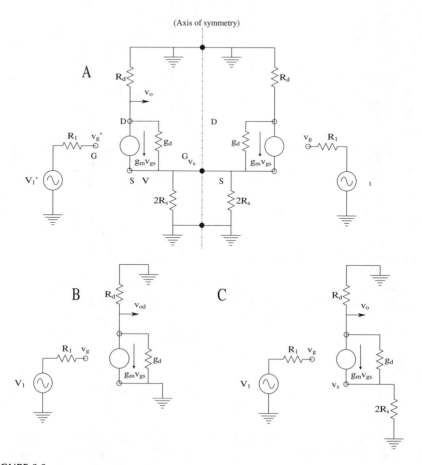

FIGURE 3.3
(A) Mid-frequency small-signal model of the FET DA in Figure 3.2. R_s on the axis of symmetry is split into two, parallel $2R_s$ resistors. (B) Left-half-circuit of the DA following application of the bisection theorem for difference-mode excitation. Note that DM excitation makes $v_s = 0$, so the FET sources can be connected to small-signal ground. (C) Left-half-circuit of the DA following application of the bisection theorem for common-mode excitation. See text for analysis.

$$\Delta v_{oc} = - v_{sc}\, g_m\, G_s/2 \qquad (3.11)$$

After some algebra is used on Equation 3.10 and Equation 3.11, the dc and mid-frequency CM gain are obtained:

$$A_C = v_{oc}/v_{sc} = \frac{-g_m r_d R_d}{r_d + R_d + 2R_s\left(1 + g_m R_d\right)} \qquad (3.12)$$

Note that $A_D \gg A_C$. The significance of this inequality is examined next.

3.3 Common-Mode Rejection Ratio (CMRR)

The common-mode rejection ratio is an important figure of merit for differential instrumentation and operational amplifiers. It is desired to be as large as possible — ideally, infinite. The CMRR can be defined as:

$$\text{CMRR} \equiv \frac{v_{1c} \text{ required to give a certain DA output}}{v_{1d} \text{ required to give the same DA output}} \quad (3.13)$$

Referring to Equation 3.2, it is clear that the CMRR can also be given by:

$$\text{CMRR} \equiv \frac{|A_D(f)|}{|A_C(f)|} \quad (3.14)$$

Note that the CMRR is a positive real number and is a function of frequency. Generally, the CMRR is given in decibels; i.e., $\text{CMRR}_{dB} = 20 \log \text{CMRR}$. For the MFSSM of the JFET DA in the preceding section, the CMRR is:

$$\text{CMRR} = \frac{\dfrac{-g_m r_d R_d}{R_d + r_d}}{\dfrac{-g_m r_d R_d}{r_d + R_d + 2R_s\left(1 + g_m R_d\right)}} = 1 + \frac{2R_s\left(1 + g_m r_d\right)}{R_d + r_d} \quad (3.15)$$

By making R_s very large by using a dynamic current source (Northrop, 1990), the CMRR of the simple JFET DA can be made about 10^4, or 80 dB.

The CMRR_{dB} of a typical commercial differential instrumentation amplifier, e.g., a Burr–Brown INA111, is given as 90 dB at a gain of 1, 110 dB at a gain of 10, and 115 dB at gains from 10^2 to 10^3, all measured at 100 Hz. At a break frequency close to 200 Hz, the $\text{CMRR}_{dB}(f)$ of the INA111 begins to roll off at approximately 20 dB/decade. For example, at a gain of 10, the CMRR_{dB} is down to 80 dB at 6 kHz. Decrease of CMRR with frequency is a general property of all DAs. Because most input common-mode interference picked up in biomedical applications of DAs is at dc or at power line frequency, it is important for such DAs to have a high CMRR that remains high (80 to 120 dB) from dc to over 120 Hz. Modern IC instrumentation amplifiers easily meet these criteria.

A major reason for the frequency dependence of the CMRR of DAs can be attributed to the frequency dependence of $A_D(f)$ and $A_C(f)$, as described

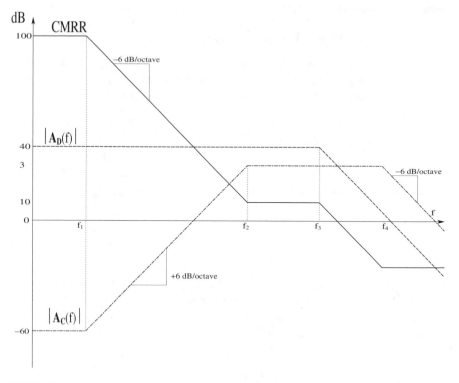

FIGURE 3.4
Typical Bode plot asymptotes for the common-mode gain frequency response, the difference-mode gain frequency response, and the common-mode rejection ratio frequency response.

in Section 3.5. Figure 3.4 illustrates typical Bode AR asymptote plots for these parameters for a DA. For example, $20 \log |A_D(f)|$ starts out at +40 dB at dc (gain of 100) and its Bode AR has its first break frequency at f_3 Hz. Starting at –60 dB at dc (gain of 0.001), $20 \log |A_C(f)|$ has a zero at approximately the open-loop amplifier's break frequency, f_1; its Bode AR increases at +20 dB/decade until it reaches a high frequency pole at f_2, where it flattens out. Because the numerical CMRR $= |A_D(f)| / |A_C(f)|$, CMRR_{dB} is simply:

$$\text{CMRR}_{dB} = 20 \log |A_D(f)| - 20 \log |A_C(f)| \qquad (3.16)$$

Thus, $\text{CMRR}_{dB} = 100$ dB at dc and decreases at –20 dB/decade from f_1 to f_2, where it levels off at 30 dB. At f_3 the CMRR_{dB} again drops off at –20 dB/decade. Good DA design tries to make f_1 as large as possible to extend the high CMRR region well into the frequency range of common-mode interference and noise.

3.4 CM and DM Gain of Simple DA Stages at High Frequencies

3.4.1 Introduction

Figure 3.7(B) and Figure 3.7(C) illustrate the small-signal, high-frequency models for a JFET DA. Note that the small-signal, high-frequency model (SSHFM) for *all* FETs includes three small fixed capacitors: the drain-to-source capacitance, C_{ds}; the gate-to-drain capacitance, C_{gd}; and the gate-to-source capacitance, C_{gs}. These capacitors, in particular C_{gd}, limit the high-frequency performance of the JFET DA. The small-signal, drain-source conductance, g_d, is also quiescent operating point dependent; it is determined by the upward slope of the FET's i_D vs. v_D curves as a function of v_{GS} (see Northrop, 1990, Section 1.6). The transconductance, g_m, of the small-signal, voltage-controlled current source is also Q-point dependent, as shown in Chapter 2.

Figure 3.5 illustrates a simple BJT DA. The hybrid-pi HFSSMs for CM and DM inputs are illustrated in Figure 3.6 after application of the bisection theorem. In the CM and DM HFSSMs, two lumped-parameter, small capacitors can be seen. C_μ is the collector-to-base capacitance, which is on the order of a single pF, and is largely due to the depletion capacitance of the reverse-biased *pn* junction between collector and base; its value is a function of the collector-to-base voltage. However, given a fixed quiescent operating point (Q-point) for the amplifier and small-signal, linear operation, it is possible to approximate C_μ with a fixed value for pencil-and-paper calculations. C_π models the somewhat larger capacitance of the forward-biased, base–emitter pn junction. It, too, depends on v_{BE} and is generally approximated by its value at V_{BEQ}. C_μ is generally on the order of 10 to 100 pF; it is larger in power transistors that have larger BE junction areas.

C_s and C_e shunting the common source or emitter resistance to ground, respectively, is on the order of a single pF, but R_s and R_e are generally the product of very dynamic current sources (with Norton resistances on the order of tens of megohms), so these capacitances can be very important in determining the high-frequency behavior of the CM gain.

3.4.2 High-Frequency Behavior of A_C and A_D for the JFET DA

It is necessary first to find an algebraic expression for the DM gain of the FET DA at high frequencies. This calculation requires the solution of two simultaneous linear algebraic node equations (Figure 3.7(B)). The node voltages are v_g and v_{od}. All the currents are summed, *leaving* these nodes as positive. After rearranging terms,

$$v_g\left[s\left(C_{gd}+C_{gs}\right)+G_1\right]-v_{od}\,sC_{gd}=v_{1d}\,G_1 \qquad (3.17A)$$

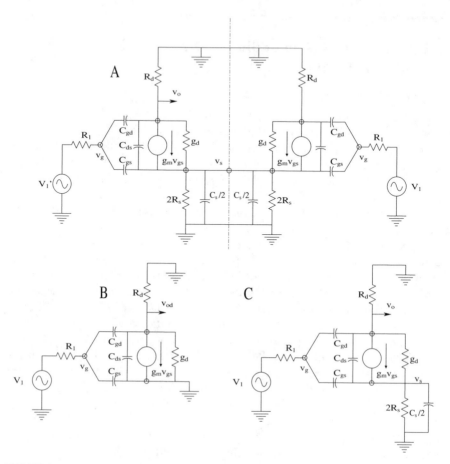

FIGURE 3.5
(A) HFSSM for the complete JFET DA. Note the axis of symmetry splits R_s and C_s symmetrically.
(B) HFSSM of the left half of the DA given DM excitation. (C) HFSSM of the left half of the DA
given CM excitation.

$$-v_g\left[sC_{gd}-g_m\right]+v_{od}\left[\left(g_d+G_d\right)+s\left(C_{ds}+C_{gd}\right)\right]=0 \qquad (3.17\text{B})$$

These two node equations are solved using Cramer's rule to find the CM
gain:

$$A_D(s)=\frac{v_{od}}{v_{1d}}=\frac{\left[-g_m r_d R_d/\left(r_d+R_d\right)\right]\left(1-sC_{gd}/g_m\right)}{s^2\left[C_{gd}\left(C_{gs}+C_{ds}\right)+C_{ds}C_{gs}\right]R_1 r_d R_d/\left(r_d+R_d\right)+s\left[\left(C_{gd}+C_{gs}\right)R_1+\right.} \cdots \qquad (3.18)$$

$$\left.\left(C_{ds}+C_{gd}\right)r_d R_d/\left(r_d+R_d\right)+C_{gd}g_m r_d R_d R_1/\left(r_d+R_d\right)+1\right]$$

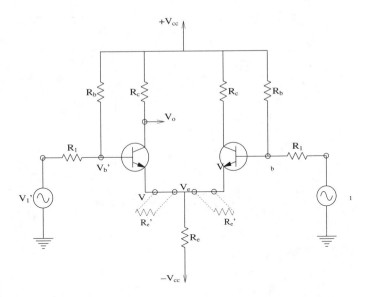

FIGURE 3.6
A BJT DA. Note symmetry. The resistors R_e' are used to raise the DM input resistance.

$A_D(s)$ is seen to have a quadratic denominator and a curious high-frequency, right-half s-plane zero at g_m/C_{gd} r/s. Its low frequency gain is the same as found in Section 3.2, i.e., $-g_m r_d R_d/(r_d + R_d)$. To find the poles, it is expedient to insert typical numerical parameter values for a JFET DA (Northrop, 1990). Let $C_{gd} = 3$ pF; $C_{gs} = 3$ pF; $C_{ds} = 0.2$ pF; $C_s = 3$ pF; $g_m = 0.005$ S; $r_d = 10^5$ ohms; $R_d = 5 \times 10^3$ ohms; $R_e = 10^6$ ohms (active current source); and $R_1 = 10^3$ ohms. After numerical calculations, the zero is found to be at 265 MHz and the two real poles are at 1.687 and 309 MHz. The dc DM gain is -23.8, or 27.5 dB. Thus $20 \log |A_D(f)|$ is down by -3 dB at 1.687 MHz.

To find $A_C(s)$ for the JFET DA, the HFSSM of Figure 3.7(C) is used. Unfortunately, according to the bisection theorem, the voltage, v_s, on the axis of symmetry is non-zero, so a third (v_s) node must have a node equation written when finding v_{oc}. The three node equations are:

$$v_g\left[G_1 + s\left(C_{gd} + C_{gs}\right)\right] - v_{oc}\left[s\,C_{gd}\right] - v_s\left[s\,C_{gs}\right] = v_{1c}\,G_1 \qquad (3.18A)$$

$$-v_g\left[s\,C_{gd} - g_m\right] + v_{oc}\left[\left(g_d + G_d\right) + s\left(C_{ds} + C_{gd}\right)\right] - v_s\left[g_m + g_d + s\,C_{ds}\right] = 0 \qquad (3.18B)$$

$$-v_g\left[g_m + s\,C_{gs}\right] - v_{oc}\left[g_d + s\,C_{ds}\right] +$$
$$v_s\left[s\left(C_s/2 + C_{ds} + C_{gs}\right) + G_s/2 + g_d + g_m\right] = 0 \qquad (3.18C)$$

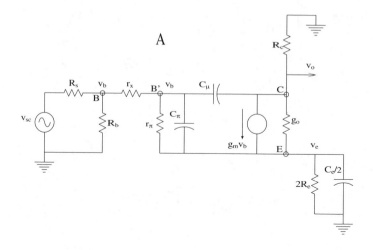

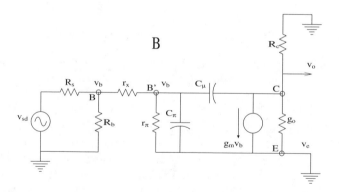

FIGURE 3.7
(A) High-frequency SSM for the left-half BJT DA given common-mode excitation. (B) High-frequency SSM for the left-half BJT DA given difference-mode excitation.

No one in his right mind would attempt an algebraic solution of a third-order system as described by Equation 3.18A through Equation 3.18C on paper. Clearly, a computer (numerical) simulation is indicated; a circuit analysis program such as pSPICE or MicroCap™ can be used. Figure 3.8 and Figure 3.9 show Bode plots of the DM and CM HFSSM frequency responses calculated by the venerable MicroCap™ III circuit analysis software (which runs under DOS, not Windows™). Note that the CM frequency response gain is approximately –46 dB at low frequencies. A zero at approximately 120 kHz causes the CM AR to rise at +20 dB/decade until a pole at approximately 10 MHz causes it to level off. A second pole at approximately 300 MHz causes the CM frequency response to fall off again.

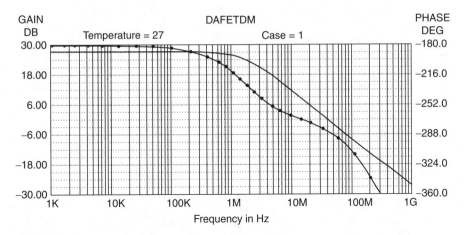

FIGURE 3.8
Difference-mode frequency response of the JFET DA of Figure 3.7A. The –3-dB frequency is approximately 1.9 MHz. See text for details.

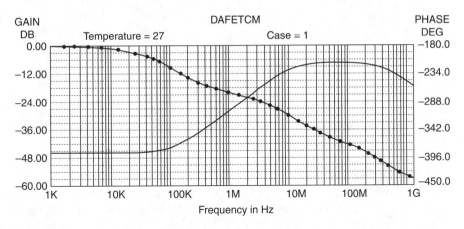

FIGURE 3.9
Common-mode frequency response of the JFET DA of Figure 3.7A. Note that the AR rises +3 dB from –46 dB at 110 kHz, then rises to a maximum of –7 dB and falls off again by 3 dB at approximately 400 MHz. Phase is bold trace with squares.

On the other hand, the DM frequency response is flat at +27.5 dB from dc out to the first real pole at approximately 1.7 MHz. The DM AR then rolls off at –20 dB/decade until the second pole, estimated to be at 310 MHz. However, the zero at 265 MHz pretty much cancels out the effect of the 310-MHz pole on the DM AR.

Note that the decibel CMRR for this amplifier is simply $20 \log |A_D(f)| -20 \log |A_C(f)|$. At low frequencies, the CMRR is 27.5 – (–46) = 73.5 dB and stays this high up to approximately 100 kHz, when it begins to drop off due to the rise in $|A_C(f)|$. At 10 MHz, the CMRR has fallen to 21 dB, etc.

3.4.3 High-Frequency Behavior of A_D and A_C for the BJT DA

Next, examine the high-frequency gain of the simple BJT DA shown in Figure 3.5 for DM and CM inputs. The hybrid-pi HFSSM for BJTs is used. Application of the bisection theorem results in the reduced CM and DM HFSSMs shown in Figure 3.6(A) and Figure 3.6(B). First, the DM HF gain will be found; the DM circuit of Figure 3.6(B) has three nodes: v_b, v_b', and v_{od}. The v_b node can be eliminated when it is noted that $R_b \gg (r_x, R_s)$, so R_b can be set to ∞, and a new Thevenin resistance, $R_s' = R_s + r_x$, is defined. Now v_b' and v_{od} must be solved for. Note that $v_e = 0$. The two node equations are written:

$$v_b' [G_s' + g_\pi + s (C_\pi + C_\mu)] + v_{od} [s C_\mu] = v_{sd} G_s' \qquad (3.19A)$$

$$v_b' [g_m - s C_\mu] + v_{od} [g_o + G_c + s C_\mu] = 0 \qquad (3.19B)$$

Even though the admittance matrix, Δ, is second order, its paper-and-pencil solution is tedious, so MicroCap will be used to solve for the linear DM HFSSM's frequency response. In this example, the parameter values are taken to be: $R_c = 6.8$ kΩ; $r_o = \infty$; $g_m = 0.05$ S; $r_\pi = 3$ kΩ; $R_e = 10^6$ Ω; $C_e = 5$ pF; $C_\mu = 2$ pF; $C_\pi = 30$ pF; $r_x = 10$ Ω; and $R_s = 50$ Ω, Thus $R_s' = 60$ Ω. Figure 3.9 shows the DM frequency response Bode plot. The low and mid-frequency gain is 50.4 dB, the –3-dB frequency is approximately 2.0 MHz, and the 0-dB frequency is approximately 410 MHz; this is a frequency well beyond the upper frequency where the hybrid-pi HFSSM is valid.

For CM excitation of the BJT DA, use the linear HFSSM schematic (Figure 3.6(A)). Note that three node equations are required because $v_e \neq 0$. Again, a computer solution is used for the CM frequency response, shown in Figure. 3.10. Figure 3.10(A) depicts the CM decibel gain and phase for the unrealistic condition of zero parasitic capacitance (C_e) from the BJT emitter to ground. Note that the CM gain is approximately –49 dB at frequencies below 10 kHz, rises to a peak of –1.3 dB at approximately 30 MHz, and then falls off again at frequencies above 40 MHz. Thus the DA's CMRR starts at 50.4 – (–49) = 99.4 dB at low frequencies and falls off rapidly above 20 kHz.

Curiously, if $C_e = 4$ pF is assumed, a radical change in the CM frequency response is seen. Figure 3.10(B) shows the low frequency CM gain to be approximately –49.5 dB; the frequency at which the CM gain is up 3 dB is approximately 14 MHz. It reaches a peak at approximately 200 MHz of –33.8 dB, giving a significant improvement in the BJT DA's CMRR at high frequencies. Now if C_e is "detuned" by only ±0.2 pF, Figure. 3.10C and Figure 3.10D show that the +3-dB frequency has dropped to approximately 750 kHz and the peak CM gain has risen to –27.2 dB at approximately 320 MHz. It is amazing that the DM gain frequency response is extremely sensitive to C_e, a parasitic parameter over which little control can be exercised; this can be shown when simulating transistor DAs with real transistor models instead of linear HFSSMs. Note that subtle changes in C_e can radically improve or ruin the high-frequency CMRR of a transistor DA.

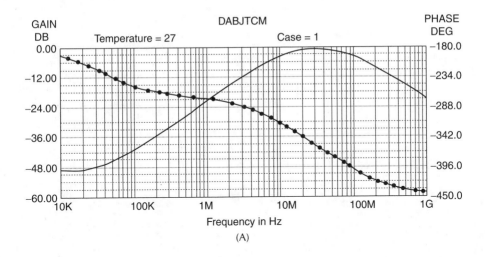

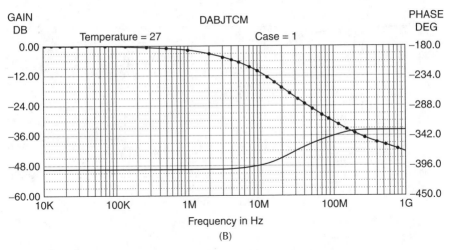

FIGURE 3.10

Common-mode gain frequency response of the BJT DA of Figure 3.6A with various values of parasitic emitter capacitance, C_e, showing how C_e can improve the DA's CMRR by giving a low CM gain at high frequencies. (A) CM gain frequency response (FR) with $C_e = 0$. (B) CM gain FR with an optimum $C_e = 4$ pF. (C) CM gain FR with $C_e = 4.2$ pF. (D) CM gain FR with $C_e = 3.8$ pF.

3.5 Input Resistance of Simple Transistor DAs

In general, simple, two-transistor DAs have much lower R_{in} for DM signals than for CM inputs; this is true over the entire frequency range of the DA. This effect is more pronounced for BJT DA stages than for JFET or MOSFET DAs. By way of illustration, consider the CM HIFSSM of the BJT amplifier

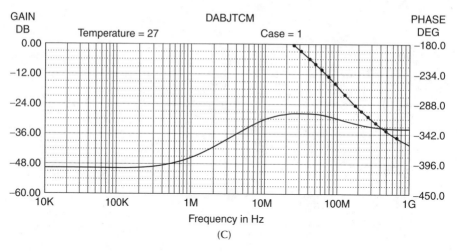

GAIN DB / PHASE DEG — DABJTCM — Temperature = 27 — Case = 1

(C)

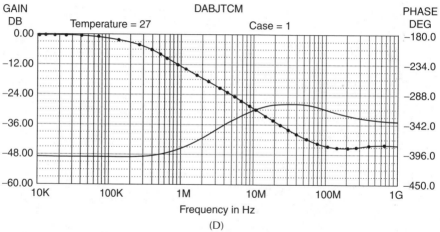

GAIN DB / PHASE DEG — DABJTCM — Temperature = 27 — Case = 1

(D)

FIGURE 3.10 (continued)

illustrated in Figure 3.6(A). When $|R_{in}(f)|_{DM} = |V_{sc}/I_{sc}|$ is plotted using Micro-Cap, at low frequencies $|R_{in}| \cong r_\pi + r_x = 3$ E3 ohms, and it begins to roll off at approximately 100 kHz. On the other hand, when the CM HIFSSM of Figure 3.6(B) is stimulated, the low frequency $|R_{in}(f)|_{CM} \cong 3$ E8 ohms, or $2R_E$ $(1 + g_m\, r_\pi)$, a sizeable increase over the DM $|R_{in}(f)|$. The low-frequency $|R_{in}(f)|_{CM}$ begins to roll off at only 200 Hz.

Ideally, the $|R_{in}(f)|$ for *both* CM and DM would be very large, to prevent loading of the sources driving the DA. High $|R_{in}(f)|_{DM}$ can be achieved in several ways. One way is to insert a resistor R_e' between the emitter of each BJT and the V_e node (see Figure 3.5). It is easy to show from the mid-frequency, common-emitter h-parameter MFSSM of the BJT DA for DM inputs (see Figure 3.11(B)) that $R_{inDM} = V_{sd}/I_b = h_{ie} + R_e'(1 + \beta)$. The practical upper bound on R_e' is set by dc biasing considerations. The small-signal input resistance, h_{ie}, can be shown to be approximated by:

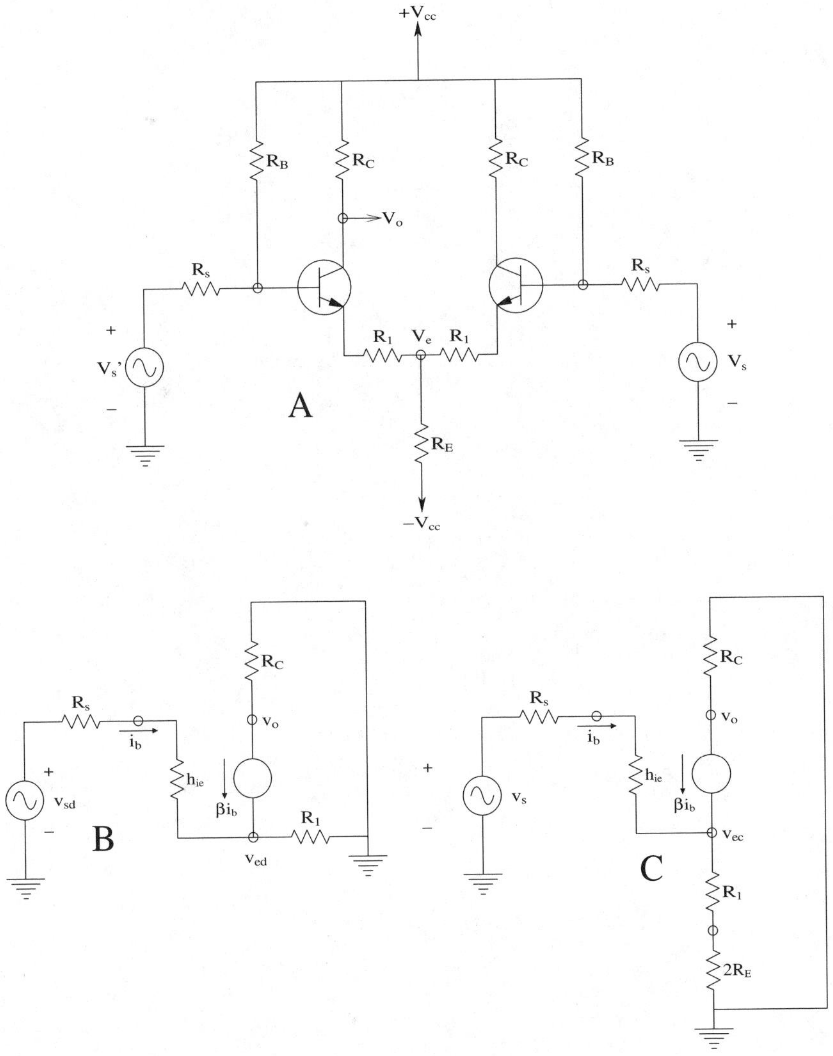

FIGURE 3.11
(A) A BJT DA with extra emitter resistances, R_1, which lower DM gain and increase DM input resistance. (B) Simplified MFSSM of the left side of the DA given DM inputs. (C) Simplified MFSSM of the left side of the DA given CM inputs.

$$h_{ie} \cong V_T \, \beta / I_{CQ} \qquad (3.20)$$

where $V_T = kT/q$; β is the transistor's current gain, h_{fe}; and I_{CQ} is the collector current at the BJT's quiescent (Q) operating point.

Another approach is to use BJT Darlington amplifiers in the DA; a Darlington circuit and its simplified MFSSM are shown in Figure 3.12. Darlingtons can easily be shown to have an input resistance of:

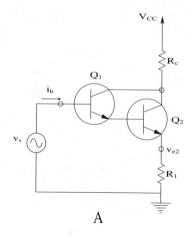

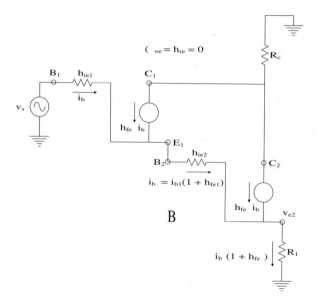

FIGURE 3.12
(A) A Darlington stage that can replace the left-hand BJT in the DA of Figure 3.11A. (B) MFSSM of the Darlington valid for DM excitation of the DA. The input resistance for the Darlington DA given DM excitation is derived in the text.

$$R_{in} = h_{ie1} + h_{ie2}(1 + \beta_1) \tag{3.21}$$

If an emitter resistor, R_1, is used as in the first case, R_{in} can be shown to be:

$$R_{in} = h_{ie1} + (1 + h_{fe1})[h_{ie2} + R_1(1 + h_{fe2})] \cong h_{fe1} \, h_{fe2} \, R_1 \tag{3.22}$$

Thus, if $h_{fe1} = h_{fe2} = 100$ and $R_1 = 200\ \Omega$, $R_{in} > 2\ M\Omega$.

Another obvious way to increase R_{in} for DM excitation (and CM as well) is to design the DA headstage using JFETs or MOSFETs. Using these devices, the low- and mid-frequency R_{in} is on the order of 10^9 to 10^{12} Ω.

3.6 How Signal Source Impedance Affects Low-Frequency CMRR

Figure 3.13 illustrates a generalized input circuit for an instrumentation DA. Note that the two Thevenin sources, v_s and v_s' can be broken into DM and CM components. As defined earlier:

$$v_{sd} \equiv (v_s - v_s')/2 \qquad (3.23A)$$

$$v_{sc} \equiv (v_s + v_s')/2 \qquad (3.23B)$$

Superposition is used to compute the effects of v_{sc} and v_{sd} on the output of the DA. When v_{sc} is considered, v_s and v_s' are replaced with v_{sc} in Figure 3.13; when v_{sd} is considered, v_s is replaced with v_{sd} and v_s' with $-v_{sd}$. Note that manufacturers usually specify a common-mode input impedance, Z_{ic}, measured from one input lead to ground under pure CM excitation, and a difference-mode input impedance, Z_{id}, measured under pure DM excitation from either input to ground. The input Zs are generally given by manufacturer's specs as a resistance in parallel with a small shunting capacitance, for example, Z_{ic} as 10^{11} Ω||5 pF. In the following development, the signal frequency is assumed to be sufficiently low so that the currents through the input capacitances are negligible compared to the parallel input resistance. Thus, only input resistances are used.

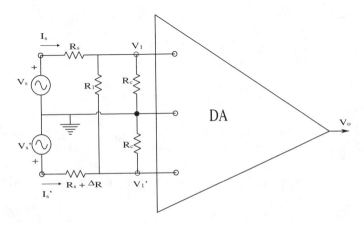

FIGURE 3.13
A generalized input equivalent circuit for a DA.

By Ohm's law, the DM current into the noninverting input node is just:

$$i_d = 2v_{sd}/R_1 + v_{sd}/R_{ic} \tag{3.24}$$

From which,

$$i_d/v_{sd} = 1/R_{sd} = 2/R_1 + 1/R_{ic} \tag{3.25}$$

can be written. Solving for the equivalent shunting resistance in Equation 3.25 yields:

$$R_1 = 2\, R_{id}\, R_{ic}/(R_{ic} - R_{id}) \tag{3.26}$$

In many differential amplifiers, $R_{ic} > R_{id}$. In others, $R_{ic} \cong R_{id}$ and, from Equation 3.26, $R_1 = \infty$. Thus,

$$Z_{ic} = Z_{id} \cong R_{ic} \tag{3.27}$$

Assume that $R_{ic} = R_{id}$. Thus, R_1 may be eliminated from Figure 3.13, which illustrates two Thevenin sources driving the DA through unequal source resistances, R_s and $R_s + \Delta R$.

Using superposition and the definitions in Equation 3.23A and Equation 3.23B, it is possible to show that a purely CM excitation, v_{sc}, produces an unwanted difference-mode component at the DA's input terminals:

$$v_{id}/v_{sc} = R_{ic}\, \Delta R/2(R_{ic} + R_s)^2 \tag{3.28}$$

Also, v_{sc} produces a large CM component; the ΔR term is numerically negligible.

$$v_{ic}/v_{sc} = R_{ic}/(R_{ic} + R_s) \tag{3.29}$$

For purely DM excitation in v_s, it can also be shown that

$$v_{id}/v_{sd} = R_{ic}/(R_{ic} + R_s) \tag{3.30}$$

and

$$v_{ic}/v_{sd} = R_{ic}\, \Delta R/2(R_{ic} + R_s)^2 \tag{3.31}$$

In order to find the CMRR of the circuit of Figure 3.13, Equation 3.2 will be used for v_o, and the definition for CMRR, Relation 3.13. Thus:

$$v_{oc} = A_D\, v_{sc}\, R_{ic}\, \Delta R/2(R_{ic} + R_s)^2 + A_C\, v_{sc}\, R_{ic}/(R_{ic} + R_s) \tag{3.32}$$

and

$$v_{od} = A_D v_{sd}\, R_{ic}/(R_{ic} + R_s) + A_C\, v_{sd}\, R_{ic}\, \Delta R/2(R_{ic} + R_s)^2 \tag{3.33}$$

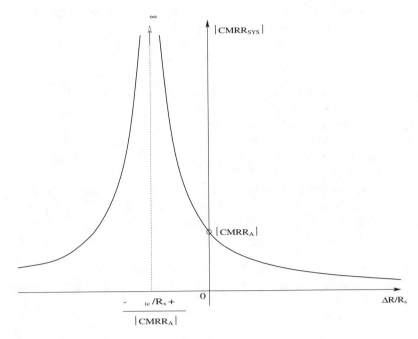

FIGURE 3.14
The CMRR of a balanced input DA as a function of the incremental change in one input (Thevenin) resistance. Note that a critical value of $\Delta R/R_s$ exists that theoretically gives infinite CMRR.

After some algebra, the circuit's CMRR, $CMRR_{sys}$, is given by

$$CMRR_{sys} = \left[A_D + A_C\, \Delta R/2\left(R_{ic} + R_s\right)\right]/\left[A_D\, \Delta R/2\left(R_{ic} + R_s\right) + A_C\right] \quad (3.34)$$

Equation 3.34 may be reduced to the hyperbolic relation:

$$CMRR_{sys} = \left[\left(A_D/A_C\right) + \Delta R/2\left(R_{ic} + R_s\right)\right]/\left[\left(A_D/A_C\right)\Delta R/2\left(R_{ic} + R_s\right) + 1\right] \quad (3.35)$$

which can be approximated by:

$$CMRR_{sys} \cong \frac{CMRR_A}{\dfrac{CMRR_A\, \Delta R}{2\left(R_{ic} + R_s\right)} + 1} \quad (3.36)$$

in which the manufacturer-specified CMRR is $CMRR_A = A_D/A_C$, and $CMRR_A \gg \Delta R/2(R_{ic} + R)$.

A plot of $CMRR_{sys}$ vs. $\Delta R/R_s$ is shown in Figure 3.14. Note that when the Thevenin source resistances are matched, $CMRR_{sys} = CMRR_A$. Also, when

$$\Delta R/R_s = -2(R_{ic}/R_s + 1)/CMRR_A, \tag{3.37}$$

the $CMRR_{sys} \rightarrow \infty$. This implies that a judicious addition of an external resistance in series with one input lead or the other to introduce a ΔR may be used to increase the effective CMRR of the system. For example, if $R_{ic} = 100$ MΩ, $R_s = 10$ kΩ, and $CMRR_A = 100$ dB, then $\Delta R/R_s = -0.2$ to give ∞ $CMRR_{sys}$. Because it is generally not possible to reduce R_s', it is easier to add a $2\ k\ \Delta R$ in series with R_s externally.

Again, it needs to be stressed that an amplifier's $CMRR_A$ is a decreasing function of frequency because of the frequency dependence of the gains, A_D and A_C. Also, the ac equivalent input circuit of a DA contains capacitances in parallel with R_1, R_{ic}, and R_{ic}' and the source impedances often contain a reactive frequency-dependent component. Thus, in practice, $CMRR_{sys}$ can often be maximized by the ΔR method at low frequencies, but seldom can be drastically increased at high frequencies because of reactive unbalances in the input circuit.

3.7 How Op Amps Can Be Used To Make DAs for Medical Applications

3.7.1 Introduction

It is true that op amps are differential amplifiers, but several practical factors make their direct use in instrumentation highly impractical. The first factor is their extremely high open-loop gain and relatively low signal bandwidth. As demonstrated in Chapter 6 and Chapter 7, op amps are designed to be used with massive amounts of negative feedback, which acts to reduce their gain, increase their bandwidth, reduce their output signal distortion, etc. When used without feedback, their extremely high open-loop gain generally produces unacceptable signal levels at their outputs, as well as dc levels that drift because of temperature-sensitive input dc offset voltage and dc bias currents. Consequently, circuits have evolved that use two- or three-op amps with feedback to make DAs with gains typically ranging from 1 to 10^3, wide bandwidths, low noise, high input Z, high CMRR, etc.

Why would one want to build a DA from op amps when instrumentation amplifiers (DAs) are readily available from manufacturers? One reason is that the builder can select ultra low-noise op amps for the circuit and can tweak resistor values to maximize the DA's CMRR. If one is building only a few DAs, a higher performance–cost ratio can be achieved by undertaking a custom design with op amps, rather than purchasing commercial IAs.

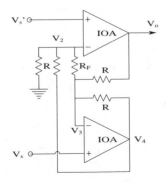

FIGURE 3.15
A two-operational amplifier DA. Resistors must be precisely matched to obtain maximum CMRR.

3.7.2 Two-OP AMP DA Designs

A two-op amp DA is shown in Figure 3.15. All resistors "R" are closely matched to <0.02% to maintain a high CMRR. Analysis is easy if ideal op amps are assumed. Node equations are written for the V_2 and V_3 nodes, which, by the ideal op amp assumption, are V_s' and V_s, respectively. The unknowns are V_o and V_4.

$$V_s' [2G + G_F] - V_s G_F - V_4 G = 0 \qquad (3.38A)$$

$$-V_s' G_F + V_s [2G + G_F] - V_o G - V_4 G = 0 \qquad (3.38B)$$

Clearly, from Equation 3.38A, $V_4 G = V_s'[2G + G_F] - V_s G_F$. This equation is substituted into Equation 3.38B, yielding:

$$V_o = (V_s = V_s')2(1 + R/R_F) = \frac{(V_s - V_s')}{2} 4(1 + R/R_F) = V_{sd} 4(1 + R/R_F) \quad (3.39)$$

Thus, the two-op amp DA configuration can have DM gains, $A_D \geq 4$. (This analysis does not treat the CM gain.)

A three-op amp DA circuit is shown in Figure 3.16. In this circuit, it is assumed that all $R_j = R_j'$, i.e., corresponding resistors are perfectly matched in order to make the CMRR $\rightarrow \infty$. Analysis of the three-op amp DA can be done with superposition, but is easier if pure CM and DM excitations are assumed and the bisection theorem is used. For pure CM excitation, $V_s' = V_s = V_{sc}$. By symmetry and the IOA assumption, $V_2 = V_2' = V_{sc}$; thus, there is no current in $R_1 + R_1'$, and $V_c = V_{sc}$. R_2 and R_2' also have no current, so no voltage drop occurs across these feedback resistors and thus $V_3 = V_3' = V_{sc}$. When the right-hand IOA circuit has matched resistors, it is a DA with gain:

$$V_o = (V_3 - V_3')(R_4/R_3) \qquad (3.40)$$

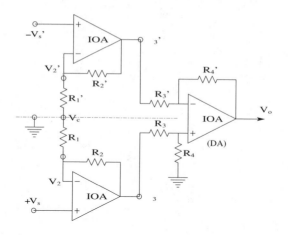

FIGURE 3.16
The symmetrical three-op amp DA. Again, for max CMRR, the primed resistors must precisely equal the corresponding nonprimed resistors.

Clearly, for CM signals:

$$A_C = \frac{V_o}{V_{sc}} = 0 \tag{3.41}$$

For pure DM excitation, $V_s' = -V_s$, $V_2 = V_s = V_{sd}$, and $V_2' = -V_s$. Thus a potential of $2V_s$ exists across resistors $(R_1 + R_1')$ and, by Kirchoff's voltage law, $V_c = 0$ on the axis of symmetry.

Because current flows through R_1 and R_2, and also R_1' and R_2', the input IOAs each have a gain of $(1 + R_2/R_1)$. Now $V_3' = -V_{sd} (1 + R_2/R_1)$ and $V_3 = V_{sd} (1 + R_2/R_1)$. Using superposition on the output IOA circuit yields:

$$\frac{V_o}{V_{sd}} = A_D = (R_4/R_3)2(1 + R_2/R_1) \tag{3.42}$$

IC versions of this DA circuit generally make $R_3 = R_4$, set the R_2s = 25 k, and replace $(R_1 + R_1')$ with a single external resistor to set A_D between 1 and 10^3. An example of such an IC DA is the Burr–Brown INA111. In practice, the OAs are not ideal and have different, finite CMRRs, and the resistors are not perfectly matched. For example, the "off-the-shelf" CMRR is 106 dB at an $A_D = 100$ for the INA111.

3.8   Chapter Summary

Because of their great importance in many aspects of analog electronic circuit design, differential amplifiers have been treated in their own chapter. DAs are essential electronic subsystems for ICs such as op amps, instrumentation amplifiers, and analog voltage comparators. DAs are widely used in instrumentation systems to condition signals because of their ability to reject, by subtraction, interference and noise that are exactly common to both inputs.

In describing DA circuit architecture, important definitions of differential and common-mode input signals, differential and common-mode gains, and common-mode rejection ratio (CMRR) as a DA figure of merit were introduced. Internal and external factors affecting the DA's CMRR at low frequencies were described.

The mid- and high-frequency behavior of DA difference-mode and common-mode gains were explored by circuit simulation and factors affecting the CMRR at high frequencies were discussed. Circuits using two- and three-op amps to make instrumentation DAs were described and analyzed.

Home Problems

3.1 A pair of matched JFETs and an ideal op amp are used to make a DA as shown in Figure P3.1. Both JFETs are described at mid-frequencies by the simple Norton (g_m, g_d) MFSSM.

a. Draw the complete MFSSM for the DA. Note that the MFSSM treats all dc voltage sources as small signal grounds and all dc current sources as open circuits.

b. Use superposition to derive an expression for $v_o = f(v_1, v_2)$. Show what happens to v_o when R_S is replaced with an ideal dc current source.

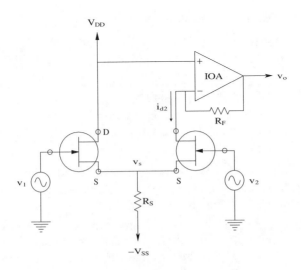

FIGURE P3.1

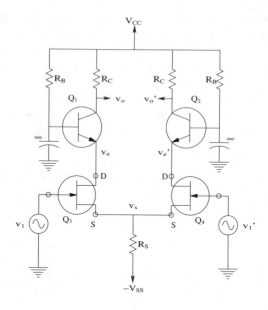

FIGURE P3.2

3.2   The schematic of a JFET/BJT cascode DA is shown in Figure P3.2. In this
      DA, $Q_1 = Q_2$ with $h_{oe} = h_{re} = 0$, $h_{fe} = 120$, $I_{CQ} = 1$ mA, $R_C = 7$ kΩ, $R_s = 25$ MΩ
      (dynamic load), and $R_B = 1.24$ MΩ. Also, $Q_3 = Q_4$ with $g_m = 5 \times 10^{-3}$ S, $g_d = 1 \times 10^{-4}$ S.

      a. Use the bisection theorem to draw the MFSSMs for pure CM and
          pure DM excitation.
      b. Find an expression for the CM gain, v_o/v_{1c}.
      c. Find an expression for the DA's DM gain, v_o/v_{1d}.
      d. Find an expression for and evaluate numerically the DA's CMRR.

3.3   Figure P3.3A shows the schematic of a 2N2369 DA given DM excitation.
      VINV is an ideal VCVS with a gain of –1. The common emitters use an active
      current sink that can be replaced by its Norton equivalent of a 2.0125-mA
      current source in parallel with a 2-MΩ resistor and a small shunt capacitance
      to ground, C_E.

      a. Use an ECAP to make a Bode plot of the DM gain, V_o/V_{1d}, vs. f
          from 10 kHz to 10 GHz. Give values for the mid-frequency gain,
          the upper –3-dB frequency, and f_T.
      b. Figure P3.3B illustrates the DA given pure CM excitation. Now
          the capacitor, C_E, will affect the CM high frequency response.
          Make a Bode plot of the CM gain, V_o/V_{1c} over 1 kHz to 1 GHz
          with $C_E \equiv 0$.

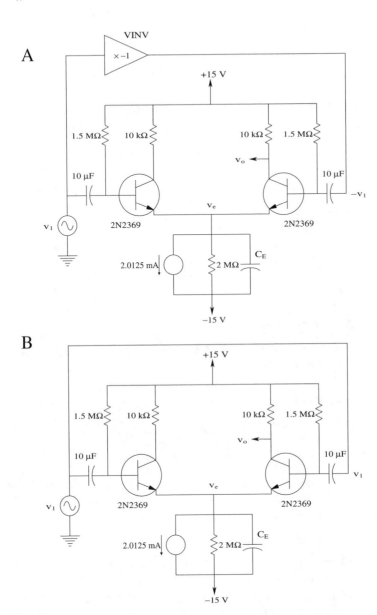

FIGURE P3.3

c. Now find a C_E value by trial and error that will *minimize* the CM frequency response. (Hint: the optimum value lies between 1 and 10 pF.)

d. The decibel CMRR for the DA is just the decibel DM gain minus the CM gain. Plot the decibel CMRR for the amplifier with $C_E = 0$, and $C_E =$ the optimum value, for 10 kHz $\leq f \leq$ 1 GHz.

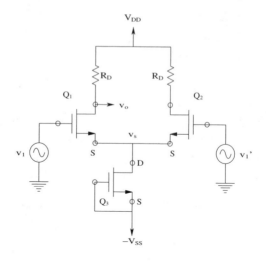

FIGURE P3.4

3.4   A MOSFET DA is shown in Figure P3.4.

   a. Draw the complete MFSSM for the DA. Use the Norton model (g_m, g_d) for the MOSFETs.

   b. Draw the left-hand MFSSM of the DA valid for DM inputs. Derive an expression for the MF $A_d = v_o/v_{1d}$.

   c. Draw the left-hand MFSSM of the DA valid for CM inputs. Derive an expression for $A_c = v_o/v_{1c}$.

   d. Give an expression for the CMRR of the DA.

3.5   Figure P3.5 illustrates a p-channel JFET DA with a pnp BJT dynamic source load. Assume $Q_1 = Q_2$ with $g_m = 0.002$ S, and $r_d = 250$ kΩ. For the BJT: $h_{fe} = 150$; $h_{oe} = 10^{-6}$ S; $h_{ie} = 1.5$ kΩ; and $h_{re} = 0$.

   a. Draw the MFSSM for the DA.

   b. Find an expression and the numerical value for the SS resistance, R_S, looking into the collector of the BJT.

   c. Find the expression and numerical value for $A_d = v_o/v_{1d}$, $A_c = v_o/v_{1c}$, and the DA's CMRR.

3.6   The DA shown in Figure P5.6 uses common-mode negative feedback between the output and the dynamic load BJT, Q_3. Assume $Q_1 = Q_2$ with $h_{fe} = 200$; $h_{ie} = 2.5$ kΩ; $h_{oe} = h_{re} = 0$; $R_1 = 70$ kΩ; and $R_C = 4$ kΩ. For Q_3: $h_{fe} = 200$; $h_{oe} = 10^{-5}$ S; $h_{ie} = 1.2$ kΩ; and $h_{re} = 0$. The numbers in parentheses are quiescent dc bias voltages. The zener diode drops 14.3 V at 0.2 mA. Treat it as an ideal DC voltage source.

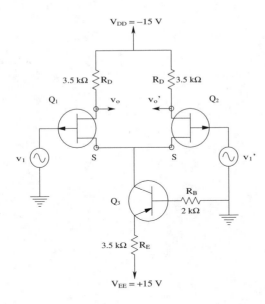

FIGURE P3.5

 a. Use the bisection theorem to draw the MFSSM for the DA given pure DM excitation.

 b. Use the bisection theorem to draw the MFSSM for the DA given pure CM excitation.

 c. Give algebraic expressions for $A_d = v_o/v_{1d}$ and $A_c = v_o/v_{1c}$. Evaluate numerically.

 d. Evaluate the DA's CMRR.

 e. By way of comparison, repeat parts a through d when the zener diode is removed and Q_3's base is tied to small-signal ground.

3.7 The DA shown in Figure P3.7 uses feedback pair amplifiers. For symmetry, $Q_1 = Q_3$ and $Q_2 = Q_4$, but $Q_1 \neq Q_2$, etc. Q_1 and Q_3 have h_{fe1}, $h_{ie1} > 0$, and $h_{re1} = h_{oe1} = 0$. Likewise, Q_2 and Q_4 have h_{fe2}, $h_{ie2} > 0$, and $h_{re2} = h_{oe2} = 0$.

 a. Draw the complete MFSSM for the DA given pure DM excitation.

 b. Draw the complete MFSSM for the DA given pure CM excitation.

 c. Find an expression for $A_d = v_o/v_{1d}$.

 d. Find an expression for $A_c = v_o/v_{1c}$.

 e. Find an expression for the DA's CMRR.

 f. Find an expression for the DA's small-signal input resistance when it is given DM input. Let $R_{ind} = v_{1d}/i_1$.

 g. Find an expression for the DA's small-signal input resistance when it is given CM input. Let $R_{inc} = v_{1c}/i_1$.

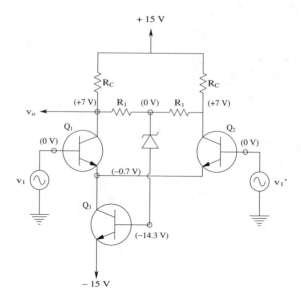

FIGURE P3.6

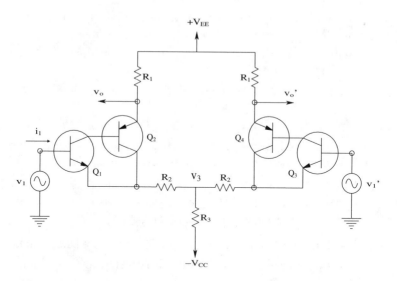

FIGURE P3.7

3.8   Figure P3.8 illustrates a DA using Darlington modules, the purpose of which
        is to raise the DM input resistance. For symmetry, $Q_1 = Q_3$ and $Q_2 = Q_4$. Q_1
        and Q_3 have h_{fe1}, $h_{ie1} > 0$, and $h_{re1} = h_{oe1} = 0$. Q_2 and Q_4 have h_{fe2}, $h_{ie2} > 0$, and
        $h_{re2} = h_{oe2} = 0$. Q_5 has h_{fe5}, h_{ie5}, and $h_{oe5} > 0$, $h_{re5} = 0$.

   a. Draw the MFSSMs for the DA for pure CM and DM excitations.

   b. Find an expression for $A_d = v_o/v_{1d}$.

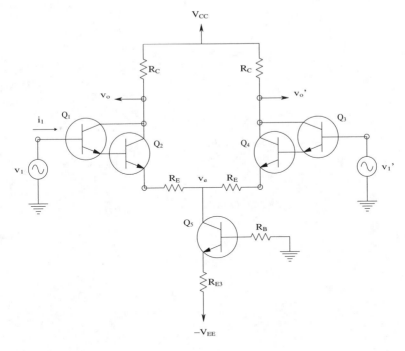

FIGURE P3.8

     c. Find an expression for $A_c = v_o/v_{1c}$.

     d. Find an expression for the DA's CMRR.

     e. Find an expression for the DA's small-signal input resistance when it is given DM input. Let $R_{ind} = v_{1d}/i_1$.

     f. Find an expression for the DA's small-signal input resistance when it is given CM input. Let $R_{inc} = v_{1c}/i_1$.

     g. Now let $h_{fe1} = 100$, $h_{ie1} = 6$ kΩ, $h_{fe2} = 50$, $h_{ie2} = 1$ kΩ, $h_{fe5} = 100$, $h_{oe5} = 10^{-5}$ S, $h_{ie5} = 2.5$ kΩ, $R_C = 5$ kΩ, $R_E = 500$ Ω, $R_{E3} = 3.3$ kΩ, and $R_B = 100$ kΩ. Calculate numerical values for parts b through f.

3.9   Two, matched, n-channel JFETs are connected as shown in Figure P3.9. They are both characterized by the saturation-region, JFET drain current relation: $I_D = I_{DSS}(1 - V_{GS}/V_P)^2$. The capacitor, C_o, blocks dc from the output signal. The circuit input is the pure difference-mode signal, $v_{gd} = v_1$. Find an algebraic expression for I_L and the ac, v_o.

3.10   Two matched 2N2222A BJTs are used to make a BJT DA shown in Figure P3.10.

     a. Simulate the circuit under CM excitation and make a Bode plot of $A_c = V_o/V_{1c}$. Let 1k Hz $\leq f \leq$ 0.1 GHz.

     b. Now make a Bode plot of the DM gain, $A_d = V_o/V_{1d}$.

     c. Plot the DA's CMRR in decibels over 1 kHz to 0.1 GHz.

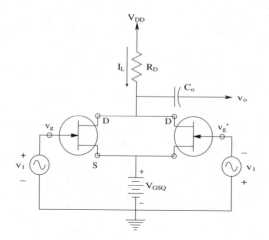

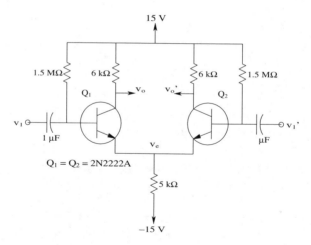

3.11 A BJT DA is shown in Figure P3.11. The circuit is symmetrical. $R_E = 10^5 \ \Omega$, $R_S = 500 \ \Omega$, $R_C = 6.8 \ \text{k}\Omega$, $R_B = 1 \ \text{M}\Omega$; BJTs: $h_{oe} = h_{re} = 0$; $h_{fe} = 100$; $h_{ie} = 2.5 \ \text{k}\Omega$. Assume C_c is a small-signal short circuit.

   a. Use MFSS analysis and the bisection theorem to find numerical values for A_D, A_C, and the CMRR. $A_D \equiv v_o/v_{1d}$ and $A_C \equiv v_o/v_{1c}$.

   b. Now the v_o output is coupled to a 10-kΩ load resistance, R_L, making the DA circuit asymmetrical, so the bisection theorem no longer can be used. Repeat a.

3.12 It is desired to measure the CMRR of a student-built differential amplifier (see Figure P3.12). First, the two inputs are shorted together and connected to a

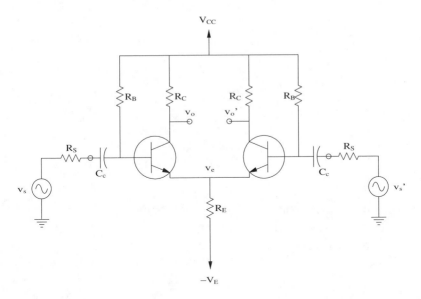

FIGURE P3.11

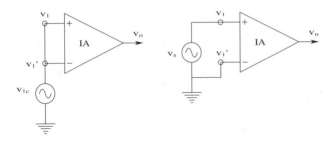

FIGURE P3.12

100-Hz sinusoidal source. The source amplitude is adjusted so that when the peak output signal is 1.0 V, the input is 10 V, peak. Then the negative input to the amplifier is grounded and the source is connected to the + input. Its amplitude is adjusted so that $V_o = 10$ V, peak, when the input is 20 mV, peak. Find numerical values for A_D, A_C, and the CMRR in decibels.

3.13 Common-mode negative feedback is applied around a DA having a differential output, shown in Figure P3.13. The amplifier follows the relations: $V_o = A_D V_{1d} + A_C V_{1c}$; $V_o' = -A_D V_{1d} + A_C V_{1c}$. Also, $V_{1c} = A_C V_{1c}$, and let $\alpha \equiv R_1/(R_1 + R_s)$ and $\beta = R_s/(R_1 + R_s)$.

a. Use superposition to find expressions for V_1 and V_1'.

b. Find an expression for V_{1c} when V_s and V_s' are such that the input is pure V_{sc}.

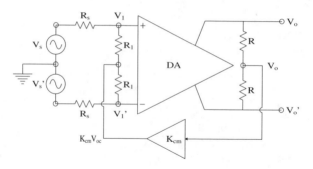

FIGURE P3.13

c. Find an expression for V_{1d} when the input is pure V_{sd}.

d. Find an expression for the CMNF amplifier's CMRR. Compare it to the CMRR of the DA alone. Let $R_1 = R_2 = 10^6 \ \Omega$; $K_{cm} = -10^3$; $A_C = 1$, and $A_D = 10^3$. Evaluate the system's CMRR numerically.

4

General Properties of Electronic Single-Loop Feedback Systems

4.1 Introduction

In electronic circuits and systems, feedback will be defined as a process whereby a signal proportional to the system's output is combined with a signal proportional to the input to form an error signal that affects the output. Nearly all analog electronic circuits use feedback — implicitly as the result of circuit design (e.g., as from an unbypassed BJT emitter resistor) or explicitly by a specific circuit network between the output and the input nodes. A circuit can have one or more specific feedback loops. However, in the interest of simplicity, the effects of a single feedback loop on circuits with single inputs will be considered. The four categories of electronic feedback and the feedback that can make an electronic system unstable (deliberately, as in the design of oscillators) or stable will be shown. The effects of feedback on amplifier frequency response, gain, noise, output and input impedance, and linearity will also be discussed.

Op amps will be used to illustrate many properties of single-input–single-output (SISO) feedback systems because all op amps use feedback and they have relatively simple dynamic characteristics. A systems approach will be used in discussing amplifier performance with feedback; little attention will be paid to the nitty-gritty of the electronic components. Block diagrams, signal flow graphs, and Mason's rule will be used to describe the systems under consideration and the root-locus technique will be used to explore feedback amplifier performance in the frequency domain.

4.2 Classification of Electronic Feedback Systems

Figure 4.1 illustrates the general architecture of a SISO feedback system. Reduction of the signal flow graph or the block diagram of Figure 4.1 yields the well-known transfer function:

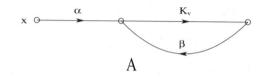

A

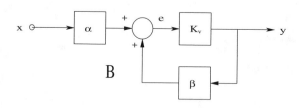

B

FIGURE 4.1
Two alternate representations for a single-input–single-output (SISO) linear feedback system.
(A) Signal flow graph notation. (B) Block diagram notation.

$$\frac{V_o}{V_s} = \frac{\alpha K_v}{1 - \beta K_v} \tag{4.1}$$

From this simple result, the following important quantities describing
feedback systems can be defined:

- Forward gain = open-loop gain = αK_v (4.2A)
- Loop gain = $A_L = \beta K_v$ (4.2B)
- Return difference = $RD = 1 - A_L$ (4.2C)
- dB of feedback = $-20 \log|1 - A_L|$ (4.2D)

Note that α, β, K_v, and A_L can be scalars or vectors (complex functions of
frequency).

A SISO system is said to have negative feedback (NFB) if it has a minus
sign associated with either K_v, β, or the summer, or with all three elements
in the block diagram. Control systems generally use NFB and it is usual to
assume a subtraction of βV_o at the summer. Electronic systems do not necessarily have a subtraction at the summer; it depends on circuit design. To
see if a SISO electronic feedback system has negative feedback, inspect the
loop gain. $A_L(j0)$ will have a minus sign (be a negative number) if the
feedback amplifier is a direct-coupled (DC) negative feedback system. If the
amplifier is reactively coupled (RC), then $A_L(j\omega)$ will have a minus sign at
mid-frequencies (its phase angle will be $-180°$). Feedback amplifier is generally a voltage, but VCCSs are encountered. Considering that feedback can
have either sign and the fed-back quantity can be voltage or current, it is

clear that four major types of feedback exist: (1) negative voltage feedback; (2) negative current feedback; (3) positive voltage feedback; and (4) positive current feedback. Negative voltage feedback is most widely encountered in electronic engineering practice. Its properties will be examined in the following sections.

4.3 Some Effects of Negative Voltage Feedback

4.3.1 Reduction of Output Resistance

Figure 4.2 illustrates a simple Thevenin amplifier circuit with NVB applied to its summing junction (input node). Assume that the amplifier's input resistor, R_{in}, $\gg R_F$ and R_s, so R_{in} can be ignored in writing the node equation for V_i. Also, in finding the NFB amplifier's open-circuit voltage gain, assume that $R_o \ll R_F$, so negligible voltage drop takes place across R_o. Thus, the node equation is:

$$V_i [G_s + G_F] - V_o G_F = V_s G_s \qquad (4.3)$$

Also,

$$V_o \cong -K_v V_i \qquad (4.4)$$

Thus:

$$V_i = -V_o / K_v \qquad (4.5)$$

and

$$-(V_o / K_v)(G_s + G_F) - V_o G_F = V_s G_s \qquad (4.6)$$

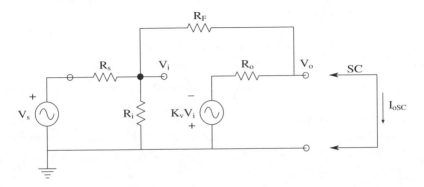

FIGURE 4.2
Schematic of a simple Thevenin VCVS with negative feedback. See text for analysis.

Thus, Equation 4.6 can be used to write the closed-loop system's transfer function:

$$\frac{V_o}{V_s} = \frac{-K_v G_s}{G_s + G_F + K_v G_F} = \frac{-K_v R_F/(R_F + R_s)}{1 + K_v R_s/(R_F + R_s)} = A_v \tag{4.7}$$

Note in comparing Equation 4.7 to Equation 4.1, that

$$A_L = -K_v [R_s/(R_F + R_s)] \text{ (Note: system has NFB.)} \tag{4.8}$$

$$\alpha = R_F/(R_F + R_s) \tag{4.9}$$

$$\beta = R_s/(R_F + R_s) \tag{4.10}$$

In op amps, K_v is numerically very large, so Equation 4.7 reduces to the well-known gain relation for the ideal op amp inverter: $V_o/V_s = -R_F/R_s$.)

There are two common ways to find the output resistance of the simple NFB amplifier of Figure 4.2. One is to set $V_s = 0$, then place an independent test source, V_t, between the V_o node and ground and calculate $R_{out} = V_t/I_t$. The other method is to measure the open-circuit output voltage using Equation 4.7, then calculate the short-circuit output current (with $V_o = 0$). Clearly, $R_{out} = V_{OC}/I_{oSC}$. Inspection of Figure 4.2 with a shorted output lets one write:

$$I_{oSC} = \frac{V_s}{(R_s + R_F)}\left[1 - \frac{K_v R_F}{R_o}\right] \cong \frac{-V_s K_v R_F}{R_o(R_F + R_s)} \tag{4.11}$$

Now R_{out} can be found:

$$R_{out} = \frac{\dfrac{-K_v R_F/(R_F + R_s)}{1 + K_v R_s/(R_F + R_s)}}{\dfrac{-V_s K_v R_F}{R_o(R_F + R_s)}} = \frac{R_o}{1 + K_v R_s/(R_F + R_s)} = \frac{R_o}{1 + \beta K_v} = \frac{R_o}{1 - A_L} \tag{4.12}$$

In general, the NFB amplifier's output impedance can be written as a function of frequency:

$$\mathbf{Z}_{out}(j\omega) = R_o/\mathbf{RD}(j\omega) \tag{4.13}$$

Note that, in general, $|\mathbf{Z}_{out}(j\omega)|$ is very small (e.g., milliohms) at dc and low frequencies, then gradually increases with ω. This property can be demonstrated by assuming K_v to have a frequency response of the form:

$$\mathbf{K}_v(j\omega) = \frac{K_{vo}}{j\omega\tau + 1} \tag{4.14}$$

Equation now yields:

$$Z_o(j\omega) = \frac{R_o}{1 + \beta K_{vo}/(j\omega\tau + 1)} = \frac{R_o(j\omega\tau + 1)}{j\omega\tau + (1 + \beta K_{vo})} = \frac{\left[R_o/(1 + \beta K_{vo})\right](j\omega\tau + 1)}{j\omega\tau/(1 + \beta K_{vo}) + 1} \quad (4.15)$$

From the preceding equation it is clear that $|Z_o| \cong R_o/\beta K_{vo}$ at dc, increasing with frequency to $|Z_o| = R_o$ at frequencies above $\beta K_{vo}/\tau$ r/s.

4.3.2 Reduction of Total Harmonic Distortion

A very important property of NFB is the reduction of total harmonic distortion (THD) at the output of amplifiers, in particular power amplifiers. First it is necessary to examine what *THD* means. Assume that a certain amplifier has a soft saturation nonlinearity modeled by:

$$y = ax + bx^2 + cx^3 + dx^4 + ex^5 + \ldots \quad (4.16)$$

Clearly, $a = K_v$, the linear gain. The $b, c, d, e, \ldots$ terms can be zero or have either sign. They give rise to the harmonic distortion that can be the result of transistor cut-off or saturation, or power supply saturation. If $x(t) = X_o \sin(\omega_o t)$, the output $y(t)$ will contain the desired fundamental frequency from the a-term, as well as unwanted harmonics. For example,

$$y(t) = a\, X_o \sin(\omega_o t) + (bX_o^2/2)\left[1 - \cos(2\omega_o t)\right] + (cX_o^3/4)$$
$$\left[3\sin(\omega_o t) - \sin(3\omega_o t)\right] + \ldots \quad (4.17)$$

The power terms approximating the nonlinear transfer characteristic of the amplifier generate dc, fundamental, and harmonics of the order of the nonlinear term in addition to the desired fundamental frequency. These can be summarized by the expression:

$$y(t) = K_v\, X_o \sin(\omega_o t) + H_2 \sin(2\omega_o t) + H_3 \sin(3\omega_o t) + H_4 \sin(4\omega_o t) + \ldots \quad (4.18)$$

The total RMS harmonic distortion is defined as:

$$\text{THD} = \sqrt{H_2^2/2 + H_3^2/2 + H_4^2/2 + \ldots} = \sqrt{\sum_{k=2}^{\infty} H_k^2/2} \quad (4.19)$$

Note that $H_k^2/2$ is the mean squared value of the kth harmonic; $(K_v^2 X_o^2/2)$ is the MS value of the fundamental frequency (desired) component of the output. In general, the larger X_o is, the larger will be the THD.

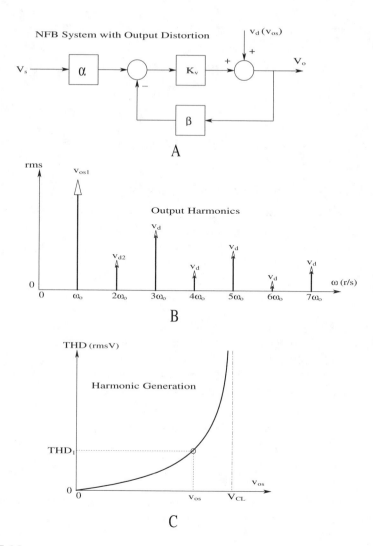

FIGURE 4.3

(A) Block diagram of a SISO negative voltage feedback system with output harmonic distortion voltage introduced in the last (power) stage. A sinusoidal input of frequency ω_o is assumed. (B) Rms power spectrum of the feedback amplifier output. v_{os1} is the RMS amplitude of the fundamental frequency output. (C) Plot of how total harmonic distortion typically varies as a function of the amplitude of the fundamental output voltage.

Figure 4.3(A) illustrates a block diagram showing how the RMS THD is added to the output of an NFB amplifier. Distortion is assumed to occur in the last stage. If there were no feedback, ($\beta = 0$), $V_o = V_s \, \alpha K_v + v_d \, (V_s \alpha K_v)$. V_s is adjusted so that the RMS output signal is v_{os1}. With feedback,

$$V_o = \frac{\overset{v_{os1}}{V_s \alpha K_v}}{1 + \beta K_v} + \frac{\overset{\text{THD}}{v_d(v_{os1})}}{1 + \beta K_v} \tag{4.20}$$

With NFB, the output THD is reduced by a factor of $1/(1 + \beta\ K_v)$, given that the signal output is the same in the nonfeedback and the feedback cases. This result has vast implications in the design of nearly distortion-free audio power amplifiers, as well as linear signal conditioning systems in general that use op amps. v_{dk} in Figure 4.3(B) is simply the kth RMS harmonic voltage; i.e., $v_{dk} = H_k/\sqrt{2}$. Figure 4.3(C) shows how the RMS THD increases as the signal output is made larger. At $v_{os} = V_{CL}$, the level of distortion increases abruptly because the amplifier begins to saturate and clip the output signal waveform.

In good low-distortion amplifier design, the input stages are made as linear as possible, and the amplifier is designed so that the output (power) stage saturates before the input and intermediate gain stages do. This allows the THD voltage to effectively be added in the last stage, and thus the THD is reduced by a factor of $1/(1 - A_L) = 1/RD$.

4.3.3 Increase of NFB Amplifier Bandwidth at the Cost of Gain

It is axiomatic in the design of electronic circuit that negative feedback allows one to extend closed-loop amplifier bandwidth (BW) at the expense of dc or mid-band gain. Another way of looking at the effect of NFB on BW is to observe that every amplifier is endowed with some gain*bandwidth product (GBWP); as a figure of merit, larger is better. GBWP remains relatively constant as feedback is applied, so when NFB reduces gain, it increases BW. The frequency-compensated (FC) op amp makes an excellent example of GBWP constancy. The open-loop gain of an FC op amp can be given by:

$$\frac{V_o}{V_i - V_i'} = \frac{K_{vo}}{s\tau_a + 1} \tag{4.21}$$

Note that the op amp is a difference amplifier and has a gain*bandwidth product:

$$\text{GBWP}_{oa} = K_{vo}/(2\pi\tau_a) \text{ Hertz} \tag{4.22}$$

Now connect the OA as a simple noninverting amplifier, as shown in Figure 4.4(A). The amplifier's output is:

$$V_o = (V_s - \beta V_o)K_{vo}/(s\tau_a + 1) \tag{4.23}$$

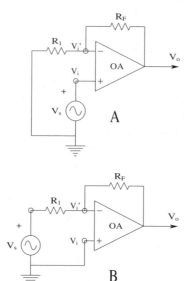

FIGURE 4.4
(A) An op amp connected as a noninverting amplifier. (B) An op amp connected as an inverting amplifier.

where

$$\beta \equiv R_1/(R_1 + R_F) \tag{4.24}$$

Solving for the voltage gain yields:

$$\frac{V_o}{V_s} = A_v(s) = \frac{K_{vo}/(1 + \beta K_{vo})}{s\tau_a/(1 + \beta K_{vo}) + 1} \tag{4.25}$$

The GBWP for this closed-loop amplifier is simply:

$$\text{GBWP}_{amp} = \frac{K_{vo}}{(1 + \beta K_{vo})} \frac{(1 + \beta K_{vo})}{2\pi\tau_a} = \text{GBWP}_{oa} \tag{4.26}$$

For the closed-loop feedback amplifier to have exactly the same GBWP as the open-loop op amp is a special case. Note that the closed-loop gain is divided by the RD and the closed-loop BW is multiplied by the RD.

Next, consider the gain, BW, and GBWP of a simple op amp inverter, shown in Figure 4.4(B). To attack this problem, write a node equation on the summing junction (V_i') node:

$$V_i'(G_1 + G_F) - V_o G_F = V_s G_1 \tag{4.27}$$

noting that:

$$V_o = -V_i' K_{vo}/(s\tau_a + 1) \qquad (4.28)$$

Equation 4.28 is solved for V_i' and substituted into Equation 4.27, and the closed-loop transfer function is found:

$$\frac{V_o}{V_s} = A_v(s) = \frac{-K_{vo}R_F/\left[R_F + R_1(1+K_v)\right]}{s\tau_a(R_F + R_1)/\left[R_F + R_1(1+K_v)\right]} \qquad (4.29)$$

The low and mid-frequency closed-loop gain is:

$$A_v(0) = -K_{vo}R_F/\left[R_F + R_1(1+K_v)\right] \qquad (4.30)$$

and the closed-loop amplifier's BW is its –3-dB frequency where $|A_v(f_b)| = |A_v(0)|/\sqrt{2}$. This is simply:

$$f_b = \left[R_F + R_1(1+K_v)\right]/\left[2\pi\tau_a(R_F + R_1)\right] \text{ hertz} \qquad (4.31)$$

Thus, its gain*bandwidth product is:

$$\text{GBWP}_{amp} = \frac{K_{vo}R_F\left[R_F + R_1(1+K_{vo})\right]}{\left[R_F + R_1(1+K_{vo})\right]\left[2\pi\tau_a(R_F + R_1)\right]} = \frac{K_{vo}}{2\pi\tau_a} \frac{R_F}{(R_F + R_1)} \qquad (4.32)$$

$$= \text{GBWP}_{oa}\, \alpha$$

where α is the feed-forward attenuation of the op amp's feedback circuit.

Thus the inverting op amp circuit with feedback has a GBWP that is lower than the GBWP of the op amp. As R_F is increased, $A_v(0)$ increases and $\text{GBWP}_{amp} \to \text{GBWP}_{oa}$. In all cases, the use of NFB extends the high-frequency half-power frequency at the expense of gain.

4.3.4 Decrease in Gain Sensitivity

Gain sensitivity is the fractional change in closed-loop gain resulting from changes in amplifier circuit component values. In the case of the basic SISO feedback system of Figure 4.3(A), the closed-loop gain is:

$$\frac{V_o}{V_s} = A_v = \frac{\alpha K_v}{1 + \beta K_v} \qquad (4.33)$$

The sensitivity of A_v with respect to the gain K_v is defined by:

$$S_{K_v}^{A_v} \equiv \frac{\Delta A_v / A_v}{\Delta K_v / K_v} \tag{4.34}$$

so now

$$\Delta A_v = \left(\frac{\partial A_v}{\partial K_v}\right) \Delta K_v \tag{4.35}$$

and the partial derivative is:

$$\frac{\partial A_v}{\partial K_v} = \frac{\alpha\left[(1+\beta K_v) - \beta K_v\right]}{(1+\beta K_v)^2} = \frac{\alpha K_v}{(1+\beta K_v)} \frac{K_v^{-1}}{RD} \tag{4.36}$$

Thus,

$$\Delta A_v = \frac{A_v \Delta K_v}{K_v [RD]} \tag{4.37}$$

and the sensitivity is:

$$S_{K_v}^{A_v} \equiv \frac{\Delta A_v / A_v}{\Delta K_v / K_v} = \frac{A_v \Delta K_v / A_v}{K_v [RD] \Delta K_v / K_v} = \frac{1}{[RD]} \tag{4.38}$$

In op amps, $1/[RD]$ is on the order of 10^{-4} to 10^{-6}, so a circuit with NFB is generally quite insensitive to variations in its dc open-loop gain, K_{vo}.

Also of interest is how sensitivity varies as a function of frequency in NFB circuits. According to Northrop (1990),

Complex algebra must be used in the calculation of such sensitivities, because the closed-loop gain [frequency response] is complex. Here we express the closed-loop gain in polar form for convenience:

$$\mathbf{A}_v(j\omega) = |\mathbf{A}_v(j\omega)| \; e^{j\theta(\omega)} \tag{4.39}$$

The gain sensitivity, given by Equation [4.38], can also be written as

$$S_x^{A_v} = \frac{d\mathbf{A}_v / \mathbf{A}_v}{dx/x} = \frac{d(\ln \mathbf{A}_v)}{d(\ln x)} \tag{4.40}$$

where x is a parameter in the NFB circuit. From Equation [4.39] we can write:

$$\ln\left[\mathbf{A}_v(j\omega)\right] = \ln\left|\mathbf{A}_v(j\omega)\right| + j\theta(\omega) \tag{4.41}$$

Substitution of Equation [4.41] into Equation [4.40] yields:

$$S_x^{A_v} = \frac{d\left(\ln\left|\mathbf{A}_v(j\omega)\right|\right)}{dx/x} + j\frac{d\theta(\omega)}{dx/x} \tag{4.42}$$

The real part of $\mathbf{S}_x^{A_v}$ is called the *magnitude sensitivity*; the imaginary part of $\mathbf{S}_x^{A_v}$ is the *phase sensitivity*. Generally, x will be a real number, which simplifies the calculation of Equation [4.42]. Sensitivity analysis using Equation [4.42] can be utilized to evaluate active filter designs.

4.4 Effects of Negative Current Feedback

The purpose of negative current feedback (NCF) is to create an approximation to a voltage-controlled current source (VCCS) so that the output current, I_L, is proportional to V_s, regardless of the load, which can be nonlinear. In NCF amplifiers, the signal fed back is proportional to the current through the load. NCF, like NVF, extends the bandwidth of the amplifier within the feedback loop. Unlike NVF, NCF raises the output resistance of the amplifier within the loop. A single op amp circuit with NCF, illustrated in Figure 4.5, will be investigated; frequency dependence will not be treated in this example. A VCCS is characterized by a transconductance, G_M, and a Norton shunt conductance, G_o.

First, it is necessary to find the circuit's $G_M = I_L/V_s$. Note that the current is given by Ohm's law:

$$I_L = \frac{V_i' K_{vo}}{R_o + R_L + R_c} \tag{4.43}$$

The summing junction node voltage is found:

$$V_i'\left[G_1 + G_F\right] - \left(-I_L R_c G_F\right) = G_1 V_s \tag{4.44}$$

$$\downarrow$$

$$V_i' = \frac{G_1 V_s - I_L R_c G_F}{G_1 + G_F} \tag{4.45}$$

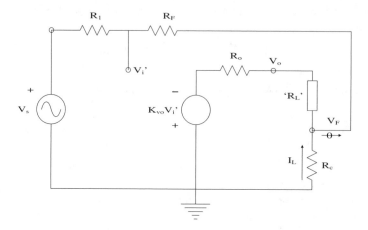

FIGURE 4.5
Schematic of a simple Thevenin VCVS with negative current feedback (NCFB).

Substituting Equation 4.45 into Equation 4.43, it is possible to solve for $I_L(V_s)$:

$$\frac{I_L}{V_s} = G_M = \frac{K_{vo}G_1}{\left(R_o + R_L + R_c\right)\left(G_1 + G_F\right) + K_{vo}R_cG_F} \tag{4.46}$$

In general, $K_{vo}\,R_cG_F \gg (R_o + R_L + R_c)(G_1 + G_F)$, so

$$G_M \cong R_F/R_c\,R_1 \text{ siemens} \tag{4.47}$$

How does NCF affect the VCCS's Norton output conductance? First, calculate the circuit's OCV, given $R_L \to \infty$. This condition also makes $I_L = V_F = 0$. Now the summing junction voltage is

$$V_i' = V_s \frac{R_F}{R_F + R_1} \tag{4.48}$$

and the OCV is:

$$OCV = V_s \frac{R_F}{R_F + R_1} K_{vo} \text{ volts} \tag{4.49}$$

Next, find the short-circuit current, i.e., the I_{Lsc} when $R_L = 0$. This condition also makes $V_F = V_o$. The SCC is:

$$I_{Lsc} = \frac{V_i'K_{vo}}{R_o + R_c} \tag{4.50}$$

where V_i' is found from:

$$V_i'[G_1 + G_F] - (-I_{Lso}R_c)G_F = V_sG_1 \tag{4.51}$$

$$\downarrow$$

$$V_i' = \frac{V_sG_1 - I_{Lsc}G_F}{G_1 + G_F} \tag{4.52}$$

Equation 4.52 is substituted into Equation 4.50 and I_{Lsc} is found:

$$I_{Lsc} = \frac{V_sG_1K_{vo}}{(R_o + R_c)(G_1 + G_F) + K_{vo}R_cG_F} \tag{4.53}$$

Now the Norton G_{out} of the amplifier with NCF is simply the ratio of I_{Lsc} to OCV:

$$G_{out} = \frac{\dfrac{V_sG_1K_{vo}}{(R_o + R_c)(G_1 + G_V) + K_{vo}R_cG_F}}{\dfrac{V_sR_FK_{vo}}{(R_F + R_1)}} = \frac{1}{(R_o + R_c) + K_{vo}R_cR_1/(R_F + R_1)} \text{ siemens} \tag{4.54}$$

The second term in the denominator of Equation 4.54 makes $G_{out} \ll G_o$, which is desirable in making an effective VCCS.

In order to see how the closed-loop VCCS's frequency response is affected by NCF, replace the op amp's open-circuit, VCVS with $K_{vo}/(j\omega\tau_a + 1)$. The transconductance is now found to be:

$$G_M(j\omega) = \frac{\dfrac{K_{vo}R_F}{(R_1 + R_F)(R_o + R_c + R_L) + K_{vo}R_cR_1}}{j\omega\dfrac{\tau_a}{\dfrac{K_{vo}R_cR_1}{(R_1 + R_F)(R_o + R_c + R_L)} + 1} + 1} \cong \frac{R_F/(R_1R_c)}{j\omega\dfrac{\tau_a(R_1 + R_F)(R_o + R_c + R_L)}{K_{vo}R_cR_1} + 1} \tag{4.55}$$

Now the approximate $\mathbf{G_M}(0) \cong R_F/(R_1R_c)$ and the −3-dB frequency is:

$$f_b \cong \frac{K_{vo}R_cR_1}{2\pi\tau_a(R_1 + R_F)(R_o + R_c + R_L)} \text{ hertz} \tag{4.56}$$

In the preceding relations, it was assumed that $K_{vo}R_cR_1 \gg (R_1 + R_F)(R_o + R_c + R_L)$. Note that the closed-loop system's bandwidth is extended by the

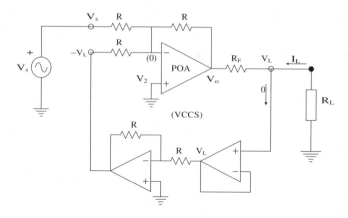

FIGURE 4.6

A three-op amp VCCS in which the load is grounded. Analysis is in the text.

NCF. The NVF circuit of Figure 4.5 is simple, but suffers the disadvantage of having the R_L "floating" between V_o and R_c. Also, the peak current is limited by the op amp used.

In Section 2.6.7 on laser diodes in Chapter 2, it was determined that an effective VCCS using NCF can be made from three op amps. The op amp that drives R_L can be made a power op amp and the load can be grounded. Figure 4.6 illustrates this NCF circuit. As in the earlier example, we will find the VCCS's $\mathbf{G_M}(j\omega)$ and $\mathbf{Z}_{out}(j\omega)$. Because the two feedback amplifiers are unity gain, they have –3-dB frequencies approaching their op amp's f_T and thus can be treated as pure gains (+1 and –1, respectively). The node equation for the summing junction is written:

$$V_i'\,[3G] - V_oG - (-V_L)G = V_sG \tag{4.57}$$

Two auxiliary equations are used:

$$V_o = -I_L\,(R_F + "R_L") \tag{4.58}$$

$$V_i' = -\frac{V_o\left(j\omega\tau_a + 1\right)}{K_{vo}} \tag{4.59}$$

Substituting the preceding equations into Equation 4.57 and rearranging terms yields:

$$\frac{\mathbf{I_L}}{\mathbf{V_s}} = \mathbf{G_M}(j\omega) = \frac{\dfrac{K_{vo}}{3\left(R_F + R_L\right) + K_{vo}R_F}}{j\omega\dfrac{\tau_a 3\left(R_F + R_L\right)}{3\left(R_F + R_L\right) + K_{vo}R_F} + 1} \tag{4.60}$$

In practical cases, $K_{vo} R_F \gg 3(R_F + R_L)$, so the VCCS's transconductance can be approximated as:

$$\mathbf{G_M}(j\omega) \cong \frac{G_F}{j\omega\tau_a 3(R_F + R_L)/(K_{vo}R_F)+1} \tag{4.61}$$

Thus, it is clear that $\mathbf{G_M}(0) \cong G_F$ and the break frequency is:

$$f_b \cong \frac{K_{vo}R_F}{2\pi\tau_a 3(R_F + R_L)} \tag{4.62}$$

which is certainly greater than the op amp's f_T.

The VCCS's $\mathbf{Z}_{out}(j\omega)$ is now of interest. Ideally, it should approach infinity. To find it, take the ratio of the circuit's OCV to SCC. Under OCV conditions, $I_L = 0$ and $V_L = V_o$. Using the node equation for V_i', it is easy to write:

$$\mathbf{OCV} = \frac{-V_s K_{vo}}{3(j\omega\tau_a + 1)} \tag{4.63}$$

Next, find the VCCS's SCC. Under SCC conditions, $R_L = 0$ and $V_L = 0$. The node equation for V_i' yields:

$$\mathbf{Z}_{out}(j\omega) = \frac{R_F(K_{vo}+3)\left[j\omega 3\tau_a/(K_{vo}+3)+1\right]}{3(j\omega\tau_a + 1)} \cong \frac{R_F K_{vo}\left[j\omega 3\tau_a/K_{vo}+1\right]}{3(j\omega\tau_a + 1)} \tag{4.64}$$

From Equation 4.64 it can be seen that, at low frequencies, $\mathbf{Z}_{out}(0) = R_F K_{vo}/3$. At frequencies above $K_{vo}/3\tau_a$ r/s, $\mathbf{Z}_{out}$(hi) $\cong R_F$, which is not very high, making a poor VCCS at high frequencies.

4.5 Positive Voltage Feedback

4.5.1 Introduction

Positive voltage feedback (PVF) is seldom used in SISO feedback amplifiers. PVF *increases* the closed-loop gain, *decreases* the closed-loop bandwidth, *increases* the R_{out} of the system, and *increases* harmonic distortion at a given output level. These activities are based on the fact that the loop gain in a simple SISO feedback amplifier with PVF is $A_L = +\beta K_v$, so for $+\beta K_v < 1$, the return difference, $(1 - \mathbf{A_L})$, is <1. PVF can be used deliberately to make a feed-back system unstable so that it oscillates. The next section illustrates the use of PVF to increase the bandwidth of an amplifier used to couple intracellular glass micropipette electrodes used in neurophysiology to further signal conditioning stages.

4.5.2 Amplifier with Capacitance Neutralization

Glass micropipette electrodes (GMEs) are used to penetrate cell membranes, allowing the measurement of the dc resting potential across the membrane and, in the case of nerve and muscle cells, the transient action potentials associated with these cells. GMEs are made by heating and pulling small-diameter, borosilicate class capillary tubing to a small diameter tip, which can range from 0.3 to 1 μm ID. The GMEs are then artfully filled with a conductive electrolyte solution such as 3 M KCl or potassium citrate, etc. A Ag|AgCl fine wire electrode is inserted in the outer (large) end of the filled GME. By the arcane arts of electrophysiology, the GME tip is caused to penetrate a cell under investigation. The cell membrane generally forms a tight seal around the tip of the GME.

A stand-alone GME with its tip immersed in a beaker of saline in which a large reference electrode is also located allows one to measure the impedance of the filled GME. At dc and very low frequencies, the resistance of the GME can be on the order of 10 to 500 megohms, depending on the GME's geometry and the filling electrolyte. There is also distributed stray capacitance between the tip lumen and the external electrolyte; the glass serves as the dielectric. Thus, the immersed tip appears as an RC transmission line giving distributed-parameter low-pass filtering to any time-varying potential seen at the tip (Webster, 1992, Chapter 5; Lavallée et al., 1969).

Rather than deal with the complexity of a transmission-line low-pass filter and include the ac characteristics of the AgCl coupling and reference electrodes, the GME will be oversimplified *in situ* by a simple RC low-pass filter; R_μ is the GME's total DC resistance and C_μ represents the total effective shunting capacitance of the GME's tip. Figure 4.7 shows the GME attached to the PVF amplifier, which uses an electrometer op amp that has a dc input bias current on the order of tens of femtoamps. It is thus characterized by an input resistance on the order of 10^{13} Ω and an input capacitance to ground, C_{in}, on the order of single pF. The PVF is applied through a variable capacitor, C_N. The noninverting gain of the amplifier, A_{vo}, is on the order 2 to 5 and is set by resistors R_F and R_1.

To begin the analysis of this PVF amplifier, consider the gain between the noninverting node and the output, V_o/V_i. This gain is found by writing the node equation for the V_i' node:

$$V_i'[G_F + G_1] - V_o\, G_F = 0 \tag{4.65}$$

and

$$\mathbf{V_o} = (\mathbf{V_i} - \mathbf{V_i'}) \frac{K_{vo}}{j\omega\tau_a + 1} \tag{4.66}$$

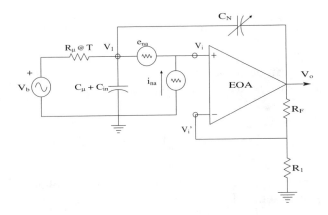

FIGURE 4.7
Schematic of a noninverting electrometer op amp with positive voltage feedback through a small neutralizing capacitor, C_N. This circuit is used with glass micropipette microelectrodes to increase system bandwidth.

Substituting Equation 4.66 into Equation 4.65 and assuming $R_1 K_{vo}/(R_1 + R_F) \geqslant 1$ reveals the frequency response function:

$$\frac{V_o}{V_i} = \frac{(1 + R_F/R_1)}{j\omega\tau_a(1 + R_F/R_1)/K_{vo} + 1} \tag{4.67}$$

Next, examine the simple low-pass frequency response function of the GME alone:

$$\frac{V_i}{V_b} = \frac{1}{j\omega R_\mu (C_\mu + C_{in}) + 1} \tag{4.68}$$

To find the frequency response of the amplifier with PVF through C_N, write the node equation for V_i:

$$V_i [G_\mu + j\omega(C_T + C_N)] - V_o j\omega C_N = V_b G_\mu \tag{4.69}$$

Note that:

$$C_T = C_\mu + C_{in} \tag{4.70}$$

and

$$\frac{V_o}{V_i} = \frac{A_{vo}}{j\omega\tau_a A_{vo}/K_{vo} + 1} \tag{4.71}$$

where $A_{vo} \equiv (1 + R_F/R_1)$. Substituting from the preceding equations, the node equation can be written:

$$\mathbf{V_o} \frac{(j\omega\tau_a A_{vo}/K_{vo}+1)}{A_{vo}}\left[G_\mu + j\omega(C_T + C_N)\right] - \mathbf{V_o} j\omega C_N = \mathbf{V_b} G_\mu \qquad (4.72)$$

Equation 4.72 can be wrestled algebraically into the transfer function of the capacitance-neutralized GME amplifier:

$$\frac{\mathbf{V_o}}{\mathbf{V_b}} = \frac{A_{vo}}{(j\omega)^2 \tau_a A_{vo}(C_T + C_N)R_\mu/K_{vo} + j\omega\left[\tau_a A_{vo}/K_{vo} + R_\mu C_T - R_\mu C_N(A_{vo}-1)\right]+1} \qquad (4.73)$$

From the standard quadratic form, the closed-loop amplifier's undamped natural frequency squared is:

$$\omega_n^2 = \frac{K_{vo}}{\tau_a A_{vo}(C_T + C_N)R_\mu} \; (r/s)^2 \qquad (4.74)$$

The amplifier's damping factor is found from the second term in the denominator of Equation 4.73

$$\xi = (\omega_n/2)\left[\tau_a A_{vo}/K_{vo} + R_\mu C_T - R_\mu C_N(A_{vo}-1)\right] \qquad (4.75)$$

It is now useful to illustrate how the capacitance-neutralized, PVF amplifier works with typical numbers. Let $K_{vo} = 10^5$; $\tau_a = 10^{-2}$ sec; $A_{vo} = 2$; $R_\mu = 10^8 \,\Omega$; $C_T = 3.05$ pF; and $C_N = 2.95$ pF. From these numbers it can be found that $\omega_n = 9.129 \times 10^4 \, r/s$, and $\xi = 0.464$ (an underdamped second-order system with good transient response). Note that if $C_N = C_T$, the system is highly underdamped and, if C_N is slightly greater than C_T, the amplifier's closed-loop poles lie in the right-half s-plane, making the amplifier oscillate. The price paid for extending the system's bandwidth can be shown to be excess noise (see Section 9.8.4 in Chapter 9).

4.6 Chapter Summary

Most electronic amplifiers use negative voltage feedback (NVF), which:

1. Reduces mid-band gain
2. Reduces total harmonic distortion at the output at a given signal output power level
3. Reduces $\mathbf{Z}_{out}$ at low and mid-frequencies
4. Decreases gain sensitivity to certain circuit parameters

5. Decreases the output signal-to-noise ratio slightly
6. Increases the closed-loop amplifier's bandwidth
7. Can increase or decrease R_{in}, depending on the circuit
8. Can make a system unstable if incorrectly applied

Negative current feedback was shown to be useful in making a VCCS out of an amplifier with normally low R_{out}. NCF is used to raise the Thevenin R_{out} so that the NCF amplifier appears to be a current source. Otherwise, its properties are similar to those resulting from NVF. Positive voltage feedback reverses properties 1 through 4 and 6 in the preceding list for NVF. It does have use for capacitance neutralization and is used in the design of certain oscillators because it can make systems unstable more easily than NVF.

Home Problems

4.1 Negative current feedback is used in a VCCS circuit used to power a laser diode (LAD), as shown in Figure P4.1. The LAD presents a nonlinear load to the VCCS. We wish the diode current to be independent of the LAD's nonlinear resistance.

   a. Assume the op amp is ideal and the differential amplifier (DA) is a VCVS in which $V_2 = K_D (V_o - V_L)$. Derive an expression for the VCVS's transconductance, $G_M = I_L/V_s$.

   b. Now assume that the power op amp is nonideal, so $V_o = K_{vo} (V_i - V_i')$. Derive an expression for the Norton output conductance seen by the LAD. (Hint: set $V_s = 0$ and replace the LAD by a test voltage source, v_T. Find $G_{out} = i_T/v_T$.)

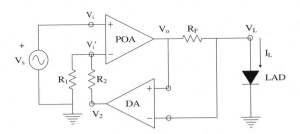

FIGURE P4.1

4.2 Negative voltage feedback is used to make an electronically regulated dc voltage source, shown in Figure P4.2. The design output voltage is 15 V at 1-A load. The power NPN BJT can be modeled by a mid-frequency h-parameter model with $h_{fe} = 19$; $h_{oe} = 2 \times 10^{-5}$ S; $h_{re} = 0$: $h_{ie} = V_T/I_{BQ}$; $V_T = 0.026$ V; and $I_{EQ} = 1$ A. DA gain is $K_D = 1 \times 10^4$; $R_L = 15\ \Omega$, neglect current through $R_F + R_1$; and $V_R = 6.2$ V, feedback attenuation $\beta = R_1/(R_1 + R_2) = 6.2/15$. The raw dc has a ripple voltage, v_r, added to it. $R_S = 50\ \Omega$.

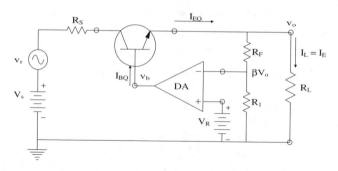

FIGURE P4.2

    a. Find an algebraic expression for and evaluate numerically the regulator's ripple gain, $A_R = v_o/v_r$. Use the MFSSM for the BJT (e.g., dc sources $\rightarrow$ ground).

    b. Now let $v_r = h_{oe} = 0$. Find an expression for and evaluate numerically the regulator's output resistance, R_{out}, seen by R_L. You can find $R_{out} = v_t/i_t$ by replacing R_L with a small-signal test voltage source, v_t.

    c. Evaluate the regulator's regulation, $\rho = \Delta V_o/\Delta R_L$.

4.3   An op amp is ideal except for a finite differential voltage gain: $v_o = K_{vo}\,(v_i - v_i')$. In the circuit of Figure P4.3, the op amp is connected to make a VCCS for R_L.

    a. What kind of feedback is used: NVFB, PVFB, NCFB, or PCFB?

    b. Give an expression for GM $= I_L/V_s$. Show what happens to GM as $K_{vo} \rightarrow \infty$.

    c. Find an expression for the Thevenin R_{out} that R_L "sees."

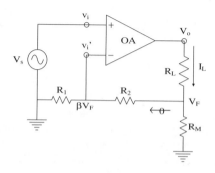

FIGURE P4.3

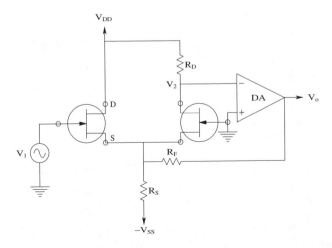

FIGURE P4.4

4.4 Figure P4.4 illustrates a source-follower–grounded-gate JFET amplifier with feedback. The JFETs are identical with the same MFSSM in which $g_m > 0$ and $g_d = 0$. The feedback voltage, $V_o = -K_D V_2$, is applied through resistor R_F to the common source node.

   a. Derive an expression for $A_v = V_2/V_1$ with no feedback (set $R_F = \infty$).

   b. Find an expression for $A_v = V_o/V_1$ with feedback. Let $K_D \to \infty$; give A_v.

4.5 A three-op amp VCCS circuit is shown in Figure P4.5. Assume that op amps OA2 and OA3 are ideal and the power op amp, OA1, is characterized by the transfer function:

$$V_o = \frac{(V_1 - V_1')K_{vo}}{(\tau s + 1)}$$

and zero output resistance.

   a. Derive an expression for the VCCS's output transadmittance, $\mathbf{Y_M}(j\omega) = \mathbf{I_L}/\mathbf{V_s}$, in time-constant form. Sketch and dimension 20 $\log|\mathbf{Y_M}(j\omega)|$ vs. ω and $\angle \mathbf{Y_M}(j\omega)$ vs. ω (Bode plot). Show what happens to $\mathbf{Y_M}(j\omega)$ as $K_{vo} \to \infty$.

   b. Derive an expression for the Norton output admittance the non-linear load sees, $\mathbf{Y}_{out}(j\omega) = \mathbf{I_L}/\mathbf{V_L}$, in time-constant form. Sketch and dimension a Bode plot of $\mathbf{Y}_{out}(j\omega)$ vs. ω. Show what happens to $\mathbf{Y}_{out}(j\omega)$ as $K_{vo} \to \infty$.

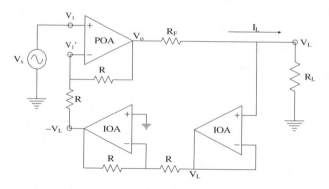

FIGURE P4.5

4.6   A DA is given a form of common-mode negative feedback, as shown in Figure P4.6. The DA has a differential output from which v_{oc} is derived by a voltage divider. The amplifier is described by the scalar equations:

$$v_o = A_D v_{1c} + A_C v_{1c}$$

$$v_o' = -A_D v_{1c} + A_C v_{1c}$$

Also, it is clear that $v_{oc} = A_C v_{1c}$. Define $\alpha = R_1/(R_1 + R_s)$ and $\beta = R_s/(R_1 + R_s)$.

a. Find expressions for v_{1c} and v_{1d} in terms of v_{sc} and $v_{sd,}$ and α, β, K, A_D, and A_C.

b. Give an expression for v_o in terms of v_{sc} and v_{sd} and circuit parameters.

c. Find an expression for the system's single-ended CMRR.

d. Let $A_D = 100$; $A_C = 0.01$; $\alpha \cong 1$; $\beta = 0.01$; and $K = 10^4$. Evaluate the single-ended CMRR numerically and compare it to the CMRR of the DA.

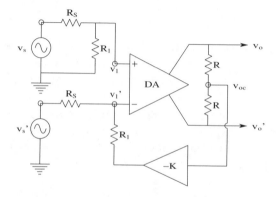

FIGURE P4.6

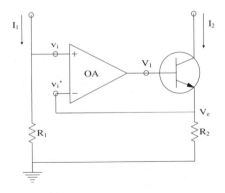

FIGURE P4.7

4.7 The op amp circuit shown in Figure P4.7 is a form of current mirror. The BJT can be modeled by its MFSSM with $h_{re} = h_{oe} = 0$. The op amp is ideal except for the gain:

$$v_o = \frac{K_v(v_i - v_i')}{(\tau s + 1)}$$

Find an expression for $I_2/I_1(j\omega)$ in time constant form.

4.8 Negative current feedback is used to make an op amp/FET VCCS, shown in Figure P4.8. MFSS analysis will be used. The FET is characterized by (g_m, g_d) and the op amp has a finite voltage gain so $v_g = K_V (v_1 - v_s)$. Assume V_{DS} is large enough to keep the FET in channel saturation.

a. Find an expression for the VCCS's small-signal transconductance, $G_M = i_d/v_1$.

b. Find an expression for the VCCS's Norton output conductance, G_{out}.

c. Let $K_v = 10^4$; $g_m = 10^{-3}$ S; $g_d = 10^{-5}$ S; and $R_S = 1$ kΩ. Find numerical values for G_M and G_{out}.

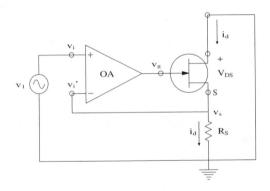

FIGURE P4.8

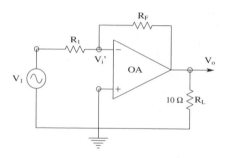

FIGURE P4.9

4.9   A certain power op amp (POA) has an open-loop gain of $V_o/V_i' = -5 \times 10^4$. When it is connected as a gain of -250 amplifier, it has a total harmonic distortion (THD) of 0.5% of the RMS fundamental output signal voltage, V_{os}, when the RMS $V_{os} = 10.0$ V. Find the percent THD when the amplifier is given a gain of -1 (unit inverter) and the V_{os} is again made 10.0 VRMS. See Figure P4.9.

4.10 The circuit of Figure P4.10 is a constant-current regulator used for charging batteries; NCFB is used. Assume the DA's gain is $K_D = 10^5$; $h_{oe} = h_{re} = 0$; $h_{fe} = 19$; $R_m = 1.0 \ \Omega$; $V_R = 5$ V (sets I_L); and $V_{BE} = 0.7$ V. Battery: $V_B = 12.6$ V (nominal); series resistance (nominal); $R_B = 0.1 \ \Omega$; $V_S = 24$ V; and $R_S = 13 \ \Omega$.

   a.   Find an expression for and evaluate numerically the small-signal transconductance of the regulator, $G_M = I_L/V_R$.

   b.   Find an expression for and evaluate numerically the small-signal Norton conductance the battery sees. (Hint: set $V_R = 0$ and use a test source, v_t, in place of the battery. $G_{out} = i_t/v_t$.)

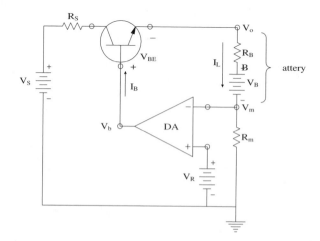

FIGURE P4.10

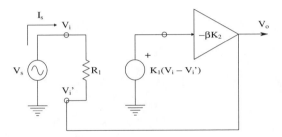

FIGURE P4.11

4.11 We have shown that NVFB reduces amplifier output impedance. In this problem, you will investigate how NVFB affects input impedance. In the schematic of Figure P4.11, an amplifier is given negative feedback as shown. Find the input resistance with feedback, $R_{in} = V_s/I_s$.

4.12 One way of additively combining feedback with the input signal in a SISO feedback amplifier is to use a difference amplifier, illustrated in Figure P4.12. The output, v_2', is given by the relation: $v_2' = K_F (v_s - v_o)$. Use a simple MFSSM for the matched BJTs in which $h_{re} = h_{oe} = 0$ and h_{fe} and $h_{ie} > 0$. A dc current source supplies the emitter currents of the two BJTs. Derive an expression for K_F in terms of circuit parameters.

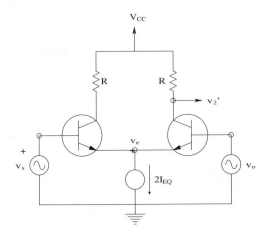

FIGURE P4.12

4.13 Both positive and negative feedback are used on an ideal op amp, shown in Figure P4.13.

a. Derive an expression for V_o/V_s in terms of the circuit parameters.

b. What vector condition on the impedances will make the system unstable?

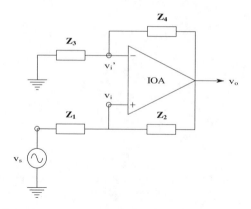

FIGURE P4.13

5

Feedback, Frequency Response, and Amplifier Stability

5.1 Introduction

This chapter explains the details of how feedback changes open-loop amplifier frequency response and examines how NVF and PVF can lead to amplifier instability. Practical use can be made of instability; tunable sinusoidal oscillators can be designed using the same analytical techniques used in the design of linear feedback amplifiers.

Over the years, many analytical techniques have been used to analyze and design feedback systems. In the author's opinion, the root-locus technique is one of the more useful ones. It allows the s-plane location of the closed-loop (CL) system's poles to be found, given the system's dc or mid-frequency loop gain and the location of the poles and zeros of the system's loop gain, $A_L(s)$. Once the closed-loop poles and zeros are known, it is a simple matter to find the CL system's frequency response or its output in time, given a transient input.

5.2 Review of Amplifier Frequency Response

5.2.1 Introduction

The steady-state sinusoidal frequency response has long been a performance criterion for linear signal conditioning systems. For example, an amplifier is given a continuous sinusoidal input of known frequency and an amplitude that does not saturate the amplifier. At the output, a sinusoidal output of the same frequency, but generally with a different amplitude from the input, and a phase shifted from the input sinusoid can be measured. The amplitude and phase shift of the output are frequency dependent. The frequency response measured experimentally can be used to define the frequency response function of the amplifier. This is the 2-D vector, $\mathbf{H}(j\omega)$. In polar form:

$$H(j\omega) = \frac{|V_o|}{|V_s|}(\omega)\angle\theta(\omega) \tag{5.1}$$

The frequency-dependent ratio of output voltage to input voltage magnitudes is called the amplitude response (AR); $\theta(\omega)$ is the phase angle between the output and the input sine waves. The frequency response junction, $H(\omega)$, whether measured or calculated, is in general a 2-D vector. (It has a magnitude and an angle as shown in Equation 5.1 or, equivalently, a real and an imaginary part.)

The two major ways to present frequency response data are (1) by Bode plot and (2) by polar (Nyquist) plot. Bode plots are much more widely used to characterize analog electronic signal conditioning systems used in biomedicine, and will be considered here. Bode and Nyquist plots are considered in detail in Section 2.4 of Northrop (2003).

5.2.2 Bode Plots

A Bode plot is a system's frequency response plot done on log-linear graph paper. The (horizontal) frequency axis is logarithmic; on the linear vertical axis is plotted $20 \log_{10}|H(f)|$, which has the units of decibels (dB) and the phase angle of $H(f)$ (the phase angle between the output and input sinusoids). One advantage of plotting $20 \log_{10}|H(f)|$ vs. f on semilog paper is that plots are made easier by the use of asymptotes giving the frequency response behavior relative to the system's break or natural frequencies. Also, using a logarithmic function causes products of terms to appear graphically as sums. Perhaps the best way to introduce the art of Bode plotting is by example.

Example 1: a simple low-pass system. Assume a system is described by the first-order frequency response function:

$$\frac{Y}{U}(j\omega) = \frac{c}{a\,j\omega + b} = H(\omega) \tag{5.2}$$

It is algebraically more convenient when creating a Bode plot to have the frequency response function in time-constant form. That is, the 0th power of ($s = j\omega$) is given a coefficient of 1 in numerator and denominator, e.g.,

$$\frac{Y}{U}(j\omega) = \frac{c/b}{j\omega(a/b)+1} = H(j\omega)\ (\text{time-constant form}) \tag{5.3}$$

The quantity (a/b) is the system's time constant, which has the units of time. One advantage of the time-constant format is that, when u is dc, $\omega = 0$, and the dc gain of the system is simply $K_{vo} = (c/b)$. The vector *magnitude* of the frequency response vector function is:

$$\left|H(j\omega)\right| = \frac{c/b}{\sqrt{\omega^2(a/b)^2 + 1}}$$ (5.4)

and its dB logarithmic value is:

$$dB = 20 \log(c/b) - 10 \log[\omega^2(a/b)^2 + 1]$$ (5.5)

For $\omega = 0$, $dB = 20 \log(c/b)$. For $\omega = (a/b)^{-1}$ r/s, $dB = 20 \log(c/b) - 10 \log[2]$, or the dc level minus 3 dB. $\omega_o = (a/b)^{-1}$ r/s is the system's break frequency. For $\omega \geq 10\omega_o$, the amplitude response is given by:

$$dB = 20 \log(c/b) - 20 \log[\omega] - 20 \log[a/b]$$ (5.6)

From the preceding equation, it is possible to see that the asymptote has a slope of –20 dB/decade of radian frequency or, equivalently, –6 dB/octave (doubling) of frequency. The phase of this system is given by:

$$\phi(\omega) = -\tan^{-1}(\omega \, a/b)$$ (5.7)

The minus sign is because the complex portion of Equation 5.3 is in its denominator. Thus, the phase goes from 0° at $\omega = 0$ to –90° as $\omega \to \infty$. Figure 5.1 illustrates the complete Bode plot for the simple first-order, low-pass system.

Example 2: this is an underdamped second-order, low-pass system described by the frequency response vector function:

$$\frac{Y}{U}(j\omega) = \frac{d}{a(j\omega)^2 + b(j\omega) + c} = \frac{B}{A} \angle \phi = H(j\omega)$$ (5.8)

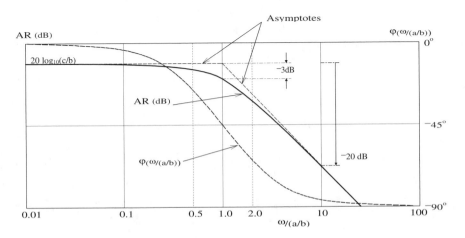

FIGURE 5.1
Normalized Bode plot for a one real pole low-pass filter. Asymptotes, AR, and phase are shown.

To put this frequency response function in time-constant form to facilitate Bode plotting, it is necessary to divide numerator and denominator by c:

$$\frac{Y}{U}(j\omega) = \frac{d/c}{(a/c)(j\omega)^2 + (b/c)(j\omega) + 1} = \frac{d/c}{(j\omega)^2/\omega_n^2 + (2\xi/\omega_n)(j\omega) + 1} \quad (5.9)$$

The constant, $c/a \equiv \omega_n^2$, is the system's undamped natural radian frequency squared and $b/c \equiv 2\xi/\omega_n$, where ξ is the system's damping factor. The system has complex-conjugate roots to the characteristic equation of its ODE if $0 < \xi < 1$. In this second example, it will be assumed that the system is under-damped, i.e., $0 < \xi < 1$. Now the Bode magnitude plot is found from:

$$db = 20 \log(d/c) - 10 \log\left\{\left[1 - \omega^2/\omega_n^2\right]^2 + \left[(2\xi/\omega_n)\omega\right]^2\right\} \quad (5.10)$$

At dc and $\omega \ll \omega_n$ and $\omega_n/2\xi$, dB $\cong 20 \log(d/c)$. The undamped natural frequency is $\omega_n = \sqrt{c/a}$ r/s. When $\omega = \omega_n$, dB $= 20 \log(d/c) - 20 \log[(2\xi/\omega_n) \omega_n] = 20 \log(d/c) - 20 \log[2\xi]$; when $\omega \gg \omega_n$, dB $= 20 \log(d/c) - 40 \log[\omega/\omega_n]$. Thus, for $\omega = \omega_n$ and $\xi < 0.5$, the dB curve rises to a peak above the intersection of the asymptotes. The high-frequency asymptote has a slope of -40 dB/decade of radian frequency, or -12 dB/octave (doubling) of radian frequency. These features are shown schematically in Figure 5.2. The phase of the second-order low-pass system can be found by inspecting the frequency response function of Equation 5.9. It is simply:

$$\phi = -\tan^{-1}\left(\frac{\omega(2\xi/\omega_n)}{1 - \omega^2/\omega_n^2}\right) \quad (5.11)$$

It can be shown (Ogata, 1970) that the magnitude of the resonant peak normalized with respect to the system's dc gain is:

$$M_p = \frac{|H(j\omega)|_{max}}{|H(j0)|} = \frac{1}{2\xi\sqrt{1-\xi^2}} \quad \text{for } 0.707 \geq \xi \geq 0. \quad (5.12)$$

and the frequency at which the peak AR occurs is given by:

$$\omega_p = \omega_n\sqrt{1 - 2\xi^2} \text{ r/s.} \quad (5.13)$$

Example 3: a lead/lag filter is described by the frequency response function:

$$\frac{Y}{X} = \frac{j\omega/\omega_1 + 1}{j\omega/\omega_2 + 1} = H(j\omega), \quad \omega_2 > \omega_1 \quad (5.14)$$

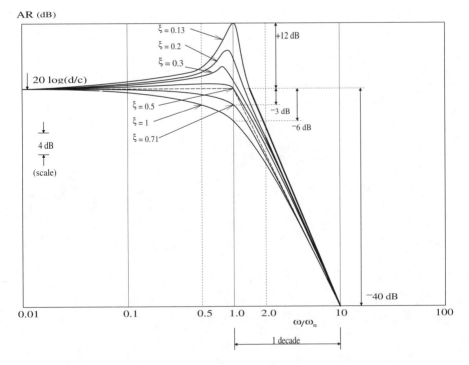

FIGURE 5.2
Normalized Bode magnitude plot of a typical underdamped quadratic low-pass filter.

For the Bode plot, at ω = dc and $\ll \omega_1, \omega_2$, dB = $20 \log|\mathbf{H}(j\omega)|$ = 0 dB. At $\omega = \omega_1$, dB $\cong 20 \log(\sqrt{2}) - 20 \log(1) = +3$ dB. For $\omega \gg \omega_2$, dB $\cong 20 \log(\omega_2/\omega_1)$. The phase of the lead/lag filter is given by:

$$\phi = \tan^{-1}(\omega/\omega_1) - \tan^{-1}(\omega/\omega_2) \qquad (5.15)$$

The Bode magnitude response and phase of the lead/lag filter are shown in Figure 5.3.

Example 4: this final example considers the frequency response of an RC amplifier with four real poles and two zeros at the origin of the s-plane. Its transfer function in Laplace format is:

$$H(s) = \frac{s^2 K_v}{(s + \omega_1)(s + \omega_2)(s + \omega_3)(s + \omega_4)} \qquad (5.16)$$

Now write the transfer function in factored time-constant form for Bode plotting and let s $\rightarrow j\omega$:

$$\mathbf{H}(j\omega) = \frac{(j\omega)^2 [K_v/(\omega_1\omega_2\omega_3\omega_4)]}{(j\omega\tau_1 + 1)(j\omega\tau_2 + 1)(j\omega\tau_3 + 1)(j\omega\tau_4 + 1)} \qquad (5.17)$$

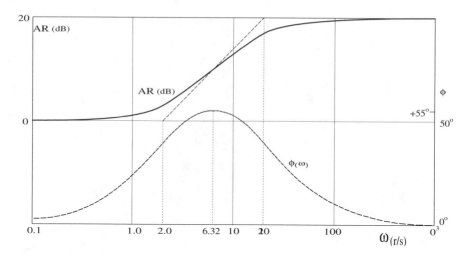

FIGURE 5.3
Bode plot of a lead-lag filter with one real pole and one real zero, magnitude and phase.

where $\tau_k = 1/\omega_k$. The algebraic expression for the Bode amplitude response is:

$$
\begin{aligned}
AR = 20 \ \log\!\left[K_v/(\omega_1\omega_2\omega_3\omega_4)\right] + 40 \ \log(\omega) - 10 \ \log\!\left[(\omega\tau_1)^2 + 1\right] \\
- 10 \ \log\!\left[(\omega\tau_2)^2 + 1\right] - 10 \ \log\!\left[(\omega\tau_3)^2 + 1\right] - 10 \ \log\!\left[(\omega\tau_4)^2 + 1\right]
\end{aligned}
\tag{5.18}
$$

At $\omega \ll 1/\tau_1$, the AR $\cong 20 \ \log[K_v/(\omega_1\ \omega_2\ \omega_3\ \omega_4)] + 40 \ \log(\omega)$, the asymptote slope is $+40$ dB/decade up to $\omega = \omega_1$. For $\omega_1 \leq \omega \leq \omega_2$, the asymptote slope is $+20$ dB/decade and for $\omega_2 \leq \omega \leq \omega_3$, the slope is 0; this is the mid-frequency range of the plot. The mid-frequency gain is:

$$
\begin{aligned}
AR_{mid} \cong 20 \ \log\!\left[K_v/(\omega_1\omega_2\omega_3\omega_4)\right] + 40 \ \log(\omega) - 10 \ \log\!\left[(\omega\tau_1)^2\right] \\
- 10 \ \log\!\left[(\omega\tau_2)^2\right]
\end{aligned}
\tag{5.19A}
$$

$$\downarrow$$

$$
\begin{aligned}
AR_{mid} \cong 20 \ \log\!\left[K_v/(\omega_1\omega_2\omega_3\omega_4)\right] + 40 \ \log(\omega) - 20 \ \log(\omega) \\
+ 20 \ \log(\omega) - 20 \ \log(\omega) + 20 \ \log(\omega_2)
\end{aligned}
\tag{5.19B}
$$

$$\downarrow$$

$$
AR_{mid} \cong 20 \ \log\!\left[K_v/(\omega_3\omega_4)\right]
\tag{5.19C}
$$

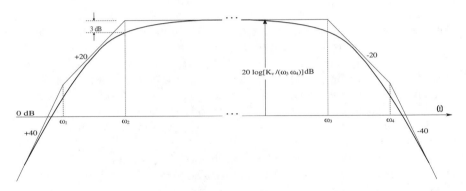

FIGURE 5.4
Typical Bode magnitude plot of a band-pass system with two zeros at the origin, two low-frequency real poles, and two high-frequency real poles.

The AR then goes down at -20 dB/decade for $\omega_3 \le \omega \le \omega_4$ and at -40 dB/decade for $\omega > \omega_4$. Figure 5.4 shows the AR plot for this amplifier. The phase is given by:

$$\phi(\omega) = + 180° - \tan^{-1}[\omega\tau_1] - \tan^{-1}[\omega\tau_2] - \tan^{-1}[\omega\tau_3] - \tan^{-1}[\omega\tau_3] \quad (5.20)$$

$\phi(\omega)$ starts at $+ 180°$ at low ω and approaches $-180°$ as $\omega \to \infty$.

Because frequency response has traditionally been used as a descriptor for electronic amplifiers and feedback control systems, many texts on electronic circuits and control systems have introductory sections on this topic with examples. (See, for example, Northrop, 1990; Ogata, 1990, Section 6-2; Schilling and Belove, 1989, Section 9.1-2; Nise, 1995, Chapter 10.) Modern circuit simulation software applications such as MicroCap™, SPICE, and Multisim™ compute Bode plots for active and passive circuits, and Matlab® and Simulink® will provide them for general linear systems described by ODEs or state equations.

5.3 What *Stability* Means

An unstable amplifier spontaneously oscillates or it produces a saturated dc output. The oscillations ideally would be sinusoidal, but they grow in amplitude until transistors in the amplifier are cut off or saturate, producing a clipped, distorted output at the oscillation frequency. A feedback amplifier can be unstable in two ways:

1. If one closed-loop pole lies in the right-half s-plane, no oscillation will occur.
2. When two complex-conjugate closed-loop poles lie in the right-half s-plane, the amplifier will begin oscillating spontaneously; the oscillations grow in amplitude until the amplifier again saturates and clips the output sine wave's peaks.

Using the root-locus technique indicates at once if a feedback amplifier will be unstable at a given gain because the RL branches locate the system's closed-loop poles as a function of the loop gain.

The describing function method of analyzing nonlinear feedback systems (Ogata, 1970; Northrop, 2000, Chapter 3) can predict if a nonlinear feedback system will oscillate, as well as give its frequency and stable amplitude. Nonlinear systems can generate a stable periodic output known as a *limit cycle*. Describing function analysis is more appropriate to control systems and will not be treated here.

Two other classic methods of testing feedback amplifier stability are the Routh–Hurwitz test and the Nyquist test. The former (Dorf, 1967; Northrop, 2000) uses an algebraic protocol to examine the roots of the numerator polynomial of the return difference (RD) of the closed-loop transfer function. Recall that the zeros of the RD are the poles of the closed-loop system. If any of the roots of the RD have positive real parts, (e.g., lie in the right-half s-plane) the closed-loop system will be unstable. It is easy today, given a linear feedback system's RD(s), to apply the ROOTS utility of Matlab® to the numerator polynomial and examine the roots for positive values, if any; therefore, the Routh–Hurwitz test appears to be obsolete.

In electronic system design, useful information about the closed-loop behavior of a feedback system may be obtained from the Nyquist test, which is based on the steady-state sinusoidal frequency response of the system's loop gain function. This test is well suited for design and stability analysis based on *experimental* frequency response data. As an introduction to the Nyquist test for closed-loop system stability, consider the conventional single-input, single-output linear feedback system shown in Figure 5.5. In this system, no minus sign assumption is made at the summing point. The closed-loop system transfer function is simply:

$$\frac{Y}{X}(s) = \frac{G(s)}{[1 - A_L(s)]} = \frac{G(s)}{RD(s)} \tag{5.21}$$

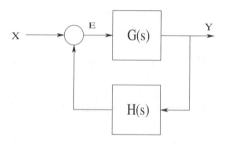

FIGURE 5.5
A simple two-block SISO feedback system.

In a negative feedback system, the loop gain $A_L(s) = -G(s)H(s)$, so:

$$\frac{Y}{X}(s) = \frac{G(s)}{[1 + G(s)H(s)]} \tag{5.22}$$

The denominator of the closed-loop transfer function is called the return difference, $RD(s) \equiv [1 + G(s)H(s)]$. If $RD(s)$ is a rational polynomial, as stated earlier, then its zeros are the poles of the closed-loop system function. The Nyquist test effectively examines the zeros of $RD(s)$ to see if any lie in the right-half s-plane. Poles of the closed-loop system in the right-half s-plane produce unstable behavior. In practice, it is more convenient to work with $A_L(s) = 1 - RD(s)$ and see if any complex (vector) $\mathbf{s}$ values make $\mathbf{A_L(s)} \to 1\angle 0°$.

The Nyquist test uses a process known as *conformal mapping* to examine the poles and zeros of $\mathbf{A_L(s)}$ — thus the zeros of $RD(s)$. In the conformal mapping process used in the Nyquist test, the vector $\mathbf{s}$ lies on the contour C_1 shown in Figure 5.6. This contour encloses the entire right-half s-plane. The infinitesimal semicircle to the left of the origin is to avoid any poles of $A_L(\mathbf{s})$ at the origin. Because the test is a vector test, $A_L(\mathbf{s})$ must be written in vector difference form. For example:

$$A_L(s) = \underset{\text{Factored Laplace form}}{\frac{K(s+a)}{(s+b)(s+c)}} \to \mathbf{A_L(s)} = \underset{\text{Vector difference form}}{\frac{-K(s-s_1)}{(s-s_2)(s-s_3)}} = \underset{\text{Vector polar form}}{\frac{K|\mathbf{A}|}{|\mathbf{B}||\mathbf{C}|}} \angle\theta_a - \theta_b - \theta_c - \pi \tag{5.23}$$

The convention used in this text places a (net) minus sign in the numerator of the loop gain when the feedback system uses negative feedback. The vectors $\mathbf{s_1} = -a$, $\mathbf{s_2} = -b$, and $\mathbf{s_3} = -c$ are negative real numbers. In practice, $\mathbf{s}$ has values lying on the contour shown in Figure 5.6. The vector differences $(\mathbf{s} - \mathbf{s_1}) = \mathbf{A}$, $(\mathbf{s} - \mathbf{s_2}) = \mathbf{B}$, and $(\mathbf{s} - \mathbf{s_3}) = \mathbf{C}$ are shown for $\mathbf{s} = j\omega_1$ in Figure 5.7. For each $\mathbf{s}$ value on the contour C_1, there is a corresponding vector value, $\mathbf{A_L(s)}$.

A fundamental theorem in conformal mapping says that if the tip of the vector $\mathbf{s}$ assumes values on the closed contour, C_1, then the tip of the $\mathbf{A_L(s)}$ vector will also generate a closed contour, the nature of which depends on its poles and zeros.

Before continuing with the treatment of the vector loop gain, it is necessary to go back to the vector return difference, $\mathbf{RD(s)} = 1 - \mathbf{A_L(s)}$, and examine the Nyquist test done on the $RD(s)$ of an obviously unstable system. Assume:

$$RD(s) = \frac{K(s-1)}{(s+2)(s+1)} \to \mathbf{RD(s)} = \frac{K(\mathbf{s}-\mathbf{s_1})}{(\mathbf{s}-\mathbf{s_2})(\mathbf{s}-\mathbf{s_3})} \tag{5.24}$$

Recall that a right-half s-plane zero of $RD(s)$ is a right-half (unstable) pole of the closed-loop system. The vector $\mathbf{s}$ assumes values on the contour C_1'

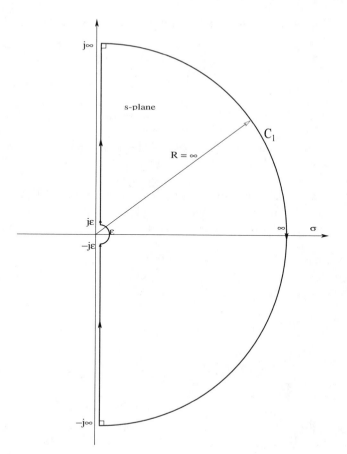

FIGURE 5.6
The contour C_1 containing **s** values traversed clockwise in the s-plane.

in Figure 5.8. Note that C_1' does not need the infinitesimal semicircle around the origin of the s-plane because RD(*s*) has no poles or zeros at the origin in this case. Note that as **s** goes from **s** = $j0+$ to **s** = $+j\infty$, the angle of the **RD(s)** vector goes from $+180$ to $-90°$ and $\left|\mathbf{RD(s)}\right|$ goes from $K/2$ to 0. When $\left|\mathbf{s}\right| = \infty$, $\left|\mathbf{RD(s)}\right| = 0$ and its angle goes from -90 to $+90°$ at **s** = $-j\infty$.

The **RD(s)** vector contour (locus) in the **RD(s)** plane is shown in Figure 5.9. Note that the vector locus for **s** = $-j\omega$ values is the mirror image of the locus for **s** = $+j\omega$ values. It can also be seen in this case that the complete **RD(s)** locus (for all **s** values on C_1' traversed in a clockwise direction in the s-plane) makes one net clockwise encirclement of the origin in the **RD(s)** vector plane. This encirclement is the result of the contour C_1' having enclosed the right-half s-plane zero of RD(*s*). The encirclement is the basis for the Nyquist test relation for the return difference:

$$Z = N_{CW} + P \qquad\qquad (5.25)$$

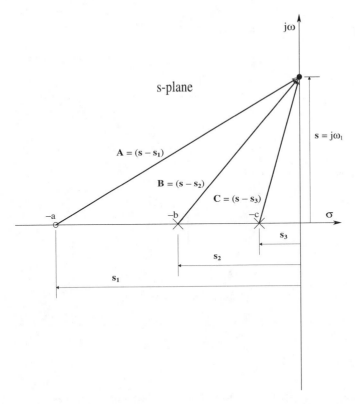

FIGURE 5.7
The s-plane showing vector differences from the real zero and two real poles of a low-pass filter to $s = j\omega_1$.

Here Z is the number of right-half s-plane zeros of RD(s) or right-half s-plane poles of the closed-loop system's transfer function. Obviously, Z is desired to be zero. N_{CW} is the observed total number of clockwise encirclements of the origin by the **RD(s)** contour. P is the known number of right-half s-plane poles of RD(s) (usually zero).

Now return to the consideration of the more useful loop gain transfer function. Recall that when **RD(s)** = 0, $A_L(s) = +1$. For the first example, take:

$$A_L(s) = \frac{-K(s-2)}{(s+5)^2(s+2)} \rightarrow A_L(s) = \frac{-K(s-s_1)}{(s-s_2)^2(s-s_3)} \tag{5.26}$$

Figure 5.10 shows the s-plane with the poles and zeros of $A_L(s)$, the contour C_1', and the vector differences used in calculating $A_L(s)$ as **s** traverses C_1' clockwise. Table 5.1 gives values of $|A_L(s)|$ and $\angle\, A_L(s)$ for **s** values on C_1'.

The polar plot of $A_L(s)$ is shown in Figure 5.11. Because $A_L(s)$ is used instead of **RD(s)**, the point $A_L(s) = +1$ is critical for encirclements, rather than the origin. The positive real point of intersection occurs for $s = j0$. It is easily

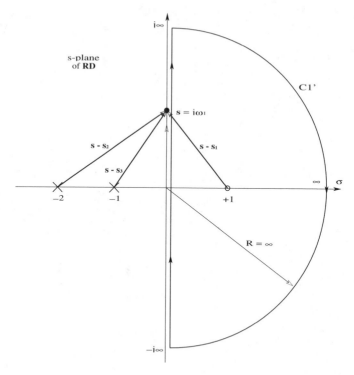

FIGURE 5.8
The vector s-plane of the return difference showing vector differences and contour C_1' for an **RD(s)** having a real zero in the right-half s-plane. **s** traverses the contour clockwise.

seen that if $K > 25$, one net CW encirclement of the +1 point will take place. The Nyquist conformal equation can be modified to:

$$P_{CL} = N_{CW} + P \qquad (5.27)$$

P_{CL} is the number of closed-loop system poles in the right-half s-plane. N_{CW} is the total number of clockwise encirclements of +1 in the $A_L(s)$ plane as **s** traverses the contour C_1' clockwise. P is the number of poles of $A_L(s)$ known *a priori* to be in the right-half s-plane. Thus, for the system of the first example, $P = 0$ and $N_{CW} = 1$ only if $K > 25$. The closed loop system is seen to be unstable with one pole in the right-half s-plane when $K > 25$.

In a second example, the system of example 1 is given positive feedback. Thus:

$$A_L(s) = \frac{+K(s-2)}{(s+5)^2(s+2)} \qquad (5.28)$$

Figure 5.12 shows the polar plot of the positive feedback system's $A_L(s)$ as **s** traverses the contour C_1'. Now if K exceeds a critical value, two clockwise

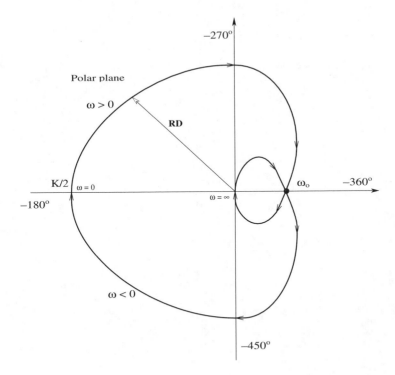

FIGURE 5.9
The vector contour in the polar (complex) plane of the **RD(s)** of Equation 5.24 as s traverses C_1' clockwise.

encirclements of +1 will occur, so two closed-loop system poles will be in the right-half s-plane. Under these conditions, the instability will be a sinusoidal oscillation with an exponentially growing amplitude. To find the critical value of K for instability, it is convenient first to find the $s = j\omega_o$ value at which the system will oscillate by examining the phase of $A_L(j\omega_o)$ where A_L crosses the positive real axis:

$$- 2\tan^{-1}(\omega_o/5) - \tan^{-1}(\omega_o/2) + [180° - \tan^{-1}(\omega_o/2)] = 0° \quad (5.29A)$$

$$\downarrow$$

$$- 2\tan^{-1}(\omega_o/5) - 2\tan^{-1}(\omega_o/2) = -180° \quad (5.29B)$$

$$\downarrow$$

$$\tan^{-1}(\omega_o/5) + \tan^{-1}(\omega_o/2) = 90° \quad (5.29C)$$

Trial and error solution of Equation 5.29C yields $\omega_o = 3.162$ r/s. Substituting this ω_o value into $|A_L(j\omega_o)| = +1$ and solving for K yields $K = 35.00$. Therefore, if $K > 35$, the positive feedback system is unstable, with two net CW encirclements of +1 and thus a complex-conjugate pole pair in the right-half

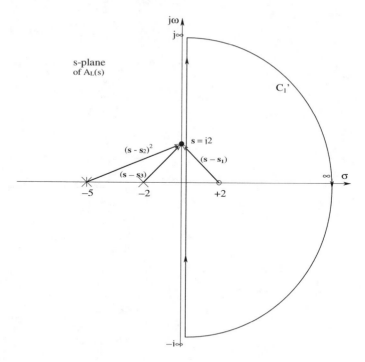

FIGURE 5.10
The vector s-plane of the loop gain showing vector differences and contour C_1' for a negative feedback system's $A_L(s)$ having a real zero in the right-half s-plane. s traverses the contour clockwise.

TABLE 5.1

Values of $A_L(s)$ as s Traverses Contour C_1' Clockwise in the s-Plane

s	$|A_L(s)|$	$\angle A_L(s)$
$\pm j0$	$+K/25$	$0°$
$j2$	$K/29$	$-133.6°$
$j5$	$K/50$	$-226.4°$
$j\infty$	0	$-360°$
$+\infty$	0	$-180°$
$-j\infty$	0	$+360°$
$-j2$	$K/29$	$+133.6°$
$-j5$	$K/50$	$+226.4°$
$-j\infty$	0	$+360°$

s-plane. Furthermore, the frequency of oscillation at the threshold of instability is $\omega_o = 3.162$ r/s.

As a third and final example of the Nyquist stability criterion, the Nyquist plot of a third-order negative feedback system with loop gain is examined:

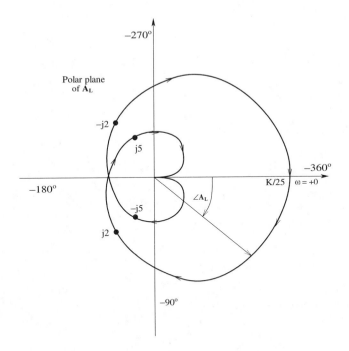

FIGURE 5.11
The Nyquist vector contour of the SISO negative feedback system's $A_L(s)$ as s traverses C_1'. Note that this type of contour is always symmetrical around the real axis, and is closed because C_1' is also closed. See text for discussion of stability.

$$A_L(s) = \frac{-K\beta}{s(s+5)(s+2)} \tag{5.30}$$

This system has a pole at the origin, so in examining $A_L(s)$, s must follow the contour C_1 with the infinitesimal semicircle of radius ε avoiding the origin. Start at $s = j\varepsilon$ and go to $s = j\infty$. At $s = j\varepsilon$, $|A_L(s)| \to \infty$ and $\angle A_L = -270°$. Because $s \to j\infty$, $|A_L(s)| \to 0$ and $\angle A_L \to -450°$. Now when s traverses the ∞ radius semicircle on C1, $|A_L(s)| = 0$ and the phase goes through $0°$ and then to $+90°$, all with $|A_L(s)| = 0$. Now as s goes from $-j\infty$ to $-j\varepsilon$, $|A_L(s)|$ grows larger and its phase goes from $+90$ to $-90°$ (or $+270°$). As s traverses the small semicircle part of C1, $|A_L(s)| \to \infty$ and the phase goes from $-90°$ to $-180°$ at $s = \varepsilon$, and then to $-270°$ at $s = j\varepsilon$.

The complete contour, $A_L(s)$, is shown in Figure 5.13. Note that if $K\beta$ is large enough, there are two CW encirclements of $+1$ by the $A_L(s)$ locus, signifying two closed-loop system poles in the right-hand s-plane and thus oscillatory instability. Because $A_L(j\omega_o)$ is real, it is possible to set the imaginary terms in the denominator of $A_L(j\omega_o) = 0$ and solve for ω_o. Thus:

$$j\omega_o (j\omega_o + 5)(j\omega_o + 2) = -j\omega_o^3 - 7\omega_o^2 + 10 j\omega_o = real \tag{5.31}$$

and $(-j\omega_o^3 + 10 j\omega_o) = 0$ or $\omega_o = 3.162$ r/s and $K\beta > 7\omega_o^2 = 70$ for instability.

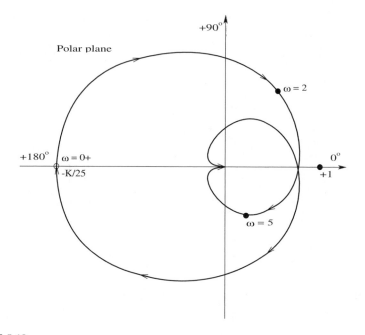

FIGURE 5.12
The Nyquist vector contour of the SISO positive feedback system's $A_L(s)$ as s traverses C_1'. This is the same system as in Figure 5.11, except it has PFB.

5.4   Use of Root Locus in Feedback Amplifier Design

Given the knowledge of the positions of the poles and zeros of the loop gain of a linear SISO single-loop feedback system, the root-locus technique allows one to predict precisely where the closed-loop poles of the system will be as a function of system gain. Thus, root locus (RL) can be used to predict the conditions for instability, as well as to design for a desired closed-loop transient response. Many texts on linear control systems treat the generation and interpretation of root-locus plots in detail (Kuo, 1982; Ogata, 1990). Root locus has also been used in the design of electronic feedback amplifiers, including sinusoidal oscillators (Northrop, 1990).

It is often tedious to construct root-locus diagrams by hand on paper, except in certain simple cases described later. Detailed quantitative RL plots can be generated using the Matlab® subroutine, "RLOCUS." Several of the examples in this section are from Matlab plots.

The concept behind the root-locus diagram is simple: Figure 5.14 shows a simple one-loop linear SISO feedback system. The closed-loop gain is:

$$\frac{Y}{X}(s) = \frac{C(s)G_p(s)}{1-A_L(s)} = \frac{C(s)G_p(s)}{1+C(s)G_p(s)H(s)} \qquad (5.32)$$

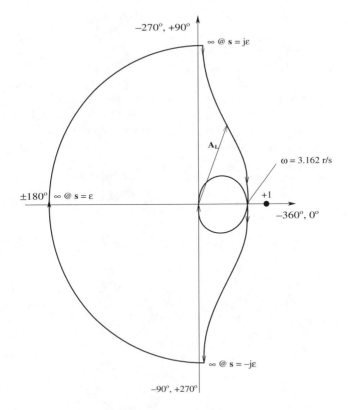

FIGURE 5.13
The Nyquist vector contour plot of the NFB $A_L(s)$ of Equation 5.30. This $A_L(s)$ has a pole at the origin.

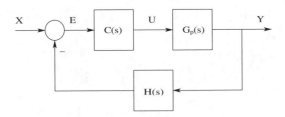

FIGURE 5.14
A three-block SISO system with negative feedback.

C(s) is the controller transfer function acting on $E(s)$; $G_p(s)$ is the plant transfer function (input $U(s)$, output $Y(s)$), and $H(s)$ is the feedback path transfer function. The system loop gain is:

$$A_L(s) = -C(s)G_p(s)H(s) \tag{5.33}$$

(The minus sign indicates that the system uses negative feedback.)

The RL technique allows one to plot complex $\mathbf{s}$ values that make the return difference $\to 0$ in the s-plane, thus making the closed-loop transfer function, $|\mathbf{F(s)}| \to \infty$. The $\mathbf{s}$ values that make $|\mathbf{F(s)}| \to \infty$ are, by definition, the poles of $\mathbf{F(s)}$. These poles move in the s-plane as a function of a gain parameter in a predictable, continuous manner as the gain is changed. Because finding $\mathbf{s}$ values that set $\mathbf{A_L(s)} = 1\angle 0°$ is the same as setting $|\mathbf{F(s)}| = \infty$, the root-locus plotting rules are based on finding $\mathbf{s}$ values that cause the angle of $-\mathbf{A_L(s)} = -180°$ and $|-\mathbf{A_L(s)}| = 1$. The root-locus plotting rules are based on satisfying the angle or the magnitude condition on $-\mathbf{A_L(s)}$. The vector format of $-\mathbf{A_L(s)}$ is used to derive the plotting rules.

For example, first assume a feedback system with the loop gain $A_L(s)$ given below. Note the three equivalent ways of writing $A_L(s)$:

$$A_L(s) = \frac{-K\beta(s\tau_1 + 1)}{(s\tau_2 + 1)(s\tau_3 + 1)} \quad \text{(time-constant form)} \tag{5.34A}$$

$$A_L(s) = \frac{-K\beta\tau_1}{\tau_2 \tau_3} \frac{(s + 1/\tau_1)}{(s + 1/\tau_2)(s + 1/\tau_3)} \quad \text{(Laplace form)} \tag{5.34B}$$

$$-\mathbf{A_L(s)} = \frac{-K\beta\tau_1}{\tau_2 \tau_3} \frac{(\mathbf{s} - \mathbf{s_1})}{(\mathbf{s} - \mathbf{s_2})(\mathbf{s} - \mathbf{s_3})} \quad \text{(vector form)} \tag{5.34C}$$

where $\mathbf{s_1} = -1/\tau_1$, $\mathbf{s_2} = -1/\tau_2$, and $\mathbf{s_3} = -1/\tau_3$.

For the magnitude criterion, $\mathbf{s}$ must satisfy:

$$\frac{|\mathbf{s} - \mathbf{s_1}|}{|\mathbf{s} - \mathbf{s_2}||\mathbf{s} - \mathbf{s_3}|} = \frac{\tau_2 \tau_3}{K\beta\tau_1} \tag{5.35A}$$

and, for the angle criterion, $\mathbf{s}$ must satisfy:

$$\theta_1 - (\theta_2 + \theta_3) = -180° \tag{5.35B}$$

Nine basic root-locus plotting rules are derived from the preceding angle and magnitude conditions and used for pencil-and-paper construction of RL diagrams:

1. Number of branches: there is one branch for each pole of $A_L(s)$.
2. Starting points: locus branches start at the poles of $A_L(s)$ for $K\beta = 0$.
3. End points: The branches end at the finite zeros of $A_L(s)$ for $K\beta \to \infty$. Some zeros of $A_L(s)$ can be at $|\mathbf{s}| = \infty$.
4. Behavior of the loci on the real axis (from the angle criterion): For a negative feedback system, on real-axis locus branches exist to the

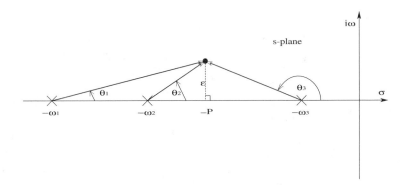

FIGURE 5.15
s-Plane vector diagram illustrating the vectors and angles required in calculating the breakaway point of complex conjugate locus branches when they leave the real axis. (See part 7 of the nine basic root-locus plotting rules in the text.)

left of an odd number of on-axis poles and zeros of $A_L(s)$. If the feedback for some reason is positive, then on-axis locus branches are found to the right of a total odd number of poles and zeros of $A_L(s)$. (See following examples.)

5. Symmetry: root-locus plots are symmetrical around the real axis in the s-plane.

6. Magnitude of gain at a point on a valid locus branch: from the magnitude criterion, at a vector point **s** on a valid locus branch:

$$K\beta = \frac{|s - s_2||s - s_3| \tau_2 \tau_3}{|s - s_1| \tau_1} \tag{5.36}$$

7. Points at which locus branches leave or join the real axis: the break-away or reentry point is algebraically complicated to find; also, there are methods based on the angle and the magnitude criteria. For example, in a negative feedback system loop gain function with three real poles, two locus branches leave the two poles closest to the origin and travel toward each other along the real axis as $K\beta$ is raised. At some critical $K\beta$, the branches break away from the real axis, one at +90° and the other at −90°. If the angle criterion at the breakaway point, as shown in Figure 5.15, is examined, it is clear that:

$$-(\theta_1 + \theta_2 + \theta_3) = -180° \tag{5.37}$$

From the geometry on the figure, the angles can be written as arc-tangents:

$$\tan^{-1}\left[\varepsilon/(\omega_1 - P)\right] + \tan^{-1}\left[\varepsilon/(\omega_2 - P)\right] + \left\{\pi - \tan^{-1}\left[\varepsilon/(P - \omega_3)\right]\right\} = \pi \tag{5.38}$$

TABLE 5.2

Asymptote Angles with the Real Axis in the s-Plane

Negative feedback		Positive feedback	
N − M	φ_k	N − M	φ_k
1	180°	1	0°
2	90°; 270°	2	0°; 180°
3	60°; 180°; 300°	3	0°; ±120°
4	45°; 135°; 225°; 315°	4	0°; 90°; 180°; 270°

For small arguments, $\tan^{-1}(x) \cong x$, so:

$$\left[\varepsilon/(\omega_1 - P)\right] + \left[\varepsilon/(\omega_2 - P)\right] - \left[\varepsilon/(P - \omega_3)\right] = 0 \qquad (5.39)$$

This equation can be written as a quadratic in P:

$$3P^2 - 2(\omega_1 + \omega_2 + \omega_3)P + (\omega_2\omega_3 + \omega_1\omega_2 + \omega_1\omega_3) = 0 \qquad (5.40)$$

The desired P-root lies between $-\omega_2$ and $-\omega_3$.

8. Breakaway or reentry angles of branches with the real axis: the loci are separated by angles of 180°/n, where n is the number of branches intersecting the real axis. In most cases, $n = 2$, so the branches approach the axis perpendicular to it.

9. Asymptotic behavior of the branches for $K\beta \to \infty$:

   (a) The number of asymptotes along which branches approach zeros at $|s| = \infty$ is $N_A = N - M$, where N is the number of finite poles and M is the number of finite zeros of $A_L(s)$.

   (b) The angles of the asymptotes with the real axis are φ_k, where $k = 1 \ldots N - M$. φ_k is given in Table 5.2.

   (c) The intersection of the asymptotes with the real axis is a value I_A along the real axis. It is given by:

$$I_A = \frac{\Sigma \ (\text{real parts of finite poles}) - \Sigma \ (\text{real parts of finite zeros})}{N - M} \qquad (5.41)$$

An example of finding the asymptotes and I_A is shown in Figure 5.16 This negative feedback system has a loop gain with four poles at $s = 0$, $s = -3$, and a complex-conjugate pair at $s = -1 \pm j2$. There are no finite zeros. Thus, $I_A = [(-3 - 1 - 1) - (0)]/4 = -5/4$. From the table, the angles are ±45° and ±135°. This RL plot was done with Matlab®.

To get a feeling for plotting RL diagrams on paper using the preceding rules, it is necessary to examine several representative examples:

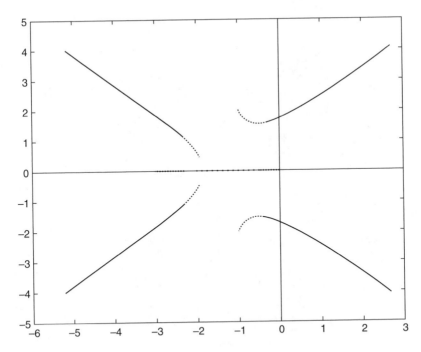

FIGURE 5.16
A Matlab RLocus plot for a negative feedback loop gain with a pole at the origin, a real pole, and a pair of C–C poles.

Example 1 examines the use of root locus in the design of a feedback amplifier using two op amp gain stages, as shown in Figure 5.17(A). This feedback amplifier can never be unstable, but its closed-loop poles can have so little damping that the system is useless. The gain for stage 1 is given by:

$$K_{v1}(s) = \frac{V_2}{(V_1 - V_1')} = \frac{10^5}{10^{-3}s + 1} = \frac{10^8}{s + 1000} \tag{5.42}$$

and the stage 2 gain is given by:

$$K_{v2}(s) = \frac{V_o}{V_2} = \frac{-10^4}{4 \times 10^{-3}s + 1} = \frac{-2.5 \times 10^6}{s + 2.5 \times 10^2} \tag{5.43}$$

The NVF system's loop gain is therefore:

$$A_L(s) = -\frac{\beta 2.5 \times 10^{14}}{(s + 10^3)(2 + 2.5 \times 10^2)} \tag{5.44}$$

The system's root-locus diagram is shown in Figure 5.17(B). The locus branches begin on the loop gain poles and move parallel to the $j\omega$ axis in

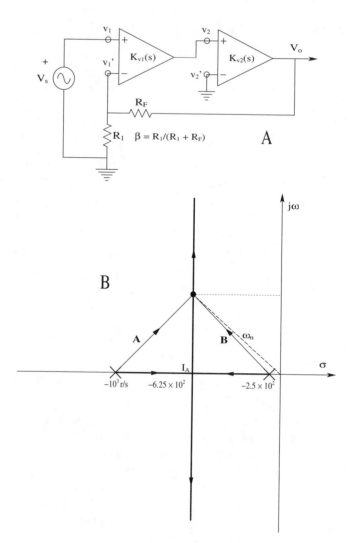

FIGURE 5.17

(A) Two op amps connected as a noninverting amplifier with overall NVFB. (B) Root-locus diagram for the amplifier. Note that unless a sharply tuned closed-loop frequency response is desired, the feedback gain, β, must be very small to realize a closed-loop system with a damping factor of 0.7071.

the s-plane to $\pm j\infty$ as β increases. The locus branches meet on the negative real axis at $\mathbf{s} = I_A$, where they become complex-conjugate:

$$I_A = \frac{\Sigma \left(\text{real parts of finite poles}\right) - \Sigma \left(\text{real parts of finite zeros}\right)}{N - M}$$

$$= \frac{-10^3 - 2.5 \times 10^2}{2} = -6.25 \times 10^2$$

(5.45)

It is desirable for the closed-loop system to have poles at **P** and **P*** so that its damping factor will be $\xi = 0.7071$. From the geometry of the RL plot, the closed-loop $\omega_n = 6.25 \times 10^2 \times \sqrt{2} = 8.84 \times 10^2$ r/s. From the RL magnitude criterion, find the β value to place the closed-loop poles at **P** and **P***:

$$\left| -\mathbf{A}_L(\mathbf{s} = \mathbf{P}) \right| = 1 = \frac{\beta_p \, 2.5 \times 10^{14}}{|\mathbf{A}||\mathbf{B}|} \tag{5.46}$$

The vectors **A** and **B** are defined in the figure and Pythagoras indicates:

$$|\mathbf{A}| = |\mathbf{B}| = \sqrt{\left(6.25 \times 10^2\right)^2 + \left(3.75 \times 10^2\right)^2} = 7.289 \times 10^2 \tag{5.47}$$

Thus, the value

$$\beta_p = \frac{\left(7.289 \times 10^2\right)^2}{2.5 \times 10^{14}} = 2.125 \times 10^{-9} \tag{5.48}$$

will give the closed-loop system a damping factor of 0.707. The feedback amplifier's closed-loop dc gain is:

$$\mathbf{A}_v(0) = +\frac{10^9}{1 + 2.125 \times 10^{-9} \times 10^9} = 3.20 \times 10^8 \tag{5.49}$$

In summary, the cascading of two compensated op amps given a single feedback loop gives a closed-loop amplifier with high gain but relatively poor bandwidth. As an exercise, consider the −3-dB bandwidth possible if two noninverting op amp amplifiers, each with its own NVF, are cascaded such that their combined dc gain is 3.20×10^8.

Example 2 examines the commonly encountered circle root locus. The negative feedback system's loop gain transfer function has two real poles and a real zero:

$$A_L(s) = \frac{-K_p \beta (s+a)}{(s+b)(s+c)} \tag{5.50}$$

where $a > b > c > 0$.

Angelo (1969) gave an elegant proof that this system's root locus does indeed contain a circle centered on the zero of $A_L(s)$. The circle's radius R is shown to be the geometrical mean distance from the zero to the poles, i.e.,

$$R = \sqrt{(a-b)(a-c)} \tag{5.51}$$

The breakaway and reentry points are easily found from a knowledge that the circle has a radius R and is centered at $\mathbf{s} = -a$. The circle root locus is shown in Figure 5.18(A).

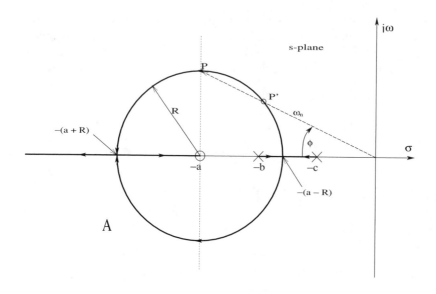

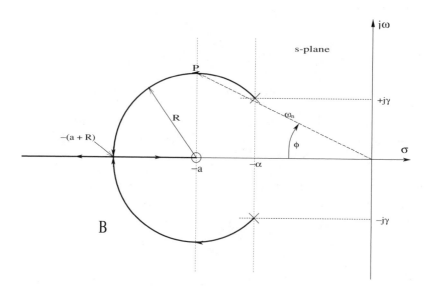

FIGURE 5.18
(A) The well-known circle root locus for a NFB system with two real poles an a high-frequency real zero. See text for discussion. (B) Interrupted circle root locus for the same NFB system with complex-conjugate poles at $s = -\alpha \pm j\gamma$.

   If the loop gain's poles are complex-conjugate, the root locus is an interrupted circle, shown in Figure 5.18(B). The circle is still centered on the zero at $s = -a$. The poles are at $s = -\alpha \pm j\gamma$. The $A_L(s)$ is:

$$A_L(s) = \frac{-K_p \beta (s+a)}{s^2 + s(2\alpha) + (\alpha^2 + \gamma^2)} \tag{5.52}$$

The circle's radius is now found from the Pythagorean theorem:

$$R = \sqrt{(a-\alpha)^2 + \gamma^2} \tag{5.53}$$

Note that as the gain, $K_p \beta$, is increased, the closed-loop system poles become more and more damped, until they become real, one approaching the zero at $s = -a$ and the other going to $-\infty$.

The damping of a complex-conjugate (CC) pole pair in the s-plane can be determined quantitatively by drawing a line from the origin to the upper-half plane pole. The damping factor, ζ, associated with the CC poles can be shown to be the cosine of the angle that the line from the origin to the CC pole makes with the negative real axis, i.e., $\xi = \cos(\phi)$. If the poles lie close to the $j\omega$ axis, $\phi \to 90°$ and $\xi \to 0$. The length of the line from the origin to one of the CC poles is the undamped natural frequency, ω_n, of that CC pole pair. Recall that the CC pole pair is the result of factoring the quadratic term, $[s^2 + s(2\xi\omega_n) + \omega_n^2]$. By way of example, the damping of the open-loop CC pole pair in Figure 5.18(B) is $\xi = \cos[\tan^{-1}(\gamma/\alpha)] = \alpha/\omega_n$.

Many other interesting examples of root-locus plots are to be found in the control systems texts by Kuo (1982) and Ogata (1970) and in the electronic circuits text by Gray and Meyer (1984). Circle root-locus plots are easy to construct graphically by hand. More complex root-locus plots should be done by computer. In closing, it should be stressed that root-locus plots show the closed-loop systems poles. Closed-loop zeros can be found algebraically; they are generally fixed (not functions of gain) and do affect system transient response. Merely locating the closed-loop poles in an apparently good position does not necessarily guarantee a step response without an objectionable overshoot.

Figure 5.19(A) through Figure 5.19(L) illustrate typical root-locus diagrams for linear SISO feedback systems. Locus branches for loop gains with NFB (left column) and for PFB (right column) are shown. The unstable systems oscillate when complex-conjugate closed-loop pole pairs move into the right-half s-plane; they saturate when one closed-loop pole moves into the right-half s-plane.

5.5 Use of Root-Locus in the Design of "Linear" Oscillators

5.5.1 Introduction

"Linear" oscillators are used to generate sinusoidal signals for many applications; probably the most important is testing the steady-state sinusoidal

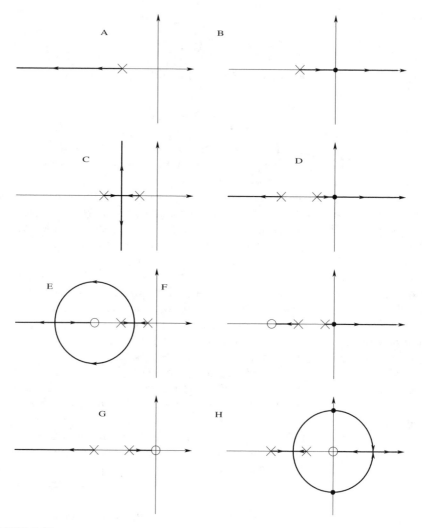

FIGURE 5.19
(A) through (L): Representative root-locus plots for six loop gain configurations for NFB and PFB conditions. PFB root-locus plots are on the right.

frequency response of amplifiers. They are also used in measurements as the signal source for ac bridges used to measure the values of circuit components R, L, and C, as well as circuits $Z(j\omega)$ and $Y(j\omega)$. Still another oscillator application is a signal source in acoustic measurements. In biomedicine, oscillators are used to power ac current sources in impedance pneumography and plethysmography (Northrop, 2002).

Linear oscillators are called "linear" because the criteria for oscillation are based on linear circuit theory and root locus, which is applied to linear systems. In reality, linear oscillators are designed to have a closed-loop, complex-conjugate pole pair in the right-half s-plane so that oscillations,

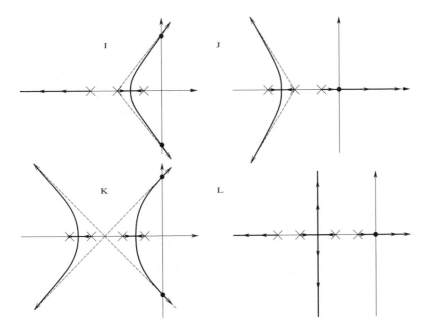

FIGURE 5.19 (continued)

when they start, will grow exponentially. Oscillations start because circuit noise voltages or turn-on transients excite the unstable system. To limit and stabilize the amplitude of the output oscillations, a nonlinear mechanism must be used to effectively lower the oscillator's loop gain to a value that will sustain stable oscillations at some design output amplitude.

Linear oscillators can be designed to use negative or positive voltage feedback. The first to be analyzed is the phase-shift oscillator, which uses NVF.

5.5.2 The Phase-Shift Oscillator

A schematic for a phase-shift oscillator (PSO) is shown in Figure 5.20. To simplify analysis, the op amps are treated as ideal. The PSO uses negative feedback applied through an RC filter with transfer function, $V_i/V_o = \beta(s)$. The second op amp provides an automatic gain control that reduces the oscillator's loop gain as a function of its output voltage, thus stabilizing the output amplitude. A small tungsten lamp is used as voltage-dependent resistance. As the voltage across the lamp, V_b, increases, its filament heats up (becomes brighter). Metals such as tungsten have positive temperature coefficients, i.e., the filament resistance increases with temperature. Filament temperature is approximately proportional to the lamp's electrical power input, so the curve of $R_b(V_b)$ is approximately square-law. As the lamp's voltage increases, so does its resistance, and the gain of the inverting op amp stage decreases as shown in the figure. The second op amp's gain is:

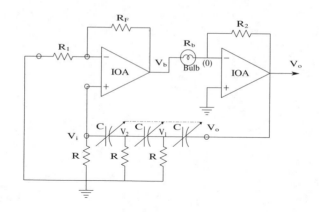

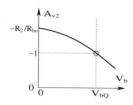 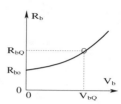

FIGURE 5.20

Top: schematic of an R–C phase-shift oscillator that uses NFB. The lamp is used as a nonlinear resistance to limit oscillation amplitude. Bottom left: gain of the right-hand op amp stage as a function of the RMS V_b across the bulb. Bottom right: resistance of the lamp as a function of the RMS V_b. The resistance increase is due to the tungsten filament heating.

$$\frac{V_o}{V_b} = A_{v2} = \frac{R_2}{R_b(v_b)} \tag{5.54}$$

R_2 is made equal to the desired $R_b = R_{bQ}$ at the desired $V_b = V_{bQ}$, so $A_{v2} = -1$ when $V_b = V_{bQ}$. If $V_b > V_{bQ}$, then $|A_{v2}| < 1$. The gain of the first (noninverting) op amp stage is simply $V_b/V_i = (1 + R_F/R_1) = A_{v1}$.

The gain of the feedback circuit is found by writing the three node equations for the circuit:

$$V_1(s2C + G) - V_2 sC + 0 = V_o sC \tag{5.55A}$$

$$-V_1 sC + V_2 (s2C + G) - V_i sC = 0 \tag{5.55B}$$

$$0 - V_2 sC + V_i (sC + G) = 0 \tag{5.55C}$$

Using Cramer's rule, solve for $\beta(s) = V_i/V_o$:

$$\beta(s) = \frac{V_i}{V_o} = \frac{s^3}{s^3 + s^2 6/(RC) + s5/(RC)^2 + 1/(RC)^3} \tag{5.56}$$

The three roots of $\beta(s)$ are real and negative, i.e., they lie on the negative real axis in the s-plane. Their vector values are found with Matlab's ROOTS utility: $s_1 = -5.0489/(RC)$, $s_2 = -0.6431/(RC)$ and $s_3 = -0.3080/(RC)$. The PS oscillator's loop gain as a function of frequency is, in vector form,

$$A_L(s) = \frac{-s^3(1+R_F/R_1)(R_2/R_b)}{(s-s_1)(s-s_2)(s-s_3)} = \frac{-A^3(1+R_F/R_1)(R_2/R_b)}{BCD} \qquad (5.57)$$

Alternately, A_L can be written as an unfactored frequency response polynomial:

$$A_L(j\omega) = \frac{(j\omega^3)(1+R_F/R_1)(R_2/R_b)}{-j\omega^3 - \omega^2 6/(RC) + j\omega 5/(RC)^2 + 1/(RC)^3} \qquad (5.58)$$

The Barkhausen criterion can be used to find the frequency of oscillation, ω_o, and the critical gain required for a pair of the oscillator's closed-loop, complex-conjugate poles to lie on the $j\omega$ axis in the s-plane. To apply the complex algebraic Barkhausen criterion, set $A_L(j\omega_o) = 1\angle 0°$ and note that, for $A_L(j\omega_o)$ to be real, the real part of its denominator must equal zero. From this condition,

$$-\omega_o^2 6/(RC) + 1/(RC)^3 = 0 \qquad (5.59)$$

The oscillation frequency is:

$$\omega_o = 1/(\sqrt{6}\ RC) = 0.40825/(RC) \quad \text{r/s} \qquad (5.60)$$

The critical gain is found by setting

$$A_L(j\omega_o) = \frac{(-j\omega_o^3)(1+R_F/R_1)(R_2/R_b)}{-j\omega_o^3 + j\omega_o 5/(RC)^2} = 1 + j0 \qquad (5.61)$$

and solving for $(1 + R_F/R_1)(R_2/R_b)$. Thus:

$$(1+R_F/R_1)(R_2/R_b) = 29 \qquad (5.62)$$

For oscillations to start, $V_b \cong 0$, and $(1 + R_F/R_1)(R_2/R_{bo})$ must be >29, so the system's poles will be in the right-half s-plane and the oscillations (and V_b) will grow exponentially. When V_b reaches V_{bQ}, $R_2/R_b = R_2/R_{bQ} = 1$, $(1 + R_F/R_1)(R_2/R_b) = 1$, and the PS oscillator's poles are at $s = \pm j\omega_o$, giving stable oscillations with $V_o = V_{bQ}$.

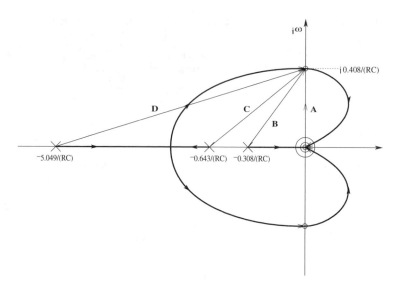

FIGURE 5.21
Root-locus diagram of the NFB phase-shift oscillator. Note that the oscillation frequency is approximately 0.408/RC r/s.

Although the root-locus diagram can be used to find the frequency of oscillation and the critical dc gain (29), in this case the application of the Barkhausen criterion saves the work of plotting the root locus to scale and doing a graphical solution. It is not necessary to factor the cubic polynomial when using the Barkhausen method; Figure 5.21 illustrates the root-locus diagram for the NVF phase-shift oscillator. Pole positions and locus break point from real axis are not to scale. In practice, a PSO can be tuned by varying a triple-ganged parallel-plate capacitor. Oscillator range can be changed by switching the three resistors in the β filter. The early (1950s) Hewlett–Packard 200CD audio oscillator used a PSO with this tuning scheme, as well as a tungsten filament lamp for amplitude control. Of course, the 200CD oscillator used vacuum tubes, not op amps.

5.5.3   The Wien Bridge Oscillator

Another commonly used oscillator that is effective in the millihertz to hundreds of kilohertz range is the Wien bridge oscillator shown in Figure 5.22. This oscillator uses PVF through a simple R–C filter. The filter's transfer function is:

$$\beta(s) = \frac{V_1}{V_o} = \frac{1/(G+sC)}{1/sC + R + 1/(G+sC)} = \frac{s/(RC)}{s^2 + s3/(RC) + 1/(RC)^2} \qquad (5.63)$$

The quadratic denominator of $\beta(s)$ is easily factored. The roots are at $s_1 = -2.618/(RC)$ and $s_2 = -0.382/(RC)$. Now the gain of the second op amp is

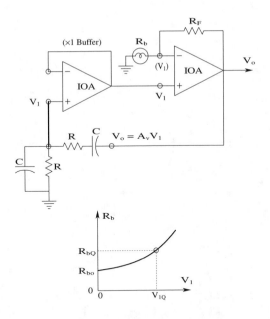

FIGURE 5.22
Top: schematic of a PFB Wien bridge oscillator. The buffer amp is not really necessary if a high input resistance op amp is used for the output. As in the case of the phase-shift oscillator, the oscillation amplitude is regulated by nonlinear feedback from a lamp. Bottom: the lamp's resistance as a function of the RMS voltage, V_1, across it.

simply $A_v = V_o/V_1 = (1 + R_F/R_{bo})$ for very small V_1. When V_1 increases as the oscillations grow, R_b increases, thus decreasing A_v to the critical value that balances the oscillator's poles on the $j\omega$ axis at $\pm j\omega_o$; $A_{vcrit} = (1 + R_F/R_{bQ})$.

The Wien bridge oscillator's loop gain in vector form is:

$$A_L(s) = \frac{+s\, A_v/(RC)}{(s - s_1)(s - s_2)} \tag{5.64}$$

The WB oscillator's root-locus diagram is, strangely, a circle, as shown in Figure 5.23. From the RL magnitude criterion, it is possible to write:

$$\left|A_L(j\omega_o)\right| = \frac{|C|A_v/(RC)}{|A||B|} = 1$$

$$= \frac{1/(RC)A_v\,1/(RC)}{\sqrt{[2.618/(RC)]^2 + 1/(RC)^2}\,\sqrt{[0.382/(RC)]^2 + 1/(RC)^2}} \tag{5.65}$$

$$\downarrow$$

$$1 = \frac{1/(RC)^2 A_v}{1/(RC)^2\,2.80249 \times 1.07048} = A_v/3 \tag{5.66}$$

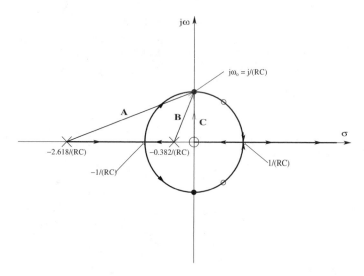

FIGURE 5.23
The Wien bridge oscillator's root-locus diagram. Oscillation frequency is near $1/RC$ r/s.

Thus, when $A_{vcrit} = 3$, the WB oscillator's poles are on the $j\omega$ axis at $s = \pm j/(RC)$, the condition that sustains steady-state output oscillations of amplitude $V_o = 3V_{1Q}$.

The Wien bridge and the phase-shift oscillators described have low total harmonic distortion (THD) in their outputs. The low distortion is the result of using the tungsten lamp in the automatic gain control nonlinearity. Other oscillators that use diode or zener diode clipping to regulate the oscillator's loop gain have outputs with greater THD.

5.6   Chapter Summary

This chapter began with a review of the frequency response as a descriptor for linear amplifier performance. The basics of Bode plotting an amplifier's frequency response were examined, including the use of asymptotes to expedite pencil-and-paper Bode plots, given an amplifier's transfer function or frequency response function. How to obtain the frequency response phase function from the frequency response function was also covered.

The concept of amplifier stability was set forth and stability was considered from the viewpoint of the location of a system's poles in the s-plane. Various stability tests were mentioned, and the root-locus (RL) technique was stressed as a useful method for characterizing a linear feedback system's closed-loop poles as a function of gain. Root-locus plotting rules were given with examples of RL plots. Application of the RL method was given in the design of feedback amplifiers with useful pole locations. The design of the phase-shift oscillator and the Wien bridge oscillator were shown to be made easier with the RL method. The venerable Barkhausen technique was introduced as an alternate to RL analysis.

Home Problems

5.1 A power op amp is used to drive a CRT deflection yoke coil as shown in Figure P5.1. Assume that the op amp is ideal except for finite differential gain, $V_o = K_v (V_i - V_i')$. Negative current feedback is used to increase the frequency response of the coil current, I_L, thus the coil's B field. Assume the current from the V_F node into R_F is negligible, $L = 0.01$ Hy; $R_L = 0.5\ \Omega$; $R_1 = 10^4\ \Omega$; $R_F = 10^4\ \Omega$; $K_v = 10^4$; $R_M = 1\ \Omega$; and $R_F, R_1 \gg R_M$.

   a. Derive an algebraic expression for the amplifier's transfer admittance, $Y_L(j\omega) = I_L/V_1$, in time V_1 constant form. Show what happens to $Y_L(j\omega)$ as K_v gets very large.

   b. Evaluate $Y_L(j\omega)$ numerically. Give the time constant of the coil with and without feedback.

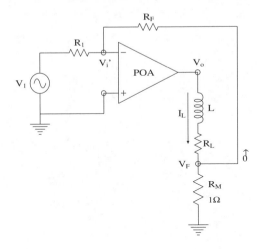

FIGURE P5.1

5.2 Negative voltage feedback is used to extend the bandwidth of a differential amplifier (not an op amp), as shown in Figure P5.2. The DA gain is given by the transfer function:

$$V_o = \frac{10^3 (V_i - V_i')}{(10^{-3}s + 1)(2 \times 10^{-4}s + 1)}$$

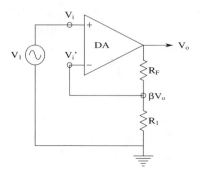

FIGURE P5.2

   a. Draw the system's root-locus diagram to scale. Let $\beta \equiv R_1/(R_1 + R_F)$.

   b. Find the numerical value of β required to give the closed-loop poles a damping factor $\xi = 0.707$.

   c. What is the system's dc gain with the β value found in part B? Give the system's f_T with this β. Compare this f_T to the f_T of the amplifier without feedback ($\beta = 0$).

   d. The same amplifier is compensated with a zero in the feedback path. Thus, $\beta = \beta_o$ ($3.333 \times 10^{-5}\, s + 1$). Repeat parts b through d.

5.3 A nonideal op amp circuit is shown in Figure P5.3. The op amp transfer function is:

$$V_o = \frac{10^4 (V_i - V_i')}{(10^{-3} s + 1)} = H_{oc}(s)(V_i - V_i')$$

Assume that $R_1 = 10^4\ \Omega$; $R_F = 90\ \text{k}\Omega$; $R_o = 100\ \Omega$; and $\beta = R_1/(R_1 + R_F)$.

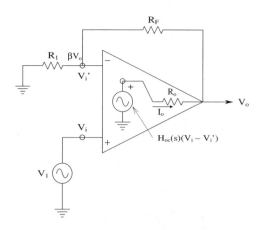

FIGURE P5.3

    a. Find an algebraic expression for the amplifier's Thevenin output impedance, $\mathbf{Z}_{out}(j\omega)$, at the V_o node, in time-constant form. (Neglect $R_F + R_1$ to ground at the output.)

    b. Sketch and dimension the Bode plot asymptotes for $|\mathbf{Z}_{out}(j\omega)|$.

5.4 Use the root-locus technique to find the range of feedback gain, β (positive and negative values), over which the cubic system of Figure P5.4 is stable. What is the minimum value of β required for oscillation? At what Hertz frequency, f_o, will the system first oscillate?

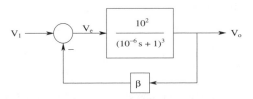

FIGURE P5.4

5.5 Positive voltage feedback is used around an op amp that is ideal except for its gain (see Figure P5.5):

$$\frac{V_o}{V_i} = \frac{+K_v}{\tau_a s + 1}$$

    a. Sketch the system's root-locus diagram to scale. Can this system oscillate?

    b. Derive an expression for $(V_o/V_1)(s)$ in time-constant form. What conditions on R_1 and R_2 determine stability?

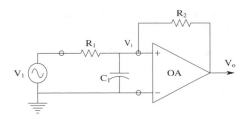

FIGURE P5.5

5.6 Two ideal op amps are used to make a "linear" oscillator, shown in Figure P5.6.

    a. Give an expression for the oscillator's loop gain, $A_L(s)$. Note that the oscillator uses positive voltage feedback.

    b. Design the oscillator to oscillate at 3.0 kHz. Use a root-locus graphical approach. Specify the required numerical values for R_F, R_1, and C_1.

    c. Illustrate a nonlinear means to limit the peak amplitude of V_o to 5.0 V.

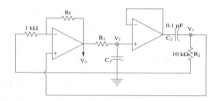

FIGURE P5.6

5.7   A certain feedback amplifier has the loop gain:

$$A_L(s) = \frac{+K_a(s-400)}{s^2 + s(1000) + 10^6}$$

   a. Assume $K_a > 0$. Draw the system's root-locus diagram to scale as
       a function of increasing K_a. Find the numerical of K_a at which the
       system is on the verge of oscillation. Find the oscillation frequency,
       ω_o r/s.
   b. Now assume $K_a < 0$. Sketch the system's root-locus to scale for
       increasingly negative K_a. Find the K_a value at which the system has
       two equal real, negative poles. (Use Matlab's® RLocus program.)

5.8   A certain feedback amplifier has the loop gain:

$$A_L(s) = \frac{-K_v}{s^2 + s2\xi\omega_n + \omega_n^2}$$

   a. Plot and dimension the root-locus for this system for $0 < K_v \le \infty$.
   b. Plot and dimension the root-locus for this system for $0 > K_v \ge -\infty$.
       Give an expression for the K_v value at which the system becomes
       unstable.

5.9   A prototype "linear" oscillator is shown in Figure P5.9. Assume the op amps
      are ideal.

   a. Find an expression for the transfer function $(V_2/V_1)(s)$.
   b. Find an expression for the circuit's loop gain. Break the loop at
       the $V_1 - V_1'$ link. $A_L(j\omega) = V_1'/V_1$.
   c. Use Matlab's RLocus program to draw the oscillator's root-locus
       diagram as a function of β for positive β. $0 < \beta \le 1$.
   d. Use the Barkhausen criterion to find an expression for the oscil-
       lation frequency, ω_o r/s, and the critical gain, β, required for
       oscillation.

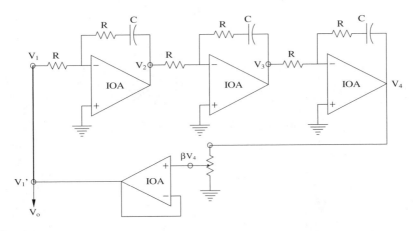

FIGURE P5.9

5.10 An otherwise ideal op amp has the gain:

$$\frac{V_o}{V_i'}(s) = \frac{-10^5}{10^{-2}s+1}$$

The op amp is connected as a simple inverting gain amplifier, as shown in Figure P5.10.

a. Find the maximum dc gain the amplifier can possess and have a −3-dB frequency of 50 kHz. That is, find the R_F required.
b. For the R_F of part a, find the inverting amplifier's f_T.

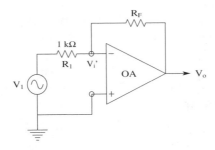

FIGURE P5.10

5.11 Figure P5.11B illustrates a "regenerative magnetic pickup circuit" as described in NASA Tech Briefs #GSC-13309. The purpose of the circuit is to present a multiturn magnetic search coil with a negative terminating impedance that, when summed with the series impedance of the coil, forms a very low Thevenin impedance. This allows more current, I_s, to flow from the

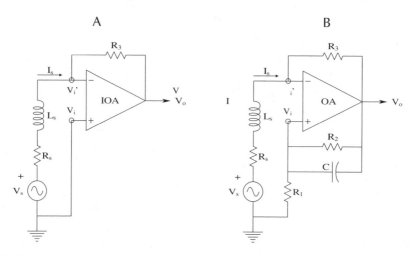

FIGURE P5.11

open-circuit induced voltage, $V_s = N\dot{\Phi}$, where N is the number of turns of the search coil and $\dot{\Phi}$ is the time rate of change of the magnetic flux linking the coil's area. The op amp, less search coil, forms what is called a *negative impedance converter circuit* (NIC) (Ghaussi, 1971, Chapter 8). Assume the op amp is ideal in this analysis.

a. Refer to Figure P5.11A. Find an expression for the transfer function, $V_o/V_s(s)$. Let $L_s = 0.01$ Hy; $R_s = 100\ \Omega$; and $R_3 = 10^4$. Also evaluate the transfer function's break frequency, $f_b = \omega_b/2\pi$ and its dc gain.

b. Refer to Figure P5.11B. Replace the search coil (L_s, R_s) with just the voltage source, V_s. Find expressions for the input current, I_s, and the input impedance looking into the V_i' node. (Note that it emulates a negative inductance.)

c. Now consider the search coil in place with open-circuit, induced EMF, V_s. Derive an expression for $V_o/V_s(s)$ in time-constant form. Comment on the conditions on the circuit parameters (R_1, R_2, R_3, and C) that will make the circuit unstable or the dc gain infinite.

5.12 Negative voltage feedback and positive current feedback are used on a power op amp circuit, shown in Figure P5.12. The op amp is ideal except for the differential gain:

$$V_o = \frac{K_{vo}\left(V_i - V_i'\right)}{\tau s + 1}$$

Assume that $(R_1 + R_2) \gg (R_3 + R_4)$; $\alpha \equiv R_2/(R_1 + R_2)$; $\beta \equiv R_1/(R_1 + R_2)$; and $\gamma \equiv R_4/(R_3 + R_4)$.

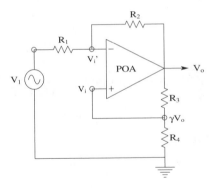

FIGURE P5.12

a. Assume op amp $R_{out} = 0$. Find an expression for V_o/V_1 in time-constant form. Comment how the PVFB affects the dc gain, corner frequency, and gain-bandwidth product.

b. Now let $R_{out} > 0$. Replace the load resistor, R_3, with a test voltage source, v_t, to find an expression for the Thevenin output resistance that R_3 "sees."

5.13 It is desired to measure the slew rate of a prototype op amp design physically. The linear small-signal behavior of the op amp is known to be $V_o = (V_i - V_i')10^5/(10^{-3} s + 1)$. The op amp is connected as a unity-gain follower, as shown in Figure P5.13A.

a. Find $V_o/V_s(s)$ in Laplace form. What is the follower's time constant?

b. A step input of 100 mV is given, i.e., $V_s(s) = 0.1/s$. Sketch and dimension $v_o(t)$ at the follower output. What is the maximum slope of $v_o(t)$?

c. The follower's response to a 10-V input step, $V_s(s) = 10/s$, is shown in Figure P5.13B. Estimate the op amp's slew rate, η, in V/μsec. Sketch and dimension $v_o(t)$ to the 10-V step when the slew rate is assumed to be infinite.

A   B

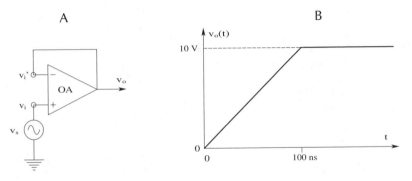

FIGURE P5.13

5.14 A certain op amp has open-loop poles at $f_1 = 100$ Hz and at $f_2 = 100$ kHz, and a negative real zero at $f_0 = 110$ kHz. Its dc gain is 10^5. The op amp is connected as a noninverting amplifier (see text Figure 6.1(C)). Plot and dimension the amplifier's root-locus diagram as a function of the closed-loop dc gain, $V_o/V_s = (R_1 + R_F)/R_1$. Let V_o/V_s range from 1 to 10^3.

6

Operational Amplifiers

6.1 Ideal Op Amps

6.1.1 Introduction

The operational amplifier (op amp) had its origins in the 1940 to 1960 era during which its principal use was as an active element in analog computer systems. Early op amp circuits used vacuum tubes; op amps were used as summers, subtractors, integrators, filters, etc. in analog computer systems designed to model dynamic electromechanical systems such as autopilots and motor speed controls. With the rise of digital computers in the 1960s, analog computers were largely replaced for simulations by software numerical methods such as CSMP™, Tutsim™, Simnon™, Matlab®, etc. However, engineers found that the basic linear and nonlinear op amp building blocks could be used for analog signal conditioning.

With the advent of semiconductors, op amps were designed with transistors as gain elements, instead of bulky vacuum tubes. The next step, of course, was to design integrated circuit (IC) op amps, one of the first of which was the venerable (but now obsolete) LM741. (Why is the LM741 obsolete? Newer op amps with gain-bandwidth products the same as or better than that of the LM741 have lower dc bias currents (I_B and I'_B); lower dc offset voltage (V_{os}) and V_{os} tempco; lower noise; higher dc gain; higher CMRR; higher Z_{in}; etc. and are often cheaper.)

At present, op amps are used for a wide spectrum of linear biomedical signal conditioning applications, including differential instrumentation amplifiers; electrometer amplifiers; low-drift dc signal conditioning; active filters; summers; etc. Nonlinear op amp applications have expanded to include true-RMS to dc conversion; precision rectifiers; phase-sensitive rectifiers; peak detectors; log converters; etc. Practical op amps come with a variety of specifications, including:

- dc Gain
- Common-mode rejection ratio (CMRR)
- (Open-loop) gain-bandwidth product (f_T)

- Slew rate (η)
- Output resistance
- Input resistance; input dc bias current (I_B)
- Input short-circuit dc offset voltage (V_{OS})
- Input current noise (i_{na})
- Input short-circuit voltage noise (e_{na}).

These specifications must be included in any detailed computer simulation of an op amp-based signal conditioning circuit for analysis and/or design. However, it is often expedient for quick, pencil-and-paper analysis to use the parsimonious ideal op amp model, as described in the next section.

6.1.2 Properties of Ideal OP Amps

The ideal op amp (IOA) model makes use of the following assumptions. It is a differential voltage amplifier with a single-ended output. It has infinite input impedance, gain, CMRR, and bandwidth, as well as zero output impedance, noise, I_B, and V_{OS}. The IOA output is an ideal differential voltage-controlled voltage source. As a consequence of the infinite differential gain assumption, a general principal of closed-loop ideal op amp operation (with negative feedback) is that both input signals are equal. Put another way, ($v_i - v_i'$) = 0; therefore, a finite output is obtained when the product of zero input and infinite differential gain is considered. In mathematical terms:

$$\left|(v_i - v_i') \, K_v\right| = \left|(0) \, \infty\right| = \left|v_o\right| < \infty \tag{6.1}$$

6.1.3 Some Examples of OP Amp Circuits Analyzed Using IOAs

The best way to appreciate how the ideal op amp model is used is to consider some examples. In the first example, consider the simple inverting amplifier shown in Figure 6.1(A). By the zero input voltage criterion described earlier, the inverting input must be at ground potential because the noninverting input is. This means that the inverting input (also called the op amp's *summing junction*) is a virtual ground; it is forced to be at 0 V by the negative feedback through the $R_F - R_1$ voltage divider. Because the summing junction (SJ) is at 0 V, the current in R_1 is, by Ohm's law, $i_1 = v_s/R_1$. i_1 enters the SJ and leaves through R_F. (No current flows into the IOA's inverting input because it has infinite input resistance.) By Ohm's law, the IOA's output voltage must be:

$$v_o = -i_1 R_F = v_s \left(-R_F/R_1\right) \tag{6.2}$$

Thus, the simple inverting op amp's gain is ($-R_F/R_1$). The minus sign comes from the fact that the SJ end of R_F is at 0 V and is the positive end of R_F.

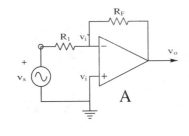

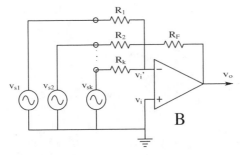

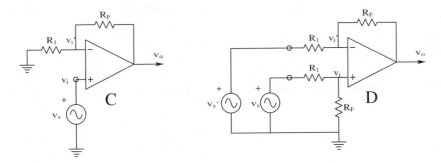

FIGURE 6.1
(A) An inverting op amp amplifier. (B) An inverting amplifier with multiple inputs. (C) A noninverting op amp amplifier. (D) An op amp difference amplifier.

In the second example, k voltage input signals are added in the inverting configuration; see Figure 6.1(B). Currents through each of $R_1, R_2, R_3, \ldots R_k$ are added at the SJ. The net current is again found from Ohm's law and Kirchoff's current law:

$$i_{net} = v_{s1}/R_1 + v_{s2}/R_2 + \ldots + v_{sk}/R_k \tag{6.3}$$

i_{net} flows through R_F, giving the output voltage:

$$v_o = -R_F \left[v_{s1}\, G_1 + v_{s2}\, G_2 + \ldots + v_{sk}\, G_k \right] \tag{6.4}$$

where it is obvious that $G_k = 1/R_k$.

In the third example, consider the basic noninverting IOA circuit, shown in Figure 6.1(C). In this case, the noninverting input is forced to be v_s by the source. Thus, the voltage at the SJ is also v_s. Now resistors R_1 and R_F form a voltage divider, the input of which is some v_o that will force the $v_i' = v_s$. The voltage divider relation, Equation 6.5,

$$v_s = v_o \frac{R_1}{R_1 + R_F} \tag{6.5}$$

can be easily solved for v_o:

$$v_o = v_s \, (1 + R_F/R_1) \tag{6.6}$$

If the output of the IOA is connected directly to the SJ (i.e., $R_F = 0$), clearly, $v_o/v_s = +1$, resulting in a unity-gain buffer amplifier with infinite R_{in} and zero R_{out}.

In the next example, Figure 6.1(D) illustrates an IOA circuit configured to make a differential amplifier. Superposition is used to illustrate how this circuit works. The output from each source considered alone with the other sources set to zero is summed to give the net output. From the first example, $v_o' = v_s' \, (-R_F/R_1)$. ($v_i$ remains zero because no current flows in the lower voltage divider with v_s set to zero.) Now $v_s' = 0$ is set and v_i due to v_s is considered. From the voltage divider at the noninverting input, $v_i = v_s R_F/(R_1 + R_F)$. Because the OA is ideal, $v_i' = v_i = v_s R_F/(R_1 + R_F)$. Using the noninverting gain relation derived in example three:

$$v_o = \left[v_s R_F/(R_1 + R_F) \right]\left(1 + R_F/R_1 \right) = v_s \left(R_F/R_1 \right) \tag{6.7}$$

Thus, the output voltage from both sources together is:

$$v_o = \left[v_s - v_s' \right]\left(R_F/R_1 \right) \tag{6.8}$$

that is, the circuit is an ideal DA with a differential gain of (R_F/R_1).

A simple DA circuit like this is impractical in the real world because (1) to get ideal DA performance, the actual DA must have an infinite CMRR and (2) the congruent resistors in the circuit must be *perfectly* matched. Also, the IOA analysis shown assumes ideal voltage sources in v_s and v_s'. Any finite Thevenin source resistance associated with either source will add to either R_1, thus destroying the match and degrading the DA's CMRR.

As a fifth example of the use of the IOA assumption in analyzing OA circuits, consider the full-wave rectifier circuit shown in Figure 6.2. This is a nonlinear circuit because it uses diodes. The volt–ampere behavior of a *pn* junction diode is often approximated by the nonlinear equation:

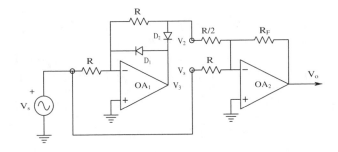

FIGURE 6.2
A full-wave rectifier or absolute value circuit using two op amps.

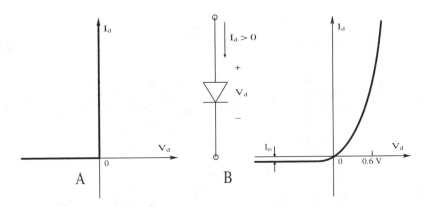

FIGURE 6.3
(A) I–V curve of an ideal diode. (B) I–V curve of a practical diode in which $i_D = I_{rs}[\exp(v_D/v_T) - 1]$.

$$i_D = I_{RS}\left[\exp(v_D/\eta V_T) - 1\right] \qquad (6.9)$$

However, in this example the ideal diode approximation in which $i_D = 0$ for $v_D < 0$ and $v_D = 0$ for $i_D > 0$ is invoked. This relation is shown in Figure 6.3(A) and the diode equation is plotted in Figure 6.3(B). Needless to say, an ideal diode complements other electrical engineering approximations such as the ideal voltage source; current source; op amp; transformer; resistor; capacitor; and inductor.

To see how this circuit works, consider the voltages V_2 and V_3 as V_s is varied. First, it is obvious that if $V_s = 0$, $V_2 = V_3 = 0$. Now let $V_s > 0$. The SJ voltage remains zero and current i_s flows inward through the SJ. It cannot exit through D_1 because current cannot flow though an ideal diode in the reverse direction. However, the current, i_s, does flow through R_F and D_1. By Ohm's law, the voltage $V_2 = (V_s/R_1)(-R_F) = -V_s(R_F/R_1)$. V_3 is infinitesimally more negative than V_2, so D_2 will conduct.

Now consider $V_s < 0$. A current V_s/R_1 leaves the SJ; D_2 does not conduct. Therefore, $V_3 = 0 + \varepsilon$. If no current flows through R_F, V_2 equals the SJ voltage, zero. In other words, V_2 sees a Thevenin OCV $= 0$ through a Thevenin resistor, R_F. To summarize: when $V_s > 0$, V_2 appears as an OCV of $-V_s (R_F/R_1)$ through a Thevenin series R of R_F ohms. When $V_s < 0$, the diodes cause the OCV, $V_2 = 0$, to appear through a Thevenin series R of R_F ohms.

V_o of the output IOA is given by:

$$V_o = -R_F [V_s \, G + V_2 \, 2G] \tag{6.10}$$

When the relations between V_2 and V_s are combined in the preceding equation and R_1 and R_F are set equal to R, it is easy to show that, in the ideal case,

$$V_o = (R_F/R)|V_s| \tag{6.11}$$

As a sixth example, consider the ideal op amp representation of a voltage-controlled current source (VCCS) circuit. Figure 6.4 illustrates one version of the VCCS. The load, R_L, has one end tied to ground and can be linear (a resistance) or nonlinear (e.g., a laser diode). It is clear from Ohm's law that $(V_o - V_L)/R_F = i_L$; thus, $V_L = V_o - i_L R_F$. From ideal op amp behavior, the SJ voltage will be held at V_s by the feedback. Now a node equation summing the currents leaving the SJ can be written:

$$V_s [2G] - V_L [G] - V_o [G] = 0 \tag{6.12}$$

The conductances cancel and $V_L = V_o - i_L R_F$ is substituted into the preceding equation. The final result is simply:

$$i_L = V_s \, G_F \tag{6.13}$$

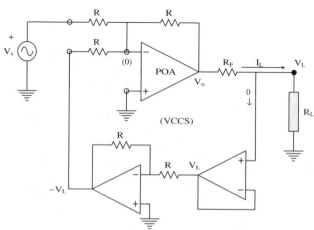

FIGURE 6.4
The three-op amp VCCS.

The transconductance of the VCCS is simply G_F of the feedback resistor. Note that the unity-gain buffer is used so that all of i_L flows into R_L to ground. (This is especially important if R_L is a glass micropipette electrode with R_L on the order of hundreds of megohms.) The inverting IOA$_3$ is required so that the voltage difference across R_F is sensed to give current feedback. IOA$_1$ supplying i_L in a practical VCCS of this architecture can be a high-voltage output type or a power op amp if high i_L is required.

Many more examples of IOA circuits can be considered. A number of them are included in this chapter's home problems.

6.2   Practical Op Amps

6.2.1   Introduction

Practical op amps are characterized by a set of parameters that describe their output dc drift, output noise, and signal-conditioning properties such as dynamic range, frequency response, and slew rate. These parameters are generally given by manufacturers on device data sheets; they include:

- Input offset voltage (V_{os})
- Input bias currents (I_B, I_B')
- Input equivalent short-circuit voltage noise (e_{na})
- Input equivalent current noise (i_{na})
- dc Differential gain (K_v)
- GBWP
- Unity gain
- –3-dB frequency (f_T)
- Lowest open-loop break frequency (f_b)
- Output voltage slew rate (η V/μs)
- CMRR
- R_{in}
- R_o

The following sections examine how a practical OA's parameters determine its behavior.

6.2.2   Functional Categories of Real Op Amps

Engineers and manufacturers group op amps into functional categories, each of which has a set of unique features that makes it suitable for a unique design application. Examples of these categories are described next.

Low noise. Signal conditioning system design with low-noise op amps in the headstage is mandatory for maximum SNR_{out}. Low-noise op amps are characterized by low values of the equivalent short-circuit input voltage noise, e_{na} nVRMS/$\sqrt{Hz}$. In the author's experience, any op amp with an $e_{na} <$ 8 nVRMS/$\sqrt{Hz}$ should be categorized as low noise. Some op amps with FET input transistors (head stages) have exceptionally low equivalent input current noise, i_{na}, as well as low e_{na}. However, some of the lowest-noise op amps have BJT head stages and boast e_{na} in the order of 1 nVRMS/$\sqrt{Hz}$. For example, the venerable OP-27 op amp has $e_{na} = 3.1$ nV/$\sqrt{Hz}$ and $i_{na} = 1$ pA/$\sqrt{Hz}$ at 30 Hz. It uses BJT head-stage architecture and has $I_B = 12$ nA.

Electrometer op amps. The two salient properties of electrometer amplifiers are their ultra-low dc bias currents and their extra-high input resistances. For example, the AD549 is an electrometer-grade JFET head-stage OA. Its I_B is rated from 60 to 200 fA (10^{-15} A), but in selected units can approach ± 10 fA. R_{in} is on the order of 10^{13} to 10^{14} Ω, $e_{na} = 35$ nV/$\sqrt{Hz}$, and $i_{na} = 0.16$ fARMS/$\sqrt{Hz}$ at 1 kHz. Electrometer op amps are used to design signal conditioning systems for pH meter glass electrodes and for intracellular glass micropipette electrodes in which source impedances can be as high as 10^9 Ω.

Chopper-stabilized op amps. This class of op amp is used to condition dc signals from devices such as strain gauge bridges (used in blood pressure sensors) and in any measurement system in which the QUM is essentially dc and minimizing long-term dc drift on the output of the analog signal conditioning system is desired. The internal chopper circuitry gives this class of OA an exceptional high dc voltage gain, on the order of 10^8. The net effect of this high gain is to minimize the effect of V_{os} and V_{os} drift with temperature change.

Another approach to canceling the effect of V_{os} drift in op amps used in dc signal conditioning applications is offered by National Semiconductor. The LMC669 auto-zero module can be used with any op amp configured as a single-ended inverting summer or as a simple noninverting amplifier. Note that the auto-zero module does not limit the dynamic performance of the op amp circuit to which it is attached; the amplifier retains the same dc gain, small-signal bandwidth, and slew rate. The effective offset voltage drift of any op amp using the auto-zero is approximately 100 nV/°C. The maximum offset voltage using the auto-zero is ± 5 μV. The auto-zero's bias currents are approximately 5 pA (and must be added to the op amp's I_B in the inverting architecture); its clock frequency can be set from 100 Hz to 100 kHz.

The LMC669 auto-zero module is very useful to compensate for dc drift in circuits using special-purpose op amps such as electrometers, which normally have large offset voltages (200 μV) and large V_{os} tempcos (5 μV/°C). The auto-zero does contribute to an increase in the circuit's equivalent input voltage noise. However, choice of sampling rate and step size, as well as the use of low-pass filtering in the feedback path, can minimize this effect. Application circuits are illustrated in Section 2.4.3 in Northrop (1997).

Wide-band and high slew rate op amps. Wide-band and high slew-rate op amps are used for conditioning signals such as ultrasound (CW and pulsed) at frequencies in the tens of megahertz, as well as pulsed signals

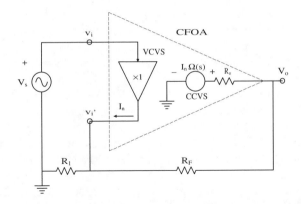

FIGURE 6.5
Simplified internal circuitry of a current-feedback op amp. The output current of the unity-gain VCVS controls the output of the Thevenin CCVS.

acquired in PET and SPECT imaging systems. A measure of op amp small-signal bandwidth is its unity gain bandwidth, f_T. In many op amps, f_T is also the device's gain-bandwidth product. As demonstrated in some detail later, under closed-loop conditions a trade-off occurs between op amp amplifier gain and bandwidth. For example, the Comlinear CLC440 voltage feedback op amp has $f_T = 750$ MHz. This means that when given a noninverting gain of 5, the –3-dB frequency will be 150 MHz using this amplifier and 75 MHz when the gain is 10, etc.

Slew rate is the maximum rate of change of the output voltage; it is basically a nonlinear, large-signal parameter. If the output voltage is a high-frequency sine wave, its will appear triangular (except for the rounded tips) if its slope magnitude ($2\pi f V_{pk}$) exceeds η. Slew rate is defined as:

$$\eta = \left| \frac{dV_o}{dt} \right|_{max} \tag{6.14}$$

The slew rate of the wide-bandwidth CLC440 op amp is 1500 V/μs. High f_T op amps all have high ηs. The AD549 electrometer op amp described previously has $f_T = 0.7$ MHz and η = 2 V/μs — definitely not a wide-band op amp. There is no need to pay for high f_T and η if an op amp circuit is not required to amplify high frequencies at high amplitudes or condition narrow fast rise-time pulses.

Current feedback op amps. Figure 6.5 illustrates the circuit architecture of a CFOA connected as a noninverting amplifier. Note that, internally, it uses a current-controlled voltage source (CCVS) to make its output Thevenin open-circuit voltage. The output voltage is given by:

$$V_o = I_c \frac{\Omega_o}{\tau s + 1} \tag{6.15}$$

Ω_o is the CFOA dc transresistance. The input to the CFOA is a unity-gain voltage-controlled voltage source (VCVS). The noninverting input (v_i) has a very high input resistance. The resistance looking into the inverting input (v_i') node is generally <50 Ω; it is the Thevenin output resistance of the unity-gain VCVS.

The output current of the VCVS, I_n, is determined by Kirchoff's current law (a node equation) written on the low-impedance inverting (v_i') node. The R_{out} of the CCVS is also < 50 Ω and generally can be neglected in pencil-and-paper analysis. The CFOA has many interesting properties, which are described in Section 6.4. One interesting property is that, unlike a voltage-input OA, the CFOA connected as a noninverting amplifier does not trade off bandwidth for closed-loop gain. Its gain can be shown to be set by R_1, while its closed-loop corner frequency is set by R_F. Its closed-loop dc gain is $(1 + R_F/R_1)$, similar to that of a conventional noninverting voltage feedback OA.

Power op amps. Power op amps are used as audio power amplifiers, drivers for small DC servo motors, drivers for LEDs, and laser diodes (as VCCSs). Most conventional op amps can source no more than about ±10 mA; also, their output voltages saturate at slightly below their dc supply voltages, usually no more than ±15 V. The most robust power op amps (e.g., Apex PA03) typically can source as much as ±30 A, given a supply voltage range of ±15/75 V, and dissipate 500 W maximum. The PA03 has a slew rate of η = 8 V/µs and f_T = 1 MHz. Other POAs, such as the Apex PA85, have extraordinary dynamic properties: namely, I_{omax} = ±350 mA(peak); a supply voltage range of ±75/600 V; a power dissipation of 40 W; a slew rate of 1000 V/µs; and f_T = 100 MHz. The PA85 is well suited to drive ultrasound transducers.

6.3   Gain-Bandwidth Relations for Voltage-Feedback OAs

6.3.1   The GBWP of an Inverting Summer

Figure 6.1(B) shows the schematic of a k-input inverting summer amplifier. The open loop op amp is assumed to have a compensated differential frequency response given by:

$$V_o = \left(V_i - V_i'\right) \frac{K_{vo}}{j\omega \tau_a + 1} \tag{6.16}$$

The gain-bandwidth product of the open-loop amplifier is:

$$GBWP_d = K_{vo} \frac{1}{2\pi \tau_a} \text{ Hz} \tag{6.17}$$

Because this is a real OA, $V_i' \neq 0$ and a node equation must be written to find V_i' to substitute into the preceding gain equation:

$$(V_i' - V_{s1})G_1 + (V_i' - V_{s2})G_2 + \ldots + (V_i' - V_{sk})G_k + (V_i' - V_o)G_F = 0 \qquad (6.18)$$

$$\downarrow$$

$$V_i' = \frac{\displaystyle\sum_{j=1}^{k} V_{sj}G_j + V_o G_F}{\left[G_F + \displaystyle\sum_{j=1}^{k} G_j\right]} \qquad (6.19)$$

Define $[G_F + \displaystyle\sum_{j=1}^{k} G_j] \equiv \Sigma G$ and note that:

$$V_i' = \frac{-V_o(j\omega\tau_a + 1)}{K_{vo}} \qquad (6.20)$$

Thus, Equation 6.19 can be solved for V_o:

$$V_o = \frac{\dfrac{-K_{vo}\displaystyle\sum_{j=1}^{k} V_{sj}G_j}{\Sigma G + G_F K_{vo}}}{\dfrac{j\omega\tau_a\Sigma G}{\Sigma G + G_F K_{vo}} + 1} \qquad (6.21)$$

The dc gain of the preceding closed-loop frequency response function for V_{sj} is simply:

$$K_{dcj} = \frac{-G_j K_{vo}}{\Sigma G + G_F K_{vo}} \qquad (6.22)$$

The closed-loop bandwidth for all V_{sj} is f_b:

$$f_b = \frac{\Sigma G + G_F K_{vo}}{2\pi\tau_a\Sigma G} \text{ Hz} \qquad (6.23)$$

and the gain-bandwidth product for the jth input is:

$$\text{GBWP}_j = \frac{K_{vo}G_j}{2\pi\tau_a\Sigma G} = \frac{\text{GBWP}_{OA}G_j}{\Sigma G} \qquad (6.24)$$

Note that $(K_{vo}/2\pi\tau_a)$ is the GBWP of the open-loop OA, and $\Sigma G \equiv G_1 + G_2 +$ ... $+ G_k + G_F$. Thus, the GBWP of the inverting OA summer is always slightly less than the GBWP of the OA alone and depends on the circuit's gains.

6.3.2   The GBWP of a Noninverting Voltage-Feedback OA

Figure 6.1(C) shows that the output of the noninverting amplifier can be written:

$$V_o = \left(V_s - V_i'\right)\frac{K_{vo}}{j\omega\tau_a + 1}$$
(6.25)

As was shown earlier, the OA alone has a GBWP given by $\mathrm{GBWP}_{ol} = K_{vo}/(2\pi\tau_a)$. The summing junction voltage is found from the node equation:

$$\left(V_i' - V_o\right)G_F + V_i'G_1 = 0$$
(6.26)

$$\downarrow$$

$$V_i' = V_o G_F \big/ \left(G_1 + G_F\right)$$
(6.27)

Equation 6.27 for V_i' is substituted into Equation 6.25 to yield the noninverting amplifier's closed-loop frequency response:

$$\frac{V_o}{V_s} = \frac{\dfrac{K_{vo}\left(R_F + R_1\right)}{R_1\left(1 + K_{vo}\right) + R_F}}{\dfrac{j\omega\tau_a\left(R_F + R_1\right)}{R_1\left(1 + K_{vo}\right) + R_F} + 1}$$
(6.28)

The noninverting amplifier's dc gain is the numerator of the preceding equation. In the limit, for very large K_{vo} (where $K_{vo} R_1 \gg R_F$), the dc gain is simply

$$K_{dc} = 1 + R_F/R_1$$
(6.29)

which is the same as for an ideal op amp. The closed-loop break frequency is:

$$f_b = \frac{R_1\left(1 + K_{vo}\right) + R_F}{2\pi\tau_a\left(R_F + R_1\right)}\ \mathrm{Hz}$$
(6.30)

The noninverting amplifier's GBWP is thus:

$$\mathrm{GBWP}_{ni} = \left[K_{vo}\big/\left(2\pi\tau_a\right)\right]\mathrm{Hz}$$
(6.31)

Therefore, GBWP$_{ni}$ is the same as the op amp and is independent of gain. Thus, an ideal hyperbolic relation exists between closed-loop –3-dB frequency (f_{bcl}) and closed-loop gain, e.g.,

$$f_{bcl} = \left[K_{vo}/(2\pi\tau_a)\right]/\left(1 + R_F/R_1\right) \text{ Hz} \tag{6.32}$$

The noninverting op amp amplifier is unique in this property.

6.4 Gain-Bandwidth Relations in Current Feedback Amplifiers

6.4.1 The Noninverting Amplifier Using a CFOA

Refer to Figure 6.5. Assume that the CCVS has a transimpedance with frequency response:

$$\frac{V_o}{I_C} = \frac{\Omega_o}{j\omega\tau_a + 1} \tag{6.33}$$

The gain-bandwidth product of the CCVS is simply $\Omega_o/(2\pi\tau_a)$ ohm Hz.

A small Thevenin source resistance appears in series with V_o from the CCVS. This R_o is $\ll R_F$, so it is neglected. There is also a small Thevenin R_o in series with the VCVS at the CFOA's input that will be neglected. A node equation is written at the V_i' node; note that

$$V_i' = V_s.$$

$$(V_s - V_o)G_F + V_s\,G_1 = I_c \tag{6.34}$$

Substituting Equation 6.34 for I_c into Equation 6.33 yields:

$$\mathbf{V_o} = \frac{\left[(\mathbf{V_a} - \mathbf{V_o})G_F + \mathbf{V_s}G_1\right]\Omega_o}{j\omega\tau_a + 1} \tag{6.35}$$

Equation 6.35 is solved for the frequency response of the closed-loop system:

$$\frac{\mathbf{V_o}}{\mathbf{V_s}}(j\omega) = \frac{(G_F + G_1)\Omega_o/(1 + G_F\Omega_o)}{j\omega\tau_a/(1 + G_F\Omega_o) + 1} \tag{6.36}$$

The closed-loop amplifier's break frequency is f_{bcl}:

$$f_{bcl} = \frac{1+G_F\Omega_o}{2\pi\tau_a} = \frac{\Omega_o + R_F}{2\pi\tau_a R_F} \cong \frac{\Omega_o}{2\pi\tau_a R_F} , \text{ because } \Omega_o \gg R_F \qquad (6.37)$$

The closed-loop break frequency is solely a function of R_F; it is independent of gain. The closed-loop gain-bandwidth product of the noninverting CFOA amplifier is easily found to be:

$$\text{GBWP} = \frac{\Omega_o}{2\pi\tau_a R_F}(1+R_F/R_1) = \frac{\Omega_o}{2\pi\tau_a}(G_F+G_1) \text{ Hz} \qquad (6.38)$$

Curiously, the GBWP depends on the absolute values of the gain-determining resistors.

6.4.2   The Inverting Amplifier Using a CFOA

Next, examine the gain-bandwidth relations in a CFOA connected as a simple inverter. Figure 6.6 shows the circuit. Note that the noninverting input node is grounded, so $v_i = v_i' = 0$. A node equation can still be written on the v_i' node:

$$(0 - V_s)G_1 + (0 - V_o)G_F - I_c = 0 \qquad (6.39)$$

$$\downarrow$$

$$I_c = -(V_s\, G_1 + V_o\, G_F) \qquad (6.40)$$

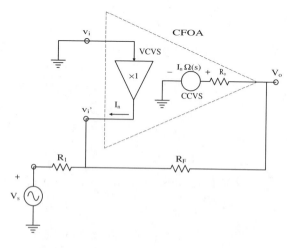

FIGURE 6.6
A CFOA connected as an inverting amplifier.

Equation 6.40 is substituted into Equation 6.33 to find the frequency response of the closed-loop amplifier:

$$\mathbf{V_o} = -\left(\mathbf{V_s}G_1 + \mathbf{V_o}G_F\right)\frac{\Omega_o}{j\omega\tau_a + 1} \tag{6.41}$$

$$\downarrow$$

$$\frac{\mathbf{V_o}}{\mathbf{V_s}} = \frac{-G_1\Omega_o/\left(1 + G_F\Omega_o\right)}{j\omega\tau_a/\left(1 + G_F\Omega_o\right) + 1} \tag{6.42}$$

Again, the closed-loop break frequency depends on the size of R_F:

$$f_{bcl} = \frac{\left(1 + G_F\Omega_o\right)}{2\pi\tau_a} \cong \frac{\Omega_o}{2\pi\tau_a R_F} \ \text{Hz} \tag{6.43}$$

The GBWP is:

$$\text{GBWP} = \frac{\left(1 + G_F\Omega_o\right)}{2\pi\tau_a}\left[G_1\Omega_o/\left(1 + G_F\Omega_o\right)\right] = \frac{\Omega_o}{2\pi\tau_a R_1} \ \text{Hz} \tag{6.44}$$

Curiously, the closed-loop break frequency depends only on R_1 and the closed-loop dc gain is

$$V_o/V_s \cong -R_F/R_1. \tag{6.45}$$

6.4.3 Limitations of CFOAs

CFOAs cannot be directly substituted into most conventional voltage feedback OA circuits. For example, consider the CFOA "integrator" circuit shown in Figure 6.7(A); the node equation on the v_i' node is written:

$$\mathbf{I_c} = (0 - \mathbf{V_s})G_1 + (0 - \mathbf{V_o})\,j\omega C \tag{6.46}$$

Equation 6.46 for I_c is substituted into Equation 6.33 for V_o:

$$\mathbf{V_o} = -\left(\mathbf{V_s}G_1 + \mathbf{V_o}\,j\omega C\right)\frac{\Omega_o}{j\omega\tau_a + 1} \tag{6.47}$$

$$\downarrow$$

$$\frac{\mathbf{V_o}}{\mathbf{V_s}} = \frac{-G_1\Omega_o}{j\omega\left(\tau_a + \Omega_o C\right) + 1} \tag{6.48}$$

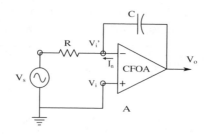

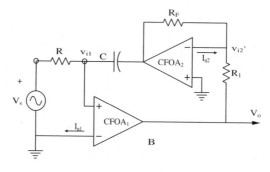

FIGURE 6.7

(A) A CFOA connected as a conventional integrator. The circuit does not work. (B) Two CFOAs connected to make a near ideal inverting integrator.

Clearly, Equation 6.48 is the frequency response of a low-pass filter, not that of an operational integrator. The closed-loop time constant will be long, however. If $\Omega_o = 10^7$ ohms and $C = 10^{-6}$ F, the closed-loop time constant will be approximately 10 sec, which means that signals with frequencies above approximately 40 mHz will be "integrated." This is a poor integrator.

By way of comparison, find the frequency response of a conventional voltage-feedback OA integrator. The VCVS op amp's open-loop gain is given by:

$$\mathbf{V_o} = -\mathbf{V_i'}\frac{K_{vo}}{j\omega\tau_a + 1} \quad \text{OLG} \tag{6.49}$$

The node equation for the summing junction is:

$$(\mathbf{V_i'} - \mathbf{V_s})G_1 + (\mathbf{V_i'} - \mathbf{V_o})j\omega C = 0 \tag{6.50}$$

from which,

$$\mathbf{V_i'} = \frac{\mathbf{V_s}G_1 + \mathbf{V_o}\,j\omega C}{G_1 + j\omega C} \tag{6.51}$$

Equation 6.51 for V_i' is substituted into Equation 6.49 to find the frequency response function for the OA integrator:

$$\frac{\mathbf{V_o}}{\mathbf{V_s}}(j\omega) = \frac{-K_{vo}}{(j\omega)^2 R_L C \tau_a + j\omega(\tau_a + K_{vo} R_1 C) + 1} \qquad (6.52)$$

The practical integrator is seen to be a two-pole low-pass filter with dc gain, $-K_{vo}$.

To appreciate what happens to the integrator's poles, substitute numerical values for the parameters and factor the quadratic denominator. Let $R_1 = 10^6 \ \Omega$; $C = 1 \ \mu F$; $K_{vo} = 10^5$; and $\tau_a = 15$ MS. The numerical frequency response function for the integrator is found to be:

$$\frac{\mathbf{V_o}}{\mathbf{V_s}}(j\omega) = \frac{-1 \text{ E5}}{(j\omega)^2 0.015 + j\omega[0.015 + 1\text{E}5] + 1}$$

$$= \frac{-6.667 \text{ E6}}{(j\omega)^2 + j\omega 6.667 \text{ E6} + 66.667} \qquad (6.53)$$

The right-hand fraction of the frequency response function is in Laplace form and is most easily factored to find its roots (poles). Thus, the integrator's frequency response function can be written in factored form:

$$\frac{\mathbf{V_o}}{\mathbf{V_s}}(j\omega) = \frac{-6.667 \text{ E6}}{(j\omega + 3 \text{ E}{-}12)(j\omega + 6.667 \text{ E6})}$$

$$= \frac{-3 \text{ E11}}{(j\omega 3.333 \text{ E11} + 1)(j\omega 1.5 \text{ E}{-}7 + 1)} \qquad (6.54)$$

Note that the integrator time constant is *enormous* (3.333 E11 sec) in this case and the high-frequency pole is at 6.667 E6 r/s, which is the GBWP of this voltage feedback OA.

As a closing note, it is possible to design an effective integrator using two CFOAs, as shown in Figure 6.7(B); however, this integrator is noninverting. If R is replaced with impedance $\mathbf{Z_1}$ and C with impedance $\mathbf{Z_2}$, then it can be shown that the circuit's transfer function is:

$$\frac{V_o}{V_s}(s) \cong \frac{\mathbf{Z_2}(s) R_A}{\mathbf{Z_1}(s) R_F} \qquad (6.55)$$

providing that $\Omega_{o1} = \Omega_{o2}$; $\tau_{a1} = \tau_{a2} \to 0$; $\Omega_{o1} G_{o1} \gg 1$; and $R_F > R_A$.

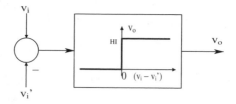

FIGURE 6.8
Block diagram of an ideal comparator I/O characteristic.

6.5 Voltage Comparators

6.5.1 Introduction

The integrated circuit analog voltage comparator (VC) is a useful circuit element with many applications in biomedical instrumentation. The VC is a simple analog/digital interface element; its input is an analog voltage difference and its output is logic HI or LO. An *ideal* VC performs the operation shown in Figure 6.8. That is, its output is logic HI when $(v_i - v_i') > 0$ and LO when $(v_i - v_i') \leq 0$. v_i or v_i' can be a dc reference voltage, ϕ.

An actual VC circuit combines the front end of an analog differential amplifier (see Chapter 3) with the output stage of an open-collector logic gate. The differential front end can be described in terms of: difference-mode gain; common-mode gain; common-mode rejection ratio; slew rate; and dc input offset voltage. Figure 6.9 illustrates the *output stage* of the well-known LM311 VC. Note that the analog DA front end has a symmetrical push–pull output coupled to the driving transistors, Q_8 and Q_9, of the output stage. To heuristically examine how this circuit works, assume that $(v_i - v_i') > 0$. Assuming a large DM gain for the DA, v_o' goes negative, turning off Q_8 and allowing v_{b10} to go positive. Positive-going v_{b10} makes v_{b11} go positive, turning off Q_{11}. When Q_{11} turns off, it turns off Q_{15}, allowing V_o at its collector to go toward V_{LL} (+5 V) or logic HI. Also, $(v_i - v_i') > 0$ causes v_o to go positive, causing Q_9 to turn on. The Q_9 emitter goes positive, forcing the Q_8 emitter to go positive and further turning it off, etc.

All this action is summarized in Figure 6.10. v_i' is the dc reference voltage, V_ϕ. Note that the static transfer curve of the comparator in Figure 6.10 shows a narrow range of finite differential voltage gain (e.g., 2×10^5 for the AD CMP04). Note that some VCs also have complementary ($\overline{Q}$) outputs for design versatility (e.g., the AD9696 TTL output VC).

A wide range of comparator switching speeds are available, given a step change in the polarity of $(v_i - v_i')$. VC switching speed has two components: (1) a pure delay time between the input step change and the beginning of output state change and (2) the time it takes for V_o to swing from LO to HI

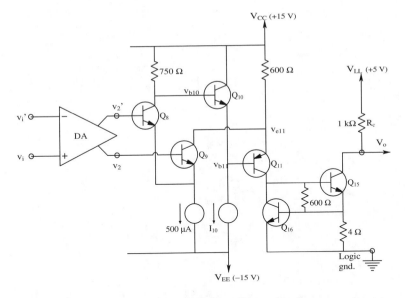

FIGURE 6.9

Partial (output circuit) schematic of an LM311 analog comparator. Note that an analog DA stage output is converted to an open-collector TTL output BJT.

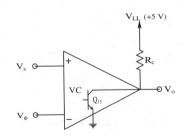

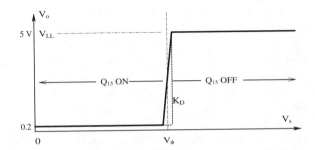

FIGURE 6.10

Top: analog comaparator. Bottom: transfer characteristic of the comparator. Comparator gain, K_D, in the linear region is as high as an op amp.

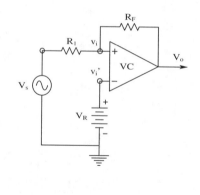

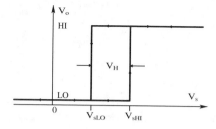

FIGURE 6.11

Top: a voltage comparator connected to have hysteresis; note PFB. Bottom: dimensions of the hysteresis I/O characteristic.

(or HI to LO). This latter delay is limited by the VC slew rate. The total time for a comparator to reach its new output state following an input step change in $(v_i - v_i')$ polarity is called the propagation delay time, t_{PD}.

The LM311 comparator output changes state about 200 ns following the input step change. Newer designs such as the AD790 change states in approximately 40 ns. The AD790 also claims a maximum offset voltage magnitude of 250 μV. The AD96685 VC claims a 2.5-ns propagation delay and has a whopping 1 mV $|V_{os}|$. Unlike the LM311, most comparators do not have a means of nulling their V_{OS}.

The input impedance of VCs is generally fairly high, about what one might expect from a fast BJT-input op amp. For example, the AD790 VC has an input impedance given as 20 megohms in parallel with 2 pF to ground. VC output impedance depends on the output state; if V_o is LO, the open-collector output transistor is saturated and R_o is in the tens of ohms. If V_o is HI, then the output transistor is cut off and R_o is basically the external pull-up resistance used with the comparator. (Some VCs put this resistor in the IC.)

VCs are often operated with hysteresis to give them noise immunity. Figure 6.11 illustrates an external positive feedback circuit that gives hysteresis, and the ideal static I/O curve for the circuit. To find an expression for the exact input voltages at which the VC's output changes state, write a node equation on the noninverting v_i node:

$$V_i[G_1 + G_F] - V_s G_1 - V_{oLO} G_F = 0 \tag{6.56}$$

At switching LO → HI, V_i is assumed to equal $V_i = V_{REF}$. Thus, from the preceding equation,

$$V_{sHI} = \frac{V_R(G_1 + G_F) - V_{oLO}G_F}{G_1} = V_R(1 + R_1/R_F) - V_{oLO}(R_L/R_F) \tag{6.57}$$

When $V_s > V_{sHI}$, $V_o = V_{oHI} = +5$ V. Now V_s must decrease to V_{sLO} before $V_o = V_{oLO} = 0.2$ V again.

Calculation of V_{sLO} uses the preceding approach, except that V_{oHI} is used in Equation 6.57:

$$V_{sLO} = V_R(1 + R_1/R_F) - V_{oHI}(R_1/R_F) \tag{6.58}$$

Consider a numerical example: let $R_1 = 10$ kΩ; $R_F = 100$ kΩ; $V_R = +1.0$ V; $V_{oHI} = +5.0$ V; and $V_{oLO} = +0.2$ V. From these values: $V_{sHI} = 1.08$ V and $V_{sLO} = 0.60$ V; the width of the hysteresis can easily be shown to be:

$$V_H = (V_{oHI} - V_{oLO})(R_1/R_F) = 0.48 \text{ V.} \tag{6.59}$$

Note that the feedback around the comparator is PVF (see Chapter 4). Not only does the VC with PFV have hysteresis for noise immunity, but the VC with hysteresis can also be used as a simple limit-cycling ON–OFF controller for a switched control system such as an oven heater (Franco, 1988, Chapter 7). It is also possible to reverse the positions of the dc reference voltage, V_R, and the input signal, V_s, in Figure 6.11 and still have hysteresis. It is left as an exercise for the reader to find expressions for V_{sLO}, V_{sHI}, and V_H under these conditions.

6.5.2. Applications of Voltage Comparators

Comparators find many applications in biomedical engineering. They are used in bar-graph (LED) display meters; flash ADC converters (see Section 10.5.5); over- and under-range alarms; static window circuits; ON–OFF controllers; and dynamic pulse-height discriminators used in nuclear medicine and neurophysiology. The first example examines a simple battery overvoltage alarm used to indicate that charging should cease. This circuit is shown in Figure 6.12. When $V_{Batt} > V_{REF}$, the output (open collector) transistor ($Q15$) in the VC is turned off, allowing the base of Q_1 to conduct through the 1-kΩ pull-up resistor, saturating Q_1. The current through the lit LED is approximately $(5 - 0.2 - 1.5)/330 = 10$ mA. If $V_{Batt} < V_{REF}$, Q_{15} is ON and saturated,

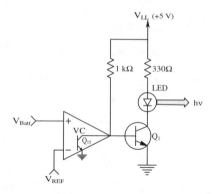

FIGURE 6.12
A comparator circuit that will light an LED when $V_{Batt} > V_{REF}$. If $V_{Batt} < V_{REF}$, then Q_{15} of the comparator is on and saturated, pulling Q_1's base low and turning it and the LED off.

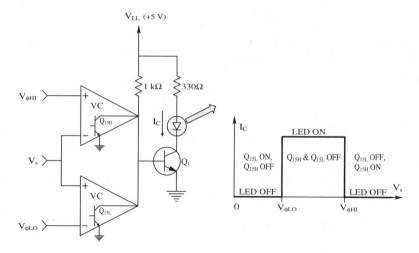

FIGURE 6.13
A comparator voltage range window that turns the LED on when V_s lies between $V_{\phi LO}$ and $V_{\phi HI}$.

pulling the base of Q_1 down to approximately 0.2 V, keeping it off and the LED unlit.

The second example of the use of VCs is a static window comparator circuit that lights an LED while the input voltage falls in a certain range, or window, of values. The circuit is shown in Figure 6.13. Note that tying the two open collector output transistors together to a common pull-up resistor effectively makes an AND gate. Both comparator outputs must be HI (Q_{15L} AND Q_{15H} are cut off) to light the LED. If either Q_{15} is ON, the base of Q_1 is pulled down to that Q_{15}'s V_{csat} and Q_1 is cut off.

In a third and final example of using VCs, examine a simple nerve spike pulse-height discriminator designed by the author. This circuit is designed to be used in neurophysiological recording; it selects only those nerve

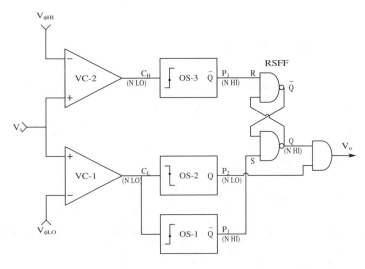

FIGURE 6.14

A nerve spike pulse-height window that produces an output pulse *only if* an input spike rises to its peak inside the window and then falls below the lower "sill." No output pulse is produced if an input spike rises through the window and exceeds the upper level, then falls below the sill.

impulses recorded with extra-cellular microelectrodes that fall within a narrow range of amplitudes (the window). This processing enables other simultaneously recorded, very large (or small) action potentials to be ignored while the desired pulses can be counted, processed, and their instantaneous frequency calculated, etc.

Figure 6.14 illustrates the organization of this window circuit. Note that this circuit involves sequential as well as combinational logic. Critical waveforms of this window circuit are shown in Figure 6.15. Note that three one-shot multivibrators are used to generate narrow (e.g., 500 ns) output pulses given input logic state transitions. The NAND gate RS flip-flop serves as a "memory" that a rising V_s has exceeded $V_{\phi LO}$. Note that, if V_s exceeds $V_{\phi LO}$, the output of VC-2, C_H, goes HI. This event triggers OS-3 to reset the RSFF Q output to LO, disabling the output AND gate.

Now when the large input again falls below $V_{\phi LO}$, the P2 pulse does not produce an output. Only the falling edge of VC-1's output, C_L, can produce an output. The second V_s pulse in Figure 6.15 lies in the window. The rising edge of C_L sets the RSFF Q output high, enabling the AND gate. When V_s falls below $V_{\phi LO}$, OS-2 produces a positive pulse that appears at V_o, signaling a pulse that occurred inside the window. (A functionally similar nerve spike pulse-height window was described by Northrop and Grossman, 1974.)

6.5.3 Discussion

The preceding sections described the basic behavior of VCs. Note that comparators are intended to signal analog voltage inequalities to appropriate

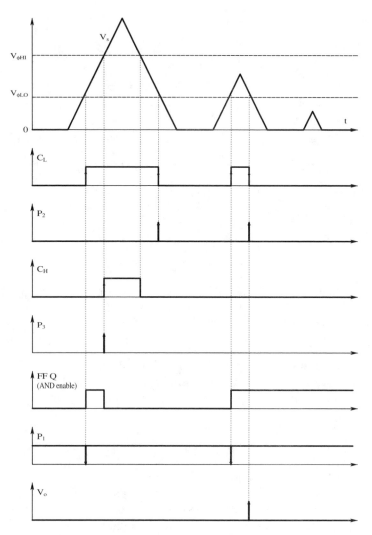

FIGURE 6.15
Critical waveforms for the pulse-height window of Figure 6.14. See text for description.

logic circuits or transistor switches; op amps are for conditioning analog signals, giving an analog output. An important point is that an open-loop op amp (one without feedback) makes a poor comparator. Yes, op amps generally have very high gain differential input gains and high CMRRs, but rapid changes in V_o are limited by the op amps' slew rate, η. η is typically on the order of 20 V/μs, which means it takes V_o roughly 250 ns to slew 5 V. Op amp outputs are generally not logic-level compatible; they swing to $\pm(V_{CC} - V_\delta)$, where V_δ is a fixed voltage by which a saturated V_o fails to reach the supply voltage. V_δ is different for different designs of op amps. It is not good design practice to use op amps for comparator applications.

6.6 Some Applications of Op Amps in Biomedicine

6.6.1 Introduction

Op amps are extremely useful in the design of all sorts of analog electronic instrumentation systems. As demonstrated in Chapter 7 and Chapter 8, op amps find great application in the design of analog active filters and as building blocks for instrumentation amplifier (differential) amplifiers and other linear and nonlinear signal conditioning systems. As the preceding sections have shown, there are a number of specialized types of op amps for specific signal processing applications. The following sections focus on four applications that often have important roles in biomedical signal processing: integrators; differentiators; charge amplifiers; and an isolated two-op amp instrumentation DA useful for measuring ECG. This amplifier also includes a band-pass filter and an analog photo-optic coupler for galvanic isolation.

6.6.2 Analog Integrators and Differentiators

A simple op amp integrator is shown in Figure 6.16. An op amp integrator is hardly ever used as a stand-alone component; it is usually incorporated as part of a feedback loop to obtain some desired dynamic characteristic for the closed-loop system. The reason for not using it alone is that it integrates its own dc bias current and offset voltage, causing its output, in the absence of an input signal, to drift into saturation slowly and linearly. In the circuit of Figure 6.16, set $V_s = 0$ and consider the op amp ideal, so $v_i' = 0$. Thus, the node voltage V_1 must equal V_{OS}. Using superposition, and considering I_B and V_{OS} to be steps applied at t = 0, the integrator's time-domain output can be written:

$$V_o(t) = -t\, I_B/C_F + V_{OS}\,(1 + t/RC_F) \tag{6.60}$$

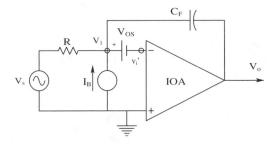

FIGURE 6.16
A dc model of a voltage op amp integrator. The op amp is assumed ideal and its offset voltage and bias current are externalized to its inverting (v_i') node. The integrator's behavior is analyzed in the text.

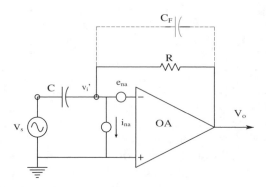

FIGURE 6.17
Circuit for an op amp differentiator. In this problem, the op amp's frequency response is considered, as well as its short-circuit input voltage noise root power spectrum, and input current noise root spectrum.

I_B and V_{OS} can have either sign, depending on the op amp design and its temperature. V_{OS} magnitude is typically in the range of hundreds of micro-volts and I_B can range from tens of faradamperes to microamperes, again depending on OA design and temperature.

If stand-alone analog integration must be done, the integrator drift must be considered. Op amps with low V_{OS} and I_B are used and a means of shorting out C_F is used to ensure zero initial conditions at the start of integration. Digital integration is no panacea; it will integrate small analog offset voltages present in the anti-aliasing filter, the sample and hold, and the ADC.

Often, when an integrator is used in a closed-loop system, it is desirable to give its transfer function a real zero, as well as the pole at the origin. The zero is used to give the system better closed-loop dynamic performance and is easily obtained by placing a resistance, R_F, in series with C_F. Assuming an ideal op amp, the transfer function is:

$$\frac{V_o}{V_s}(s) = -\frac{R_F + 1/sC_F}{R} = -\frac{(sR_FC_F + 1)}{sRC_F} = -\frac{K_i(s\tau_f + 1)}{s} \tag{6.61}$$

which is what is desired.

Figure 6.17 illustrates a conventional op amp analog differentiator. If the op amp is treated as ideal and C_F is neglected, then the transfer function is:

$$\frac{V_o}{V_s}(s) = -sRC \tag{6.62}$$

which is the transfer function of an ideal time-domain differentiator with gain $-RC$.

Now consider what happens to the differentiator's transfer function when a real frequency-compensated op amp is modeled by the open-loop gain:

$$\frac{V_o}{V_i'}(s) = \frac{-K_{vo}}{\tau_A s + 1} \tag{6.63}$$

Now the node equation on the V_i' node is:

$$V_i'(G + sC) - V_o G = V_s s C \tag{6.64}$$

Using Equation 6.63, V_i' in Equation 6.64 can be eliminated and the overall transfer function written:

$$
\begin{aligned}
\frac{V_o}{V_s}(s) &= \frac{-s\, RC\, K_{vo} / (1 + K_{vo})}{s^2 \tau_A\, RC / (1 + K_{vo}) + s(\tau_A + RC) / (1 + K_{vo}) + 1} \\
&\cong \frac{-s\, RC}{s^2 \tau_A RC / K_{vo} + s(\tau_A + RC) / K_{vo} + 1}
\end{aligned}
\tag{6.65}
$$

Note that Equation 6.65 has the form of the transfer function of a quadratic band-pass filter shown in the following equation:

$$\frac{V_o}{V_s}(s) = \frac{-sK}{s^2 / \omega_n^2 + s\, 2\xi / \omega_n + 1} \tag{6.66}$$

From Equation 6.66 and Equation 6.65, the resonant frequency is:

$$\omega_n \cong \sqrt{K_{vo} / (\tau_A RC)} \ \text{r/s} \tag{6.67}$$

and the damping factor is:

$$\xi = \frac{(\tau_A + RC)}{2\, K_{vo}} \frac{\sqrt{K_{vo}}}{\sqrt{\tau_A RC}} \tag{6.68}$$

When typical numerical values are substituted for the op amp and circuit parameters ($K_{vo} = 10^6$; $\tau_A = 0.001$ sec; $R = 10^6\ \Omega$; and $C = 10^{-6}$ F), $\omega_n = 3.16 \times 10^4$ r/s and $\xi = 1.597 \times 10^{-2}$. This damping is equivalent to a quadratic BPF $Q = 1/(2\xi) = 31.3$, which is a sharply tuned filter. Thus, any fast transients in V_s will excite a poorly damped sinusoidal transient at the differentiator output.

Another problem with the simple R–C differentiator is the differentiation of the op amp's short-circuit equivalent voltage noise, e_{na}. The transfer function for e_{na} is easily shown to be:

$$V_o = E_{na}\,(1 + s\,RC) \tag{6.69}$$

Because e_{na} has a broadband spectrum, the differentiator's output noise has a spectrum that increases with frequency, making the output very noisy. (Note that the i_{na} component in V_o is not differentiated.) When a feedback capacitor, C_F, is added in parallel with R, the differentiator's frequency response is found from the new node equation:

$$V_i'\left[G + s\left(C + C_F\right)\right] - V_o\left(G + sC_F\right) = V_s\,sC \tag{6.70}$$

Using Equation 6.63, V_i' in the preceding equation can be eliminated and the transfer function written:

$$\frac{V_o}{V_s}(s) = \frac{-s\,RC}{s^2\,\tau_A R\left(C + C_F\right)/K_{vo} + s\left[\left(\tau_A + RC\right)/K_{vo} + RC_F\right] + 1} \tag{6.71}$$

The differentiator transfer function still has the format of a BPF. Examine its ω_n and damping: all parameters are the same as the preceding ones and $C_F = 6.7 \times 10^{-11}$ F (67 pF).

$$\omega_n^2 = \frac{K_{vo}}{\tau_A R\left(C + C_F\right)} = \frac{10^6}{10^{-3} \times 10^6 \times \left(10^{-6} + 6.7 \times 10^{-11}\right)} = 9.99933 \times 10^8 \tag{6.72}$$

$$\downarrow$$

$$\omega_n = 3.1622 \times 10^4 \text{ r/s} \tag{6.73}$$

The damping factor is now found from:

$$2\xi/\omega_n = \frac{\tau_A + RC}{K_{vo}} + RC_F \tag{6.74}$$

$$\xi = 0.5 \times 3.1622 \times 10^4 \left(\frac{10^{-3} + 1}{10^6} + 6.7 \times 10^{-11} \times 10^6\right) = 1.075 \tag{6.75}$$

The ω_n has changed little, but now the system is slightly overdamped, i.e., both poles are close on the real axis in the s-plane. The differentiator's frequency response is still band pass with its peak gain at the same frequency,

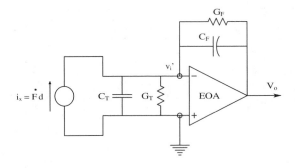

FIGURE 6.18
An electrometer op amp is used to make a charge amplifier to condition the output of a piezoelectric force transducer. See text for analysis.

but is no longer severely underdamped. Making C_F larger will make the system more overdamped; it will have two real poles, one below ω_n and the other above it. Thus, for practical reasons, an op amp, analog differentiator should have a small feedback capacitor in parallel with the feedback R to limit its bandwidth and give it reasonable damping so that input noise spikes will not excite "ringing" in its output.

6.6.3 Charge Amplifiers

A charge amplifier is used to condition the output of a piezoelectric transducer used in such applications as accelerometers, dynamic pressure sensors, microphones, and ultrasonic receivers. Figure 6.18 illustrates the schematic of an electrometer op amp used as a charge amplifier. The shunt capacitance, C_T, includes the capacitance of the piezotransducer, the connecting coax (if any), and the input capacitance of the op amp. Similarly, the conductance G_T includes the leakage conductance of the transducer, the connecting cable, and the op amp's input conductance. The op amp is assumed to have a finite gain and frequency response, i.e., it is nonideal in this respect. Thus, the summing junction voltage, v_i', is finite. The op amp's gain is modeled by:

$$V_o = -V_i' \frac{K_{vo}}{\tau s + 1} \tag{6.76}$$

The node equation for the summing junction is:

$$V_i' \left[s\left(C_F + C_T\right) + G_T + G_F \right] - V_o \left[s C_F + G_F \right] = F(s)d = sF(s)d \tag{6.77}$$

from which:

$$V_i' = \frac{sF(s)d + V_o\left[sC_F + G_F\right]}{\left[s(C_F + C_T) + C_T + G_F\right]} \tag{6.78}$$

$$\downarrow$$

$$V_o[\tau s + 1] = -K_{vo}\frac{sF(s)d + V_o\left[sC_F + G_F\right]}{\left[s(C_F + C_T) + G_T + G_F\right]} \tag{6.79}$$

$$\downarrow$$

$$\frac{V_o}{F}(s) = \frac{-sK_{vo}d}{s^2\tau(C_F + C_T) + s\left[\tau(G_F + G_T) + C_F + C_T + K_{vo}C_F\right] + K_{vo}G_F} \tag{6.80}$$

To put Equation 6.80 into time-constant format, divide top and bottom by $K_{vo} G_F$ and note that certain terms in the denominator are negligibly small. Let $s = j\omega$ in order to write the charge amplifier's frequency response:

$$\frac{V_o}{F}(j\omega) \cong \frac{-j\omega d R_F}{(j\omega)^2 \tau(C_F + C_T)R_F/K_{vo} + j\omega C_F R_F + 1} \tag{6.81}$$

The frequency response function of Equation 6.81 is band pass with two real poles. The low-frequency one is set by the feedback R and C and is $s_1 \cong -1/(R_F C_F)$ r/s; the high-frequency pole can be shown to be approximately $s_2 \cong -(K_{vo}/\tau)[C_F/(C_F + C_T)] = \omega_T C_F/(C_F + C_T)$ r/s. ω_T is the op amp's radian gain-bandwidth product. For example, set $K_{vo} = 10^6$; $\tau = 10^{-3}$ sec; $C_F = 10^{-9}$ F; $C_T = 10^{-9}$ F; $G_F = 10^{-10}$ S; and $G_T = 10^{-12}$ S. Now the low break frequency is at $f_{lo} = 1.59 \times 10^{-2}$ Hz and the high break frequency is at $f_{hi} = 80$ MHz, which is adequate for conditioning 5-MHz ultrasound.

6.6.4   A Two-Op Amp ECG Amplifier

Op amps can be used to make high-gain differential amplifiers with high common-mode rejection ratios, as described in Section 3.7.2 in Chapter 3. The two-op amp DA was found to have a DM gain:

$$V_o = (V_s - V_s')\, 2(1 + R/R_F) \tag{6.82}$$

R and R_F should be chosen so that the amplifier's DM gain is 10^3. To use this amplifier as an ECG system front end, it is necessary to define the ECG band pass with a high- and low-pass filter. An easy design is to cascade the Sallen and Key high-pass and low-pass filters, as shown in Figure 6.19. The *HPF* is given complex-conjugate poles with an $f_n = 0.1$ Hz and a damping factor of $\xi = 0.707$. Using the design formulas given in Section 7.2.2 in Chapter 7, $C_1 = C_2 = C$ and, for $\xi = 0.707$, $R_1 = 2\, R_2$. $f_n = 1/(2\pi C\sqrt{R_1 R_2}) = 0.1$,

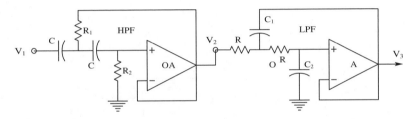

FIGURE 6.19
A band-pass filter for electrocardiography made from cascaded Sallen and Key high-pass filter and low-pass filters.

so one can solve for R_1 and R_2 after choosing $C = 3.3$ μF. A little algebra gives $R_2 = 3.31 \times 10^5$ and $R_1 = 6.821 \times 10^5$ Ω.

The parameters for the S and K *LPF* are found from $\xi = \sqrt{C_2/C_1} = 0.707$ and $f_n = 1/(2\pi R\sqrt{C_1 C_2}) = 100$ Hz. Clearly, $C_2 = 2C_1$ for the desired damping. Choose $C_1 = 0.1$ μF, so $C_2 = 0.2$ μF. Using the f_n relation, $R = 1.125 \times 10^4$ Ω. The op amps need not be special low-noise or high f_T designs, the ECG signal has limited bandwidth, and the noise performance is set by the differential front end amplifier having the gain of 10^3.

Now that the ECG signal has been amplified and its bandwidth defined, it is necessary to consider patient galvanic isolation. One easy way to achieve isolation is to run the DA and filter op amps on isolated battery power with no ground connection common with the power line mains. A pair of 12-V batteries can be used with IC voltage regulators to give ±8 V to run the four signal conditioning op amps. One cannot simply connect the output of the filter to an oscilloscope or computer to view the ECG. The common ground from the oscilloscope or computer destroys patient galvanic isolation, so some means of coupling the signal without the necessity of a common ground must be used. One means is to sample the isolated ECG and convert it with a serial output isolated ADC and then couple the digitized ECG to the outside using a photo-optic coupler (POC). (A transformer can also be used.) The digitized ECG must then be converted to analog form with a serial input DAC in order to be viewed on an oscilloscope or be an input to a strip-chart recorder.

A simpler form of galvanic isolation that uses POCs and gives an analog output is shown in Figure 6.20. OA1 is run from the isolated battery power supply of the signal conditioner. The top LED in the dual POC IC is biased on with the 3-mA dc current source, causing an average light intensity, I_{1o}, to be emitted. The isolated conditioned ECG output, V_3, causes the light intensity to vary proportionally around the average level, I_{1o}. The light from LED_1 is transmitted through a plastic light guide to photodiode, PD_2. An increase in the light hitting the photojunction of PD_1 causes a proportional increase in its (reverse) photocurrent. PD_1's increased photocurrent is the base current of the top *npn* BJT, so its collector current increases, causing the inverting input of op amp OA2 to go negative and making OA2's output go positive. The positive increment on OA2's output increases the current in

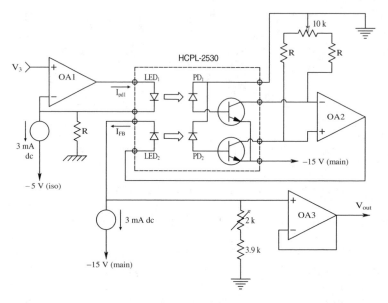

FIGURE 6.20

A linear analog photo-optic coupler used to provide galvanic isolation between the battery-operated ECG measurement differential amplifier and band-pass filter, and the output recording and display systems.

LED$_2$ above its 3-mA bias, increasing its light output and, in turn, increasing the photocurrent in PD$_2$. This increases the base current in its BJT, causing the positive input of OA2 to go negative, closing a negative feedback path that compensates for LED and PD nonlinearities. Note that the ECG ground is completely isolated from the output ground, as is the analog ECG signal, V_3, from V_{out}. The output of the feedback POC system is taken as the voltage across the 2 k + 3.9 k resistors.

6.7   Chapter Summary

This chapter has been all about op amps; it began by reviewing the properties of the ideal op amp and showing how it can be used to facilitate heuristic analysis of op amp circuits.

Practical conventional op amps were shown to be characterized by finite frequency-dependent difference-mode gains and finite input and output resistances. Their inputs were also characterized by two dc bias currents, a dc offset voltage, a short-circuit input noise voltage, and an input noise current. The various types of op amps were described, including: high frequency; high slew rate; low noise; electrometer; chopper stabilized; etc.

The effects of negative voltage feedback on a closed-loop op amp amplifier's frequency response was described in terms of the op amp's gain-bandwidth product, or unity gain frequency. The amplifier's gain-bandwidth product was shown to be constant for the special case of the noninverting amplifier configuration and to be a function of the amplifier's gain at low gains for the inverting amplifier configuration.

The current feedback amplifier (CFOA) was described and analyzed; in the noninverting gain configuration. The closed-loop amplifier's break frequency was found to be independent of the closed-loop gain and to depend only on the absolute value of the feedback resistance. The same situation obtains for the inverting amplifier configuration using the CFOA. CFOAs were also shown to be unsuitable for integrators unless a special 2-CFOA circuit is used.

Voltage comparators were described and shown to have DA front ends and TTL or ECL logic outputs. Comparators are useful in biomedical applications, including pulse height windows used in neurophysiology and in nuclear medicine. Finally, applications of op amps as differentiators, integrators, charge amplifiers, and ECG signal conditioning were examined.

Home Problems

6.1 An Apex™ PA08A high-voltage power op amp is used to drive a resistive load. This op amp can output up to ±150 mA and swing its output voltage up to ±145 V. Its slew rate is 30 V/μs. What is the maximum Hertz frequency of a sinusoidal input it can amplify to get a 100-VRMS sinusoidal output without slew rate distortion?

6.2 Figure P6.2(A) and Figure P6.2(B) illustrate a commutating auto-zero (CAZ) op amp connected as a noninverting amplifier with voltage gain $(1 + R_F/R_1)$. This is an Intersil ICL7605/7606 CAZ amplifier intended for nondrifting dc amplification applications such as strain gauge bridges and electronic scales. The over-all bandwidth is made about 10 Hz. Note that the CAZ op amp has two matched op amps internally and a number of analog MOS switches to change periodically its input circuitry and switch its output. Two matched external capacitors are used to store dc offset voltages. Assume the two internal op amps are ideal except for their offset voltages. Describe how this circuit works to realize an amazing overall offset voltage tempco of ±10 nV/°C.

6.3 Two cascaded noninverting voltage op amps are shown in Figure P6.3. Each op amp has an open-loop transfer function given by:

$$\frac{V_o}{\left(V_i - V_i'\right)} = \frac{10^5}{10^{-3}s + 1}$$

a. Give the Hertz gain*bandwidth product of the op amps alone.

b. Find an expression for the transfer function of the cascaded amplifiers, $(V_3/V_1)(s)$, in time-constant form.

c. Give numerical values for the −3-dB frequency and the f_T of the amplifier.

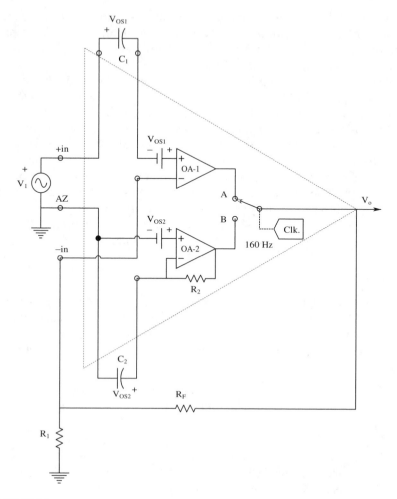

FIGURE P6.2A

6.4   Use an ECAP to simulate the response of a simple inverting op amp amplifier
      with a gain of −100 to a 1.0 kHz, 10 mV peak square wave. A TI TL071 op
      amp is used.

6.5   Examine the frequency dependence of a noninverting op amp amplifier's
      output impedance, $\mathbf{Z_o}(j\omega)$. The circuit is shown in Figure P6.5. Let $R_o = 50\ \Omega$;
      $R_F = 99\ \mathrm{k}\Omega$; $R_1 = 1\ \mathrm{k}\Omega$; and $V_{oc} = (V_i - V_i')\ 10^4/(10^{-3}\ j\omega + 1)$.

      a. Write an expression for $\mathbf{Z_o}(j\omega) = \mathbf{I_t}/\mathbf{V_t}$ in time-constant form.
      b. Make a dimensioned Bode plot of $\mathbf{Z_o}(j\omega)$ (magnitude and phase).

6.6   A 6.2-V zener diode is used in the feedback path of an ideal op amp as shown
      in Figure P6.6. A simplified ZD I–V curve is shown. $R_1 = 1\ \mathrm{k}\Omega$. Plot and
      dimension $V_o = f(V_1)$.

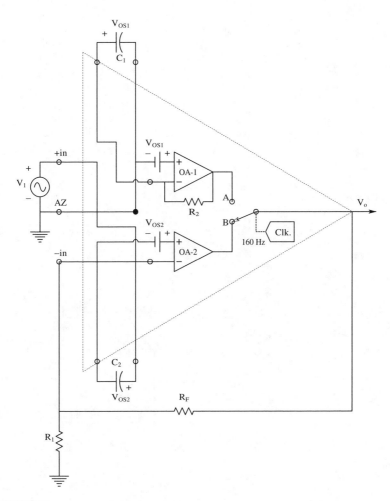

FIGURE P6.2B

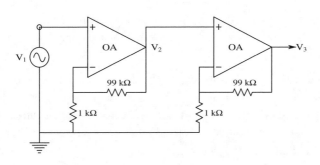

FIGURE P6.3

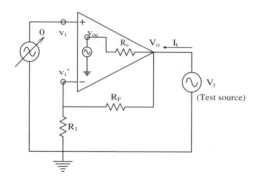

FIGURE P6.5

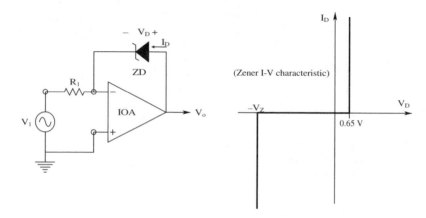

FIGURE P6.6

6.7 A version of a diode bridge is shown in Figure P6.7. Assume $v_1(t) = 1.4 \sin(377t)$ and $R_L = 1 \text{ k}\Omega$. Plot and dimension several cycles of $V_o(t)$ and $V_2(t)$. Assume the diodes have the I–V characteristic shown.

6.8 Another precision rectifier bridge is shown in Figure P6.8. $v_1(t)$ and the diodes are the same as in the preceding problem. Plot and dimension several cycles of $V_o(t)$ and $V_2(t)$.

6.9 An *npn* BJT is used in the feedback path of an ideal op amp as shown in Figure P6.9. The BJT is forward-biased; its collector current can be modeled by $I_C \cong I_s \exp(V_{BE}/V_T)$, where I_s is the collector saturation current $= 0.25 \text{ pA}$; V_{BE} is the base–emitter voltage; and $V_T = \eta kT/q \cong 26 \text{ mV}$ at room temperature. Plot and dimension $V_o = f(V_1)$.

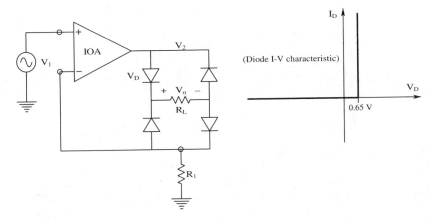

FIGURE P6.7

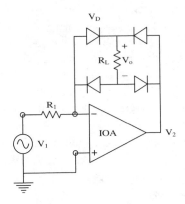

FIGURE P6.8

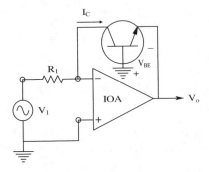

FIGURE P6.9

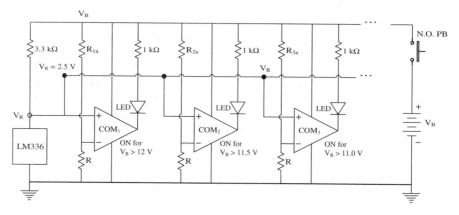

FIGURE P6.10

6.10 A laptop computer uses a nominal 12-V battery. It is desired to design a bar graph type of LED voltmeter display that will measure the battery voltage over the range of 9 to 12 V. A partial schematic of the voltmeter is shown in Figure P6.10. An LM336 IC reference voltage chip supplies a constant 2.5 Vdc as long as $V_B > 6$ V. The comparators also run off V_B as long as $V_B > 6$ V. Comparator 1 lights its LED when the voltage at its inverting terminal exceeds $V_R = 2.5$ V; this makes its logic output low and allows current to flow through its LED. The comparator 1 inverting terminal voltage is $\alpha_1 V_B$. $\alpha_1 = R/(R + R_{1a})$. $R \equiv 10$ kΩ. Comparator 1's LED lights only for $V_B > 12$ V. Comparator 2 lights its LED for $V_B > 11.5$ V; comparator 3's LED lights for $V_B > 11.0$ V; comparator 4's LED lights for $V_B > 10.5$ V; the comparator 5 LED lights for $V_B > 10.0$ V; comparator 6's LED lights for $V_B > 9.5$ V; and comparator 7's LED lights for $V_B > 9.0$ V. Thus, a fully charged battery will light all seven LEDs when the button is pushed and, if $10.0 < V_B < 10.5$, only LEDs 5, 6, and 7 will light. Calculate the necessary values of R_{1a} through R_{7a} required to make the LED voltmeter work as described.

6.11 Figure P6.11 shows a noninverting op amp amplifier and its equivalent input resistance circuit. Find an algebraic expression for the input admittance, $G_{in} = I_s/V_s$ S. Assume that $V_o = V_s (1 + R_F/R_1)$ for the amplifier. Assume that R_i and $R_{cm} \gg R_F$ and R_1. Evaluate G_{in} numerically: let $R_i = 10$ MΩ; $R_{cm} = 400$ MΩ; and $R_F = R_1 = 3.3$ kΩ.

6.12 Find an expression for the transfer function of the filter of Figure P6.12 in time-constant form. The op amp is ideal.

6.13 Find an expression for the frequency response function of the filter of Figure P6.13 in time-constant form. What function does this circuit perform on V_s?

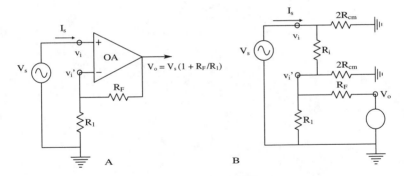

FIGURE P6.11

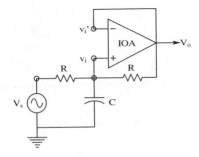

FIGURE P6.12

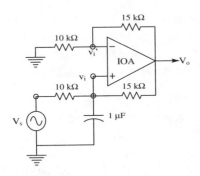

FIGURE P6.13

6.14 The circuit of Figure P6.14 is a dc millivoltmeter. Find the value of R required so that the dc microammeter reads full scale ($100\ \mu A$ dc) when $V_s = 100$ mV dc. The op amp is ideal.

6.15 Derive an expression for $V_o = f(V_s, R, \Delta R)$ for the one active arm Wheatstone bridge signal conditioner of Figure P6.15. An ideal op amp is used.

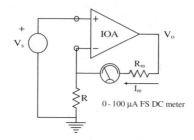

FIGURE P6.14

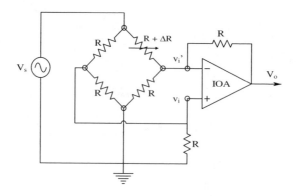

FIGURE P6.15

6.16 In Figure P6.16, an ideal op amp is used control the collector current of a power BJT that supplies a relay coil. The relay coil has an inductance of 0.1 Hy and a series resistance, R_L, of 30 ohms. Model the BJT by its MFSS *h*-parameter model with $h_{oe} = 0$. Derive expressions for the transfer functions, V_b/V_s, and V_c/V_s in time-constant form. Note that $V_e/V_s = 1$ because of the ideal op amp assumption. Let $h_{fe} = 19$; $h_{ie} = 10^3 \ \Omega$; and $R_E = 100 \ \Omega$.

a. Find an expression for V_b/V_s. Evaluate numerically.

b. Find an expression for the transfer function V_c/V_s in Laplace form. Evaluate numerically.

c. Let $V_s(t)$ be an ideal voltage pulse that jumps to 2 V at $t = 0$ and to zero at $t = 1$ sec. Sketch and dimension $V_c(t)$ for this input.

d. Considering the results of the preceding part of this problem, what nonlinear component can be added to the circuit to protect the transistor? Sketch the modified circuit.

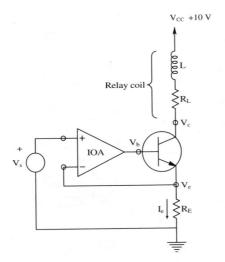

FIGURE P6.16

7

Analog Active Filters

7.1 Introduction

Filter (noun) is an electrical engineering term having a broad definition. Filters are generally considered to operate on signals in the frequency domain; that is, they attenuate, stop, pass, or boost certain frequency regions in the input signal's spectrum. These operations are called *filtering* (verb). They may be classified as low pass (LP); band pass (BP); high pass (HP); or band reject (BR or notch). Band-pass and band-reject filters can have narrow-pass bands or reject bands. One descriptor of such sharply tuned filters is their Q, which can be defined as the BP filter's center frequency divided by its half-power bandwidth; the narrower the bandwidth is, the higher the Q. (Bandwidth is generally measured as the frequency span between half-power frequencies, where the filter's frequency response function is down −3 dB or to 0.7071 times the peak pass gain.)

Filter transfer functions can be expressed in general as rational polynomials in the complex variable, **s**. The rational polynomials can be factored to find the poles and zeros of the transfer function. The filter's poles are the roots of the denominator polynomial; its zeros are the roots of the numerator polynomial. Roots are the complex values of **s** that make a polynomial equal zero. If the highest power of s in the denominator polynomial is n, n poles will be in the complex s-plane. If the filter is stable (and all should be), all of the filter's poles will lie in the left-half s-plane; however, in limiting cases, conjugate pole pairs can lie on the $j\omega$ axis.

Likewise, if the highest power of s in the numerator polynomial is m, m zeros will be in the s-plane. The zeros can lie anywhere in the s-plane; if some lie in the right-half s-plane, the filter is called *nonminimum phase.* If all the zeros lie in the left-hand s-plane, the filter is called *minimum phase.* The poles and zeros can have real values or occur in complex-conjugate pairs of the form, $\mathbf{s} = \alpha \pm j\beta$, where β is nonnegative and $-\infty < \alpha < \infty$. Conjugate zeros on the $j\omega$ axis are found in notch filters. A filter's frequency response is found by letting $\mathbf{s} = j\omega$ in the filter's transfer function and then finding 20 times the log of the magnitude of the frequency response function vs. f in Hertz and the angle of the frequency response function vector vs. f.

Analog active filters use feedback around op amps to realize desired transfer functions for applications such as band-pass and low-pass filtering to improve signal-to-noise ratios. AFs use only capacitors and resistors in their circuits. Inductors are not used because they are generally large, heavy, and imperfect, i.e., they have significant losses from coil resistance and other factors. AFs are also used to realize sharp cut-off low-pass filters (LPFs) for anti-aliasing filtering of analog signals before periodic, analog-to-digital conversion (sampling). Active notch filters are often used to eliminate the coherent interference that accompanies ECG, EMG, and EEG signals.

Some disconcerting news is that since EEs first discovered that op amps can be used to realize filters, a plethora of different AF design architectures have been developed. In, fact, several excellent texts have been written on the specialized art of active filter design (Schaumann and Van Valkenburg, 2001; Lancaster, 1996; Huelsman, 1993; Deliyannis, Sun, and Fidler, 1998). In some AF designs, filter parameters such as mid-band gain, break frequency, Q, or damping factor cannot be designed for with unique R and C components. For example, all the filter's Rs and Cs interact, so no single component or set of components can independently determine mid-band gain, break frequency, etc.

The good news is that high-order active filters are generally designed on a modular cascaded basis using certain preferred circuit architectures that allow exact pole and zero placement in the s-plane by simple component value choice. Some examples of these preferred AF architectures will be examined, beginning with the simple controlled-source, Sallen and Key quadratic low-pass filter.

7.2   Types of Analog Active Filters

7.2.1   Introduction

In the AF designs described next, the op amps will be assumed to be ideal. For serious design evaluation, computer modeling must be used with op amp dynamic models. Note that a filter's transient response can be just as important as its frequency response. The band-pass filtering of an ECG signal is an example of a biomedical application of an active filter that is transient response sensitive. The fidelity of the sharp QRS spike must be preserved for diagnosis; there must be little rounding of the R-peak and no transient "ringing" following the QRS spike. The linear phase Bessel filter is one class of AF that is free from ringing and suitable for conditioning ECG signals. The exact position of the poles of a high-order ($n > 2$) Bessel filter determine its characteristics; this filter will be examined in detail later.

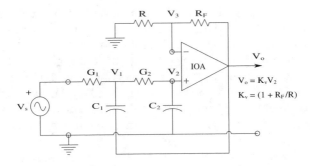

FIGURE 7.1
A Sallen and Key quadratic low-pass filter.

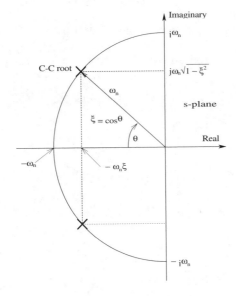

FIGURE 7.2
Complex-conjugate pole geometry in the s-plane, showing the relations between pole positions and the natural frequency and damping factor.

7.2.2 Sallen and Key Controlled-Source AFs

A basic filter building-block for AFs is the Sallen and Key (S & K), quadratic (two-pole), controlled source (VCVS) architecture. S & K AFs can be cascaded to make high-order low-pass, high-pass, or band-pass filters.

A low-pass S & K filter is shown in Figure 7.1. S & K AFs are quadratic filters, i.e., they generally have a pair of complex-conjugate (C-C) poles, as shown in Figure 7.2. Their transfer function denominators are of the form

$s^2 + s2\xi\omega_n + \omega_n^2$ (in Laplace format). The real part of the C-C poles is negative $(-\xi\omega_n)$ and the imaginary parts are $\pm j\omega_n\sqrt{1-\xi^2}$. ω_n is called the undamped natural frequency (in radians/sec) and ξ is the damping factor. For C-C poles, $0 < \xi < 1$. The damping factor is the cosine of the angle between the negative real axis in the s-plane and the vector connecting the origin with the upper pole. The closer the poles are to the $j\omega$ axis, the less damped is the output response of the filter to transient inputs. Also, LPFs with low damping exhibit a peak in their steady-state sinusoidal frequency response (Bode magnitude response) around ω_n.

To find the S & K LPF's transfer function, write node equations for the V_1 and V_2 nodes:

$$V_1\left[G_1 + G_2 + sC_1\right] - V_2 G_2 - V_o sC_1 = V_s G_1 \tag{7.1A}$$

$$-V_1 G_2 + V_2\left[G_2 + sC_2\right] = 0 \tag{7.1B}$$

Now V_2 can be replaced with V_o/K_v and the node equations rearranged:

$$V_1\left[G_1 + G_2 + sC_1\right] - V_o\left[sC_1 + G_2/K_v\right] = V_s G_1 \tag{7.2A}$$

$$-V_1 G_2 + V_o\left[G_2 + sC_2\right]/K_v = 0 \tag{7.2B}$$

Using Cramer's rule, it is possible to solve for V_o:

$$\Delta = s^2 C_1 C_2/K_v + s\left[C_2 G_1/K_v + C_2 G_2/K_v + C_1 G_2/K_v - C_1 G_2\right] + G_2^2/K_v \tag{7.3}$$

$$\Delta V_o = + V_s G_1 G_2 \tag{7.4}$$

Thus, the LPF's transfer function can be written:

$$\frac{V_o}{V_s}(s) = \frac{G_1 G_2}{s^2 C_1 C_2/K_v + s\left[C_2 G_1/K_v + C_2 G_2/K_v + C_1 G_2/K_v - C_1 G_2\right] + G_1 G_2/K_v} \tag{7.5}$$

Now multiply top and bottom by $R_1 R_2 K_v$ to put the filter's transfer function in time-constant form:

$$\frac{V_o}{V_s}(s) = \frac{K_v}{s^2 C_1 C_2 R_1 R_2 + s\left[R_1 C_2 + R_2 C_2 + C_1 R_1(1 - K_v)\right] + 1} \tag{7.6}$$

The denominator of the S & K AF's transfer function can be written in the standard underdamped quadratic form: $s^2/\omega_n^2 + s\,2\,\xi/\omega_n + 1$. By inspection, $\omega_n = 1/\sqrt{R_1 R_2 C_1 C_2}$ r/s. The filter's dc gain is K_v, and its damping factor is:

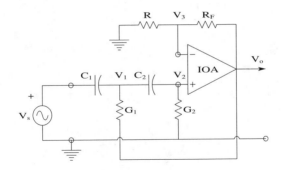

FIGURE 7.3
A Sallen and Key quadratic high-pass filter.

$$\xi = \frac{\left[C_2\left(R_1+R_2\right)+C_1R_1\left(1-K_v\right)\right]}{2\sqrt{R_1R_2C_1C_2}} \tag{7.7}$$

For reasons of simplicity, practical S & K active LPF design generally sets $K_v = 1$ and $R_1 + R_2 = R$. Under these conditions, the damping factor is set by the ratio of the capacitor values:

$$\xi = \sqrt{\left(C_2/C_1\right)} \tag{7.8}$$

The dc gain is unity and the undamped natural frequency is:

$$\omega_n = 1/\left(R\sqrt{C_1C_2}\right) \text{ r/s} \tag{7.9}$$

To execute an S & K LPF design, given a ω_n and damping factor ξ, first set C_2/C_1, then pick absolute values for C_1 and C_2 and set R to get the desired ω_n. Several S & K LPFs can be cascaded to create a high-order LPF. Pole pair positions in the s-plane can individually be controlled (ξ_k, ω_{nk}) to realize a specific filter category such as Butterworth, Bessel, Chebychev, etc.

Next, consider the design of the S & K high-pass filter, shown in Figure 7.3. Analysis proceeds in the same manner used for the S & K LPF, except that it is assumed that $K_v = 1$ to begin; thus, $V_2 = V_o$. The node equations are:

$$V_1\left[G_1+s\left(C_1+C_2\right)\right]-V_o\left[G_1+sC_2\right]=V_ssC_1 \tag{7.10A}$$

$$-V_1sC_2+V_o\left[G_2+sC_2\right]=0 \tag{7.10B}$$

Thus,

$$\Delta = G_1 G_2 + sC_2 C_1 + sC_1 G_2 + sC_2 G_2 + s^2 C_1 C_2 + s^2 C_2^2 - sC_2 G_1 - s^2 C_2^2$$
$$= G_1 G_2 + s[C_1 G_2 + C_2 G_2] + s^2[C_1 C_2] \tag{7.11}$$

and:

$$\Delta V_o = V_s\, s^2\, C_1 C_2 \tag{7.12}$$

The S & K HPF transfer function is thus:

$$\frac{V_o}{V_s}(s) = \frac{s^2 C_1 C_2}{s^2[C_1 C_2] + s[C_1 G_2 + C_2 G_2] + G_1 G_2} \tag{7.13}$$

When top and bottom are multiplied by $R_1 R_2$,

$$\frac{V_o}{V_s}(s) = \frac{s^2 C_1 C_2 R_1 R_2}{s^2 C_2 C_1 R_1 R_2 + sR_1[C_1 + C_2] + 1} \tag{7.14}$$

Now if $C_1 = C_2 = C$, the final form of the HPF transfer function is obtained:

$$\frac{V_o}{V_s}(s) = \frac{s^2 C^2 R_1 R_2}{s^2 C^2 R_1 R_2 + sR_1 2C + 1} \tag{7.15}$$

where $\omega_{nh} = 1/[C\sqrt{R_1 R_2}]$ r/s, and $\xi_h = \sqrt{R_1 R_2}$.

An S & K LPF put in series with an S & K HPF yields a fourth-order band-pass filter with two low-frequency C-C poles at ω_{nh}, a mid-band gain of 1, and a pair of C-C poles from the LPF at ω_{nlo}. Clearly, $\omega_{nh} < \omega_{nlo}$. (The BPF is fourth order because it has four poles.) The damping factors, ξ_h and ξ_{lo}, determine the amount of ringing or transient settling time when the BPF is presented with a transient input such as an ECG QRS spike. ξ is usually set between 0.707 and 0.5.

A final S & K filter to consider is the quadratic BPF shown in Figure 7.4. The filter's transfer function is found by first writing the node equations on the V_1 and $V_2 = V_o$ nodes:

$$V_1[G_1 + G_3 + sC_1] - V_o[G_3 + sC_1] = V_s G_1 \tag{7.16A}$$

$$-V_1 sC_1 + V_o[G_2 + s(C_1 + C_2)] = 0 \tag{7.16B}$$

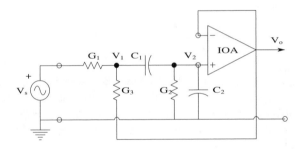

FIGURE 7.4
A Sallen and Key quadratic band-pass filter.

The determinant is:

$$\Delta = G_1 G_2 + s C_1 G_1 + s C_2 G_1 + G_3 G_2 + s C_1 G_3 + s C_2 G_3 + s C_1 G_2$$
$$+ s^2 C_1^2 + s^2 C_1 C_2 - s C_1 G_3 - s^2 C_1^2 \tag{7.17}$$
$$= G_2 (G_1 + G_3) + s[C_1 (G_1 + G_2) + C_2 (G_1 + G_3)] + s^2 C_1 C_2$$

and V_o is found from:

$$\Delta V_o = V_s \, s \, C_1 G_1 \tag{7.18}$$

The BP transfer function is written first as:

$$\frac{V_o}{V_s}(s) = \frac{s C_1 G_1}{s^2 C_1 C_2 + s[C_1 (G_1 + G_2) + C_2 (G_1 + G_3)] + G_2 (G_1 + G_3)} \tag{7.19}$$

To simplify, let $C_1 = C_2 = C$ and multiply top and bottom by $R_1 R_2 R_3$:

$$\frac{V_o}{V_s}(s) = \frac{s C R_2 R_3}{s^2 C^2 R_1 R_2 R_3 + s C R_2 [2R_3 + R_1] + (R_3 + R_1)} \tag{7.20}$$

Next, to put the transfer function in time-constant form, divide top and bottom by $(R_3 + R_1)$:

$$\frac{V_o}{V_s}(s) = \frac{s C R_2 R_3 / (R_3 + R_1)}{s^2 C^2 R_1 R_2 R_3 / (R_3 + R_1) + s C R_2 [(2R_3 + R_1)/(R_3 + R_1)] + 1} \tag{7.21}$$

The filter's $\omega_n = 1/[C\sqrt{(R_1 R_2 R_3)/(R_3 + R_1)}]$ r/s; its peak gain at $\omega = \omega_n$ is $R_3/(2 R_3 + R_1)$ and the BPF's Q is:

$$Q = 1/2\xi = \frac{\sqrt{R_1 R_2 R_3 (R_3 + R_1)}}{R_2 (2R_3 + R_1)} \tag{7.22}$$

The S & K BPF's peak gain and Q are independent of C; C can be used to set ω_n, once the three resistors are chosen to find the desired Q and peak gain. This is not as easy to design as the S & K LPF and HPF filter.

Before closing this section on Sallen and Key controlled (voltage)-source quadratic filters, it should be noted that the designer must simulate the filter's behavior with an accurate model of the op amp to be used in order to predict the filter's behavior at high frequencies (near the op amp's fT), as well as how the filter behaves with transient inputs.

7.2.3   Biquad Active Filters

For many filter applications, the biquad architecture offers ease in design when two-pole filters are desired; independent setting of ω_n, ξ and mid-band gain, K_{vo}, are possible with few components (Rs and Cs). There are two biquad AF architectures: one-loop and two-loop. One cost of the biquad AFs is that they use more than one op amp (three or four) to realize that which an S & K AF can do with one op amp. The benefit of the biquad architecture is ease in design. Figure 7.5 shows the one- and two-loop configurations.

The two-loop biquad's transfer functions will be analyzed at the V_3, V_4, and V_5 output nodes. The output at the V_5 node is low pass; this can be shown by writing the transfer function using Mason's rule (Northrop, 1990, Appendix A):

$$\frac{V_5}{V_S}(s) = \frac{(-R/R_1)(-R/R_2)(-1/sR_3C)(-1/sR_3C)}{1 - \left[(-1)(-R/R_2)(-1/sR_3C) + (-1)(-1/sR_3C)^2\right]} \tag{7.23}$$

This LPF transfer function can be simplified algebraically to time-constant form:

$$\frac{V_5}{V_S}(s) = \frac{R^2/R_1 R_2}{s^2 R_3^2 C^2 + s\left[RR_3 C/R_2\right] + 1} \tag{7.24}$$

By comparison with the standard quadratic polynomial form,

$$\omega_n = 1/R_3 C \text{ r/s} \quad (\omega_n \text{ set by } R_3 \text{ and } C) \tag{7.25A}$$

$$\xi = R/2R_2 \quad \text{(damping factor set by } R_2) \tag{7.25B}$$

$$K_{vo} = R^2/R_1 R_2 \quad \text{(dc gain set by } R_1, \text{ once } R_2 \text{ is chosen)} \tag{7.25C}$$

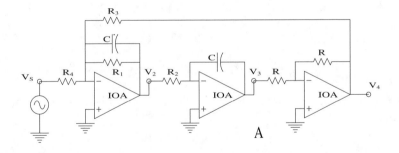

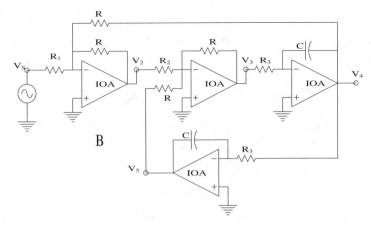

FIGURE 7.5
(A) The three-op amp, one-loop biquad active filter. (B) The four-op amp, two-loop biquad active filter.

Next, consider the transfer function for V_4. Note that the denominator is the same as for the V_5 transfer function:

$$\frac{V_4}{V_S}(s) = \frac{(-R/R_1)(-R/R_2)(-1/sR_3C)}{1-\left[(-1)(-R/R_2)(-1/sR_3C)+(-1)(-1/sR_3C)^2\right]} \tag{7.26}$$

Multiplying the numerator and denominator of Equation 7.26 by $(-1/sR_3C)^2$ yields:

$$\frac{V_4}{V_S}(s) = \frac{-sR^2R_3C/(R_1R_2)}{s^2R_3^2C^2+s\left[RR_3C/R_2\right]+1} \tag{7.27}$$

which is a quadratic BPF. The filter parameters are:

$$\omega_n = 1/R_3 C \text{ r/s} \quad (\omega_n \text{ set by } R_3 \text{ and } C) \tag{7.28A}$$

$$Q = R_2/R \qquad (Q \text{ set by } R_2: Q = 1/2\, \xi) \tag{7.28B}$$

$$K_{vo} = R/R_1 \qquad (\text{peak gain at } \omega_n \text{ set by } R_1) \tag{7.28C}$$

Finally, examine the transfer function to the V_3 node. By Mason's rule,

$$\frac{V_3}{V_S}(s) = \frac{\left(-R/R_1\right)\left(-R/R_2\right)}{1 - \left[(-1)\left(-R/R_2\right)\left(-1/sR_3C\right) + (-1)\left(-1/sR_3C\right)^2\right]} \tag{7.29}$$

Again, divide numerator and denominator of Equation 7.29 by $(-1/sR_3C)^2$ and obtain the transfer function of a quadratic high-pass filter:

$$\frac{V_4}{V_S}(s) = \frac{s^2 R^2 R_3^2 C^2 / \left(R_1 R_2\right)}{s^2 R_3^2 C^2 + s\left[RR_3 C/R_2\right] + 1} \tag{7.30}$$

As before:

$$\omega_n = 1/R_3 C \text{ r/s} \tag{7.31A}$$

$$\xi = R/2R_2 \tag{7.31B}$$

$$K_{vhi} = R^2/(R_1 R_2) \tag{7.31C}$$

An interesting benefit from the biquad AF design is the ability to realize quadratic notch and all-pass configurations with the aid of another op amp adder. An ideal notch filter has a pair of conjugate zeros on the $j\omega$ axis in the s-plane; its transfer function is of the form:

$$\frac{V_n}{V_S}(s) = \frac{s^2/\omega_n^2 + 1}{s^2/\omega_n^2 + s/(Q\omega_n) + 1} \tag{7.32}$$

Clearly, when s = $j\omega_n$, $|V_n/V_S(j\omega_n)| = 0$. Figure 7.6 illustrates how a biquad AF and an op amp adder can be used to realize a notch filter of the form modeled by Equation 7.32.

The biquad + op amp summer architecture can also be used to realize a quadratic all-pass filter in which a pair of complex-conjugate zeros is found in the right-half s-plane with positive real parts the same magnitude as the C-C poles in the left-half s-plane. The general form of this filter is:

$$\frac{V_{ap}}{V_S}(s) = \frac{s^2/\omega_n^2 - s2\xi/\omega_n + 1}{s^2/\omega_n^2 + s2\xi/\omega_n + 1} \tag{7.33}$$

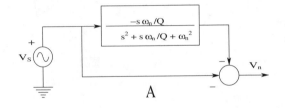

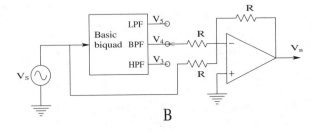

FIGURE 7.6
(A) Block diagram showing how a notch filter can be formed from a quadratic BF. (B) A practical circuit showing how a two-loop biquad's V_4 BPF output can be added to V_s to make the notch filter.

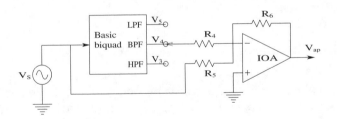

FIGURE 7.7
A practical circuit showing how a two-loop biquad's V_4 BPF output can be added to V_s to make a quadratic all-pass filter.

Figure 7.7 illustrates the circuit architecture used to realize a symmetrical APF. The APF output is given by:

$$V_{ap} = R_6[V_S/R_5 + V_4/R_4] \tag{7.34}$$

Now substitute the transfer function for the BPF into Equation 7.34 to get the APF transfer function:

$$\frac{V_{ap}}{V_S}(s) = -\left[R_6/R_5 + \frac{(R_6/R_4)(-sR^2R_3C/R_1R_2)}{s^2R_3^2C^2 + s[RR_3C/R_2] + 1}\right] \tag{7.35}$$

$$= -\left[\frac{(R_6/R_5)s^2R_3^2C^2 + (R_6/R_5)s[RR_3C/R_2] + (R_6/R_5) - (R_6/R_4)(sR^2R_3C/R_1R_2)}{s^2R_3^2C^2 + s[RR_3C/R_2] + 1}\right]$$

To obtain the symmetric APF, let $R_1 = R$; $R_5 = 2R_4$; and $R_6 = R_5$. The desired transfer function is then:

$$\frac{V_{ap}}{V_S}(s) = -\frac{s^2 R_3^2 C^2 - s R_3 CR/R_2 + 1}{s^2 R_3^2 C^2 + s R_3 CR/R_2 + 1} \tag{7.36}$$

The natural frequency of poles and zeros is:

$$\omega_n = 1/R_3 C \text{ r/s} \tag{7.37A}$$

$$\xi = R/2R_2 \tag{7.37B}$$

$$K_{vo} = -1, -\infty \le \omega \le \infty \tag{7.37C}$$

The purpose of all-pass filters is to generate a phase shift with frequency with no attenuation; the phase of the APF described earlier can be shown to be:

$$\varphi = -\pi - 2\tan^{-1}\left[\frac{\omega R_3 CR/R_2}{1 - \omega^2 R_3 2C^3}\right] \text{ radians} \tag{7.38}$$

7.2.4 Generalized Impedance Converter AFs

Often one wishes to design AFs that work at very low frequencies, e.g., below 20 Hz. Such filters can find application in conditioning low-frequency physiological signals such as the ECG, EEG, and heart sounds. If a conventional biquad AF is used to make a high-pass filter whose $f_n = 1$ Hz, for example, it is necessary to obtain very large capacitors that are expensive and take up excessive volume on a PC board. For example, the capacitor required for $f_n = 1$ Hz and $R_3 = 100$ kΩ is:

$$C = \frac{1}{2\pi f_n R_3} = 1.59 \text{ μF} \tag{7.39}$$

The GIC circuit, shown in general format in Figure 7.8, allows the size of a small capacitor, e.g., 0.001 μF, to be magnified electronically, transformed into a large, equivalent, very high-Q inductor, or made into a D-element that can be shown to have the impedance, $Z_D(\omega) = 1/(\omega^2 D)$, where D is determined by certain R_s and C_s as shown next.

Find an expression for the driving point impedance of the general GIC circuit, $\mathbf{Z_{11}} = \mathbf{V_1}/\mathbf{I_1}$. Clearly, from Ohm's law:

$$\mathbf{Z_{11}} = \mathbf{V_1}/\mathbf{I_1} = \frac{\mathbf{V_1}}{(\mathbf{V_1} - \mathbf{V_2})/\mathbf{Z_1}} \tag{7.40}$$

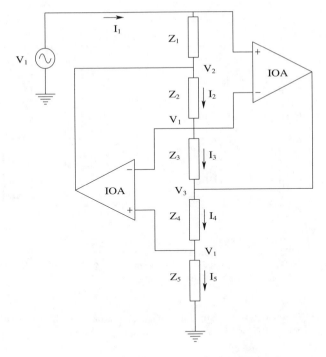

FIGURE 7.8
General architecture for a generalized impedance converter (GIC) circuit. The Z_k can be resistances or capacitances $(1/j\omega C_k)$, depending on the filter requirement.

Also, from the ideal op amp assumption and Ohm's law, it is possible to write the currents:

$$I_2 = (V_2 - V_1)/Z_2 = I_3 = (V_1 - V_3)/Z_3 \qquad (7.41)$$

$$I_4 = (V_3 - V_1)/Z_4 = I_5 = V_1/Z_5 \qquad (7.42)$$

From the Equation 7.40, Equation 7.41, and Equation 7.42, it is easy to show:

$$V_3 = V_1(1 + Z_4/Z_5) \qquad (7.43)$$

$$V_2 = V_1\left(\frac{Z_3 Z_5 - Z_2 Z_4}{Z_3 Z_5}\right) \qquad (7.44)$$

and the GIC driving point impedance is given compactly as:

$$Z_{11} = V_1/I_1 = Z_1 Z_3 Z_5/(Z_2 Z_4) \text{ complex ohms} \qquad (7.45)$$

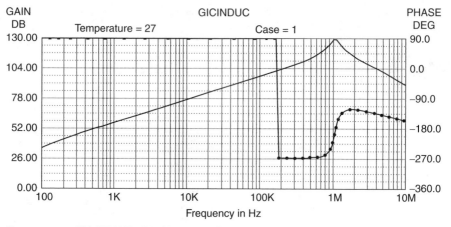

Frequency   = 100.00000E + 05   Hz   Gain   = 89.003 Db
Phase angle = –158.263   Degrees   Group delay = 0.00000E + 00
Gain slope   = –114.36240E – 01 Db/Oct   Peak gain   = 128.556 Db/F = 107.01700E + 04
1: Another run   2: Analysis limits   3: Quit   4: Dump

FIGURE 7.9
Magnitude and phase of $Z_{11}(f)$ looking into a GIC emulation of a 0.1-HY inductor. In this MicroCap simulation, TL072 op amps were used. Smooth line is magnitude.

Now if Z_2 or $Z_4 = 1/j\omega C$ (a capacitor) and the other elements are resistors, Z_{11} has the form:

$$Z_{11} = j\omega \, [C_4 \, R_1 R_3 R_5/R_2] \text{ reactive (inductive) ohms} \qquad (7.46)$$

that is, the GIC emulates a low-loss inductor over a wide range of frequency. The inductance of the emulated inductor is:

$$L_{eq} = [C_4 \, R_1 R_3 R_5/R_2] \text{ Hy} \qquad (7.47)$$

Figure 7.9 illustrates the magnitude and phase response of an inductive Z_{11} vs. frequency. Using MicroCap™, $20 \log |Z_{11}(f)|$ and $\angle \, Z_{11}(f)$ vs. f are plotted. The circuit used in this simulation is the same as in Figure 7.8, with $Z_1 = Z_3 = Z_4 = Z_5 = 1 \text{ k}\Omega$ and $Z_2 = 1/j\omega C_2$; $C_2 = 0.1 \text{ μF}$.

Equation 7.47 shows that the simulated inductance is 0.1 Hy. (Op amp output current saturation effects are not included in this simple simulation.) Note that $|Z_{11}(f)|$ increases linearly with frequency until about 180 kHz, at which its phase abruptly goes from the ideal +90 to –270°, and $20 \log |Z_{11}(f)|$ exhibits a tall peak at approximately 1 MHz. Clearly, the circuit model emulates a 0.1-Hy inductor below 180 kHz. A simple nonsaturating, two-time-constant model of the TL082 op amp was used in the MicroCap simulation.

Because the GIC inductive Z_{11} is referenced to ground, it must be used in active filters that require inductors with one end tied to ground. Figure 7.10(A) illustrates an inductive GIC used in a simple high-Q, quadratic BPF.

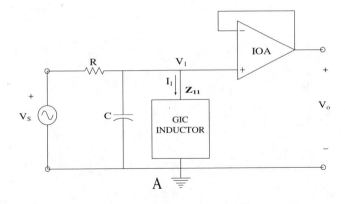

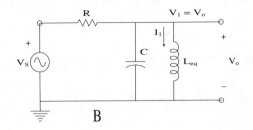

FIGURE 7.10

(A) Circuit of an *RLC* band-pass filter using the GIC inductor. The GIC circuit allows emulation of a very large, high-*Q* inductor over a wide range of frequencies and is particularly well suited for making filters in the subaudio range of frequencies. (B) The actual BPF.

Figure 7.10(B) illustrates a simple *R–L–C* BPF suitable for circuit analysis. A node equation gives the BPF's transfer function:

$$\frac{V_o}{V_S}(s) = \frac{s L_{eq}/R}{s^2 C L_{eq} + s L_{eq}/R + 1} \tag{7.48}$$

In this filter:

$$\omega_n = 1/\sqrt{C L_{eq}} \ \ \text{r/s} \tag{7.49A}$$

$$Q = 1/(2\xi) = R\sqrt{C/L_{eq}} \tag{7.49B}$$

$$\frac{V_o}{V_S}(j\omega_n) = 1\angle 0° \tag{7.49C}$$

L_{eq} is given by Equation 7.47.

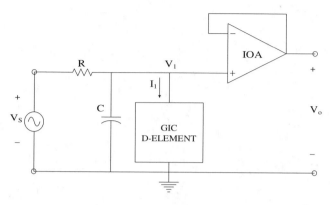

FIGURE 7.11
Circuit showing how a GIC "D" element can make a low-frequency, low-pass filter.

The GIC "D element" Z_{11} is a frequency-dependent negative resistance (FDNR) that can be made by putting capacitors in the Z_1 and Z_3 positions in the GIC circuit. Thus, the driving point impedance is real and negative:

$$Z_{11} = \frac{(1/j\omega C_1)(1/j\omega C_3)R_5}{R_2 R_4} = \frac{-R_5}{\omega^2 C_1 C_3 R_2 R_5} = \frac{-1}{\omega^2 D} \text{ ohms} \qquad (7.50)$$

$$D = C_1 C_3 R_2 R_4 / R_5 \qquad (7.51)$$

Figure 7.11 shows that the D element can make a quadratic LPF. Write the node equation for V_o in terms of the Laplace complex variable, s:

$$V_o [G + sC + s^2 D] = V_S G \qquad (7.52)$$

Solving for V_o yields:

$$\frac{V_o}{V_S}(s) \equiv \frac{1}{s^2 DR + sCR + 1} \qquad (7.53)$$

Clearly, for the GID FDNR LPF,

$$\omega_n = 1/\sqrt{DR} \text{ r/s} \qquad (7.54A)$$

$$\xi = (C/2)\sqrt{R/D} \qquad (7.54B)$$

By using relation Equation 7.44 for V_2/V_S, it is possible to realize notch and all-pass filters from the basic GIC circuit. Figure 7.12 and Figure 7.13 illustrate examples of these filters. Readers can develop their transfer functions as exercises.

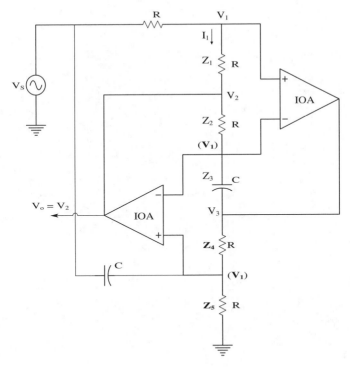

FIGURE 7.12
A GIC all-pass filter.

In summary, note again that the major reason for using the GIC architecture is to realize AFs that are useful at very low frequencies, e.g., 0.01 to 10 Hz, without having to use expensive, very large capacitances.

7.3 Electronically Tunable AFs

7.3.1 Introduction

In many biomedical instrumentation systems, a conditioned (by filtering) analog signal is periodically sampled and digitized. The digital number sequence is then further processed by certain digital algorithms that can include, but are not limited to: signal averaging; computation of signal statistics (e.g., mean, RMS value, etc.); computation of the discrete Fourier transform; convolution with another signal or kernel; etc. The computer is often used to change the input filter's parameters (half-power frequencies or center frequency; damping factor or Q) to accommodate a new sampling rate or changes in the analog signal's power spectrum.

A particular application of a computer-controlled analog filter is the anti-aliasing (A-A) low-pass filter. In order to prevent aliasing and the problems

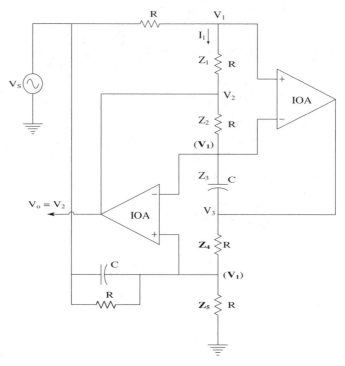

FIGURE 7.13
A GIC notch filter.

this creates for the signal in digital form, the A-A filter must pass no significant signal spectral power to the analog-to-digital converter at frequencies above one half the sampling frequency, f_s. $f_s/2$ is called the *Nyquist frequency, f_n.* (See Section 10.2 in Chapter 10 for a complete treatment of sampling and aliasing.)

The key to designing a digitally tuned filter is the variable gain element (VGE) (Northrop, 1990, Section 10.1). The design of digitally-controlled variable gain elements (DCVGEs) has several approaches: one uses a digital-to-analog converter (DAC) configured to produce 0 to 10 Vdc output, V_C, which is the input to an analog multiplier IC; the other input to the analog multiplier is the time-variable analog signal, $v_k(t)$, whose amplitude is to be adjusted. The output of the analog multiplier is then $v_k'(t) = v_k(t)V_C/10$. $V_C/10$ varies from 0 to 1 in steps determined by the quantization set by the number of binary bits input to the DAC. Another VGE is the digitally programmed gain amplifier (DPGA), with a gain digitally selected in 6-dB steps (i.e., 1, 2, 4, 8, 16, 32, 64, and 128) using a 3-bit input word (e.g., the MN2020). Still another class of DCVGE is represented by the AD8400, 8-bit, digitally controlled potentiometer (DCP) connected as a variable resistor. The DCP resistance is given by:

$$V_j' = R_{total} \sum_{k=1}^{N} B_k 2^{k-(1+N)} = R_{total} A_k \qquad (7.55)$$

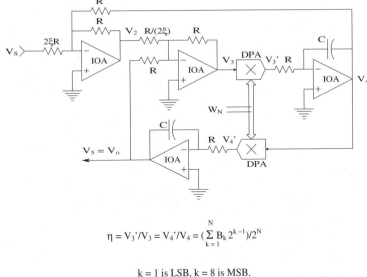

$$\eta = V_3'/V_3 = V_4'/V_4 = (\sum_{k=1}^{N} B_k 2^{k-1})/2^N$$

$k = 1$ is LSB, $k = 8$ is MSB.

$W_N = \{B_k\}$ input (control) word

FIGURE 7.14
The use of two parallel digitally controlled attenuators to tune the break frequency of a two-loop biquad low-pass filter at constant damping. See text for analysis.

where N is the number of bits controlling the DCP and B_k is the kth bit state (0 or 1). Note that the DCP is similar in operation to a 2-quadrant multiplying digital-to-analog converter (MDAC), which also can be used as a DCVGE (Northrop, 1990).

The following sections examine how DCVGEs can tune a two-loop biquad A-A LPF's ω_n and Q.

7.3.2 The Tunable Two-Loop Biquad LPF

Figure 7.14 illustrates the schematic of a 2-loop biquad LPF with digital control of its natural frequency at constant damping using 8-bit digitally controlled attenuators (DCAs). (One form of a DCA that uses DPP is shown in Figure 7.15.) It is easy to derive this digitally tuned LPF's transfer function using Mason's rule:

$$\frac{V_o}{V_S}(s) = \frac{(-1/2\xi)(-2\xi)(\eta)(-1/sRC)(\eta)(-1/sRC)}{1 - \left[(-1)(-2\xi)(\eta)(-1/sRC) + (-1)(\eta)(-1/sRC)(\eta)(-1/sRC)\right]} \quad (7.56A)$$

$$\downarrow$$

$$\frac{V_o}{V_S}(s) = \frac{1}{s^2(RC/\eta)^2 + s(RC/\eta)(2\xi) + 1} \quad (7.56B)$$

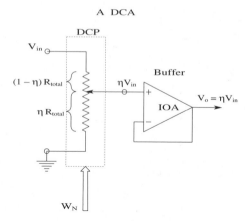

FIGURE 7.15
Schematic of a digitally controlled attenuator (DCA).

From the standard quadratic format:

$$\omega_n = \eta/RC \text{ r/s} \tag{7.57}$$

The constant damping, ξ, is set by the size of the input resistor ($2\,\xi R$) and the resistor size V_2 sees ($R/2\,\xi$). Thus, with 1 LSB in, $W_n = \{0,0,0,0,0,0,0,1\}$, $\omega_n = (1/256)(1/RC)$ r/s; with $W_N = \{1,1,1,1,1,1,1,1\}$, $\omega_n = (255/256)(1/RC)$ r/s. The dc gain of the filter is +1.

As a second example, consider the digitally controlled band-pass filter shown in Figure 7.16 in which two N-bit, serial binary words (W_{N1} and W_{N2}) are used to set the filter's natural frequency, ω_n, and a third variable gain element is used to adjust the filter's Q. In this example, digitally controlled amplifier gains are used. Using Mason's rule as before, the transfer function can be written as:

$$\frac{V_4}{V_S}(s) = \frac{(-1)\mathbf{A_1}(-1/128)\mathbf{A_2}(-1/sRC)}{1-\left[(-1)\mathbf{A_1}(-1/128)\mathbf{A_2}(-1/sRC)+(-1)\mathbf{A_2}(-1/sRC)\mathbf{A_2}(-1/sRC)\right]} \tag{7.58}$$

$$\downarrow$$

$$\frac{V_4}{V_S}(s) = \frac{-s(\mathbf{A_1}/\mathbf{A_2})RC/128}{s^2(RC/\mathbf{A_2})^2+sRC(\mathbf{A_1}/\mathbf{A_2})/128+1} \tag{7.59}$$

where the resonant frequency is set by $\mathbf{A_2}$ and the Q by $1/\mathbf{A_1}$:

$$\omega_n = \mathbf{A_2}/RC \text{ r/s} \tag{7.60A}$$

$$Q = 128/\mathbf{A_1} \tag{7.60B}$$

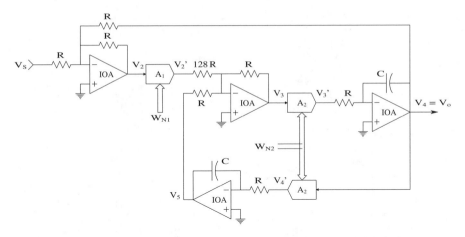

FIGURE 7.16
In this digitally tuned biquad BPF, digitally controlled amplifier gains are used to set ω_n and the Q.

$$\frac{V_4}{V_S}(\omega_n) = -1 \; (\text{peak gain}) \qquad (7.60\text{C})$$

Note that the $\mathbf{A_1}$ digitally controlled variable-gain amplifier drives a resistor of 128R so that the effective gain from V_2 to V_3 is $(-\mathbf{A_1}/128)$. $\mathbf{A_1}$ values are typically (1, 2, 4, 8, 16, 32, 64, 128), so the BPF's Q values are (128, 64, 32, 16, 8, 4, 2, 1). Thus, the digital word, W_{N2}, can be used to scan the filter's center frequency over a 1:128 range under constant Q conditions or the BPF's Q can be adjusted independently with W_{N1}.

7.3.3 Use of Digitally Controlled Potentiometers To Tune a Sallen and Key LPF

Digitally controlled potentiometers (DCPs) are IC devices based on the nMOS and CMOS transistor switch technology used in certain ADCs. Figure 7.17(A) illustrates the schematic of a simple analog (mechanical) potentiometer. Note that the potentiometer has three leads: two to the fixed resistor (CW and CCW) and the third (variable) connection called the *wiper* (W). In Figure 7.17(B), the potentiometer is connected as a variable resistor. Figure 7.17(C) illustrates a digitally programmed IC potentiometer. Only one MOS transistor switch is closed at a time connecting a node in the series resistor array to the wiper. The resistors are generally polycrystalline silicon deposited on an oxide layer for electrical isolation. They can have equal values (linear potentiometer) or be given values to approximate logarithmic attenuation.

Typically, DCPs have 256 (discrete) taps and thus an 8-bit serial input word is needed to select the wiper position. Like mechanical (analog) potentiometers, DCPs can be given the potentiometer (voltage divider) configuration

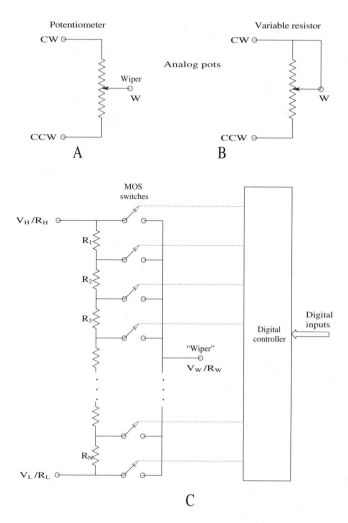

FIGURE 7.17

(A) Schematic of a conventional mechanically tuned analog potentiometer. (B) A potentiometer connected as a variable resistor. (C) A digitally programmed analog potentiometer. Only one MOS switch is closed at a time. An 8-bit digital pot has 256 taps.

or be used as variable resistances. Manufacturers of DCPs include Analog Devices, Maxim, and Xicor.

A DCP connected as a variable resistor can be used to set an AF's filtering parameters (ω_n, gain, and Q or damping). Figure 7.18 illustrates the use of two DCPs (with the same control input) to tune an S & K LPF at constant damping by varying R. Recall that the natural frequency of an S & K LPF's poles is at $\omega_n = 1/(R\sqrt{C_1 C_2})$ r/s, and its damping factor is solely determined by the square root of the ratio of the capacitors; e.g., $\xi = \sqrt{C_2 C_1}$. Thus, for this LPF, $\omega_n = 1/(R_{dp}\sqrt{C_1 C_2})$ r/s. Note that ω_n varies hyperbolically with R_{dp}.

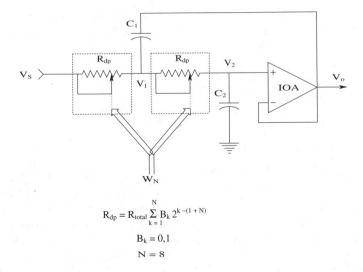

$$R_{dp} = R_{total} \sum_{k=1}^{N} B_k 2^{k-(1+N)}$$

$$B_k = 0,1$$

$$N = 8$$

FIGURE 7.18

A pair of digitally controlled potentiometers are used as variable resistors in a digitally tuned Sallen and Key low-pass filter.

Many examples exist of electronically tuned AFs (see Chapter 10 in Northrop, 1990). Analog voltages or currents derived from DACs, or serial or parallel digital words can be used to set resistors or gains in DCVGEs. (A classic example of adaptive filter design is the venerable Dolby B™ audio noise reduction system; this system is treated in detail in Chapter 10 of Northrop (1990)).

7.4 Filter Applications (Anti-Aliasing, SNR Improvement, etc.)

Most analog active filters used in biomedical signal conditioning are intended to restrict the amplifier pass band to that of the signal spectrum, thereby cutting off broadband noise outside the signal spectrum and improving the signal-to-noise ratio at the filter output over that at the input to the signal conditioning system. Another major application of active filters is anti-aliasing, i.e., attenuating signal and noise power at the input to an analog-to-digital converter to a negligible level at frequencies of half the sampling frequency and greater.

In modern ECG and EEG data acquisition systems, one often finds an optional notch filter that can be used to attenuate coherent interference (hum) at line frequency (60 Hz). All-pass filters are used to generate a phase shift between the input and output signal without attenuation. These filters are used to adjust synchronization signal phase in lock-in amplifiers and synchronous rectifiers, and to correct for phase lags inherent in data transmission on coaxial cables and other transmission lines.

7.5   Chapter Summary

7.5.1   Active Filters

There are many op amp active filter architectures. Some are easier to use in designing than others. This chapter focused on the easy ones: the controlled-source Sallen and Key filters; the biquad active filter family; and filters based on the generalized impedance converter circuit (GIC). Also covered were the design and analysis of electronically tunable active filters using variable-gain elements such as analog multipliers, multiplying DACs, digitally controlled potentiometers, and digitally controlled gain amplifiers. Electronically tuned filters have application as anti-aliasing filters and tuned filters that can track a coherent signal's frequency — to compensate for Doppler shift, for example.

Although not covered in this chapter, a family of active filters called *switched-capacitor filters* (SCFs) are primarily used in telecommunications. The SCFs use MOS switches to commute capacitors in what would otherwise be an op amp, R–C filter design. The switched capacitor can be shown to emulate a resistor of value $R_{eq} = T_c/C_s$, where T_c is the period of the commutation and C_s is the switched capacitor value. The interested reader can consult Section 9.2 in Northrop (1990).

7.5.2   Choice of AF Components

Because most analog AFs used in biomedical applications operate on signals in the 0- to 5-kHz range, overall filter high-frequency response is often not an important consideration. Instead, concern is with noise, linearity, dc drift, and stability of parameter settings (dc gain, ω_n, and damping, ξ). To minimize noise and maximize parameter stability, metal film resistors (or wire-wound resistors) with low tempcos are generally chosen.

Choice of capacitors is important in determining filter linearity. Some capacitor dielectrics exhibit excessive losses, unidirectional dc leakage, and dielectric hysteresis; thus they can distort filtered signals. In particular, electrolytic and tantalum dielectric capacitors *are not* recommended for AF components; they are usually used for bypassing applications where they are operated with a fixed dc voltage bias. Polycarbonate dielectric capacitors can also distort signals. The best capacitor dielectrics are air, mica, ceramic, oiled paper, and mylar. Again, low tempcos are desired. Do not be tempted to use electrolytic or tantalum capacitors in an AF design that requires large capacitor values in order to realize a low ω_n. Instead, use a GIC design for the filter that uses smaller Cs.

Op amps used in AFs also must be chosen for dc stability (low offset voltage tempco), low noise, and high dc gain. Filters used at high frequencies (>10 kHz) generally require op amps with appropriately high f_Ts. All high-frequency filters should be simulated with an electronic circuit analysis program such as MicroCap or a flavor of SPICE™ to ensure that no surprises will occur at high frequencies.

Home Problems

7.1 The active filter circuit of Figure P7.1 is a version of a notch (band reject) filter. Assume the op amps are ideal.

    a. Find an expression for the transfer function of the filter in time-constant form. Let $RC = \tau$.

    b. Find the β value that will make the filter an ideal notch filter, i.e., put conjugate zeros exactly on the $j\omega$ axis. Give an expression for the center frequency of the notch. What is the dc gain of the filter?

    c. Now make the op amps be TI TL072. Use an ECAP to simulate the frequency response of the notch filter. Set the notch frequency to 60 Hz. Use the ideal β value. Explain why the notch does not go to $-\infty$ at 60 Hz. At what frequencies is the filter down -3 dB?

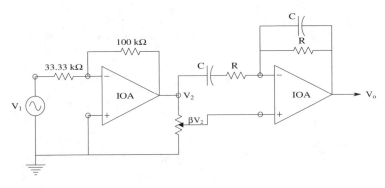

FIGURE P7.1

7.2 Consider the Sallen and Key high-pass filter shown in text Figure 7.3.

    a. Design an HPF with pass-band gain of unity, $f_n = 100$ Hz, and $\xi = 0.707$. Use a TL071 op amp. Specify circuit parameters.

    b. Use an ECAP Bode plot to verify your design. Give the -3-dB frequencies of the filter and its high- and low-frequency f_Ts.

7.3 Derive an expression for the transfer function of the active filter of Figure P7.3 in time constant form. Give expressions for the filter's ω_n, dc gain, and damping factors of the numerator and denominator.

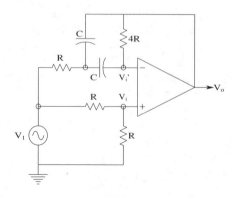

FIGURE P7.3

7.4   Design a band-pass filter for neural spike signal conditioning using two cascaded quadratic Sallen and Key active filters (1 LP, 1 HiP) with the following specifications: mid-band gain = 0 dB; −3 dB f_{LO} = 300 Hz; ξ_{LO} = 0.5; −3 dB f_{HI} = 4 kHz; and ξ_{HI} = 0.5. (Note that the filter −3dB-frequencies are not necessarily their f_ns.) Use OP-27 op amps. Specify the R and C values. Note: all Rs must be between 10^3 and 10^6 Ω and C values must lie between 3 pF and 3 µF. Verify your design with a PSpice or MicroCap Bode plot.

7.5   Design a quadratic GIC band-pass filter for geophysical applications to condition a seismometer output having f_n = 1 Hz and Q = 10. Verify your design with a Bode plot done with MicroCap or PSpice. Use the same ranges of Rs and Cs as in the preceding problem.

7.6   For the three-op amp biquad AF shown in Figure P7.6

   a. Write the transfer function, V_4/V_1 in time-constant form.

   b. Write the transfer function, V_2/V_1, for the AF in TC form. Give expressions for ω_n, Q, and V_2/V_1 at ω_n.

   c. Write an expression for the transfer function, V_5/V_1, in time constant form. Use an ECAP to make a Bode plot of V_5/V_1. Let R = 1 kΩ; R_1 = 10 kΩ; R_4 = 1 kΩ; and C = 10 nF. Op amps are TL074s.

7.7   Find an expression for V_4/V_1 in time-constant form for the biquad AF shown in Figure P7.7. Give expressions for ω_n, Q and $|V_4/V_1|$ at ω_n. Assume ideal op amps.

7.8   Figure P7.8 illustrates a voltage-tunable, 1-pole LPF. An analog multiplier is used as the variable-gain element (VGE). The analog multiplier output V_3 = $-V_2 V_c/10$.

   a. Derive an expression for V_o/V_1 in time-constant form.

   b. Make a dimensioned Bode plot of V_o/V_1. Give expressions for the dc gain and the break frequency.

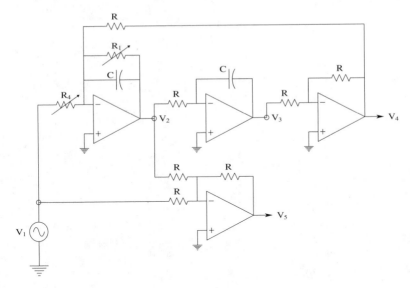

FIGURE P7.6

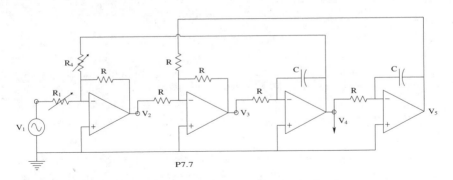

FIGURE P7.7

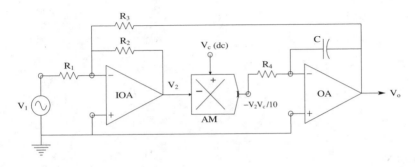

FIGURE P7.8

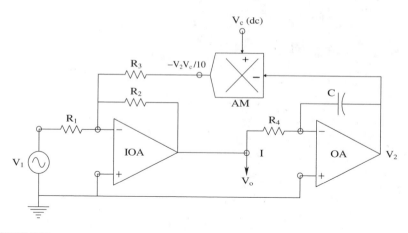

FIGURE P7.9

7.9   Figure P7.9 illustrates another voltage-tuned active filter.

    a.   Derive an expression for V_o/V_1 in time-constant form.

    b.   Make a dimensioned Bode plot of V_o/V_1. Give expressions for the dc gain and the break frequency.

7.10   The circuit of Figure P7.10 is an op amp AF realization of a Dolby B™ audio noise reduction system recording encoder. It is designed to boost the high-frequency response of magnetic tape-recorded signals containing little power at high frequencies in order to improve playback signal-to-noise ratio (when used in conjunction with a Dolby B™ decoder filter). (Magnetic tape has an omnipresent high-frequency background "hiss" on playback, regardless of signal strength.)

    a.   Derive an expression for V_o/V_1 in time-constant form.

    b.   Make a dimensioned Bode plot of V_o/V_1. Give expressions for the dc gain and the break frequencies.

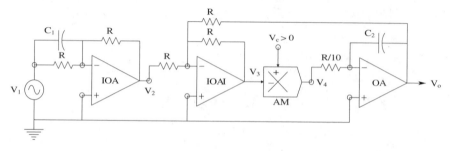

FIGURE P7.10

7.11 The circuit of Figure P7.11 is an op amp AF realization of a Dolby B™ audio noise reduction system decoder. It is designed to attenuate the high-frequency response of recorded signals containing high frequencies in order to improve playback signal-to-noise ratio (when used in conjunction with a Dolby B encoder filter).

a. Derive an expression for V_o/V_1 in time-constant form.

b. Make a dimensioned Bode plot of V_o/V_1. Give expressions for the dc gain and the break frequencies.

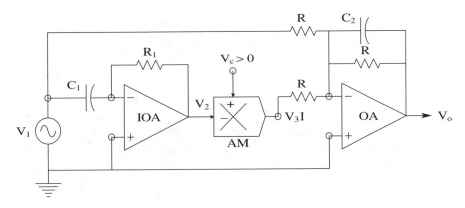

FIGURE P7.11

7.12 The circuit of Figure P7.12 is a digitally tunable biquad band-pass filter. MDACs are used as variable gain elements (VGEs). The analog input signal to the MDAC is multiplied by a fraction determined by the digital word input to the MDAC. For example, for MDAC1, its output is the analog signal:

$$V_3 = V_2 \frac{\displaystyle\sum_{1}^{N} D_{1k} 2^{k-1}}{2^N}$$

where N is the number of binary bits in the word, $D_{1k} = 0,1$; for $N = 8$, the maximum gain is 255/256 (All $D_{1k} = 1$) and the minimum gain is 0/256 (all $D_{1k} = 0$).

a. Find the transfer function, $(V_o/V_1)(s)$ in Laplace format.

b. Give expressions for the filter's ω_n, Q, and peak gain in terms of $\{D_{1k}\}$, $\{D_{2k}\}$, and system parameters. What is the range of Q? Assume $N = 8$ bits and the op amps are ideal.

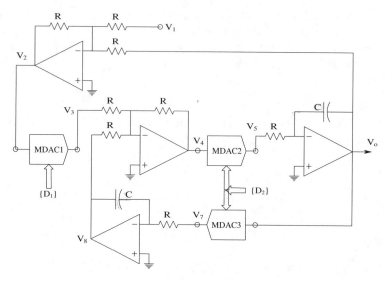

FIGURE P7.12

7.13 Derive the transfer function in time-constant form for the GIC all-pass filter of Figure 7.12 in the text.

7.14 Derive the transfer function in time-constant form for the GIC notch filter of Figure 7.13 in the text.

8

Instrumentation and Medical Isolation Amplifiers

8.1 Introduction

Instrumentation amplifiers (IAs) are basically differential amplifiers characterized by very high input impedance, very high common-mode rejection ratio (CMRR), and differential gain set by a single resistor, generally in the range from ×1 to ×1000. In addition, IAs also have low noise, offset voltage, bias current, and offset current.

Medical isolation amplifiers (IsoAs) provide an ultra-low conductive pathway between the input (patient) terminals and the output terminals and ground. This pathway provides what is called ohmic or galvanic isolation for a patient. In medical applications, this isolation is required for reasons of patient safety. The dc resistance between input and output terminals is typically on the order of gigaohms (thousands of megohms); at ac, capacitance between input and output terminals is on the order of single picofarad. There are five established isolation architectures

1. Transformer isolation in which power is coupled to the (isolated) input stage by high-frequency current and signal is coupled to the output stage also by transformer, by modulating the power supply oscillator frequency

2. Photo-optic coupling in which the isolated conditioned input signal is coupled to the output by means of photo-optic couplers (using an LED and a photodiode or photoresistor). Power is still supplied through high-frequency isolation transformer.

3. Capacitive coupling of a signal-modulated, high-frequency digital carrier from the isolated input stage through a pair of 1-pF capacitors to a demodulator in the output stage

4. Magnetic coupling using giant magnetoresistive resistors (GMRs) in a Wheatstone bridge. A GMR's resistance is altered by its local magnetic field. The isolated input signal is converted to a current

that is passed through coils in close proximity to two GMRs in a bridge. The ΔRs unbalance the bridge, which is on the output side of the IA. The unbalance is detected by a DA, which generates a current used to re-null the bridge. The renulling current is sensed and is proportional to the input voltage. Isolation is maintained by the ohmic isolation between the input coils and the GMR bridge resistors.

5. The flying capacitor chopper circuit uses a small capacitor charged up by the signal voltage and then switched by a high-speed DPDT relay to an output amplifier that reads the voltage across the capacitor. Such switched-capacitor IAs have ohmic isolation set by the relay structure and are useful only for dc or very low-frequency signals.

8.2   Instrumentation Amps

IAs, *per se*, are not suitable for medical applications because medical amplifiers require severe ohmic (galvanic) isolation. Medical amplifiers can use IAs in their front ends, however. Several IC manufacturers make IAs, e.g., Burr–Brown and Analog Devices.

This section first examines some of the properties of a low-cost, low-power IA, the AD620. This device can have its differential gain set from 1 to 10^3 by a single resistor. The −3-dB bandwidth (BW) varies with gain in accordance with the gain × bandwidth constancy relation. At $A_v = 10^3$, the BW is approximately 10 kHz; at $A_v = 100$, the BW is approximately 120 kHz; at $A_v = 10$, the BW is approximately 400 kHz; and at $A_v = 1$, the BW is approximately 1 MHz.

The equivalent short-circuit input voltage noise root power spectrum depends on A_v. For $A_v = 100$, 10^3, $e_{na} = 9$ nV/√Hz at 1 kHz. The input noise increases as the gain A_v decreases. Input current noise $i_{na} = 100$ fA RMS/√Hz, regardless of gain. The AD620's CMRR varies with gain, ranging from 90 dB at $A_v = 1$ to 130 dB at $A_v = 10^3$. This IA's input bias current, I_B, = 0.5 nA; the input offset voltage, V_{os}, is 15 µV. The input impedance is 10 GΩ ‖ 2 pF for common-mode and difference mode inputs (see Chapter 3).

A low-noise precision IA, the AMP01 by Analog Devices, offers slightly different specifications. The gain is set between 1 and 10^3 by a single resistor. The −3-dB bandwidths are approximately 26, 82, 100, and 570 kHz for gains of 10^3, 10^2, 10, and 1, respectively. The short-circuit input voltage noise root spectrum is 5 nV/√Hz at $A_v = 10^3$, and 1 kHz, and the current noise spectrum is 0.15 pA/√Hz at $A_v = 10^3$, and 1 kHz. The AMP01's input resistance is 1 GΩ for difference-mode signals at $A_v = 10^3$ and 20 GΩ for common-mode inputs at $A_v = 10^3$. The input bias current is typically 1 nA and the input offset

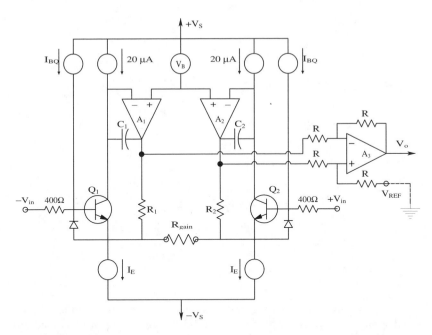

FIGURE 8.1
Simplified schematic of an Analog Devices' AD620 instrumentation amplifier.

voltage is typically ±20 µV. The AMP01's CMRR is 130, 130, 120, and 100 dB for gains of 10^3, 10^2, 10, and 1, respectively.

The advantage of using a "boughten" IA instead of a "homebrew" IA made from three op amps (see Section 3.7.2 in Chapter 3) is that, in order to meet the out-of-the-box CMRR specifications of the commercial IA, the designer needs resistors matched to at least 0.02% and the input op amps also need to be matched. Components matched to 0.02% are expensive in terms of time or of money. Figure 8.1 illustrates a simplified schematic of the AD620 from its data sheet supplied by Analog Devices. Super-beta transistors Q_1 and Q_2 connected as a differential pair are the input elements of this IA. The 400-Ω resistors and diodes at each transistor base serve to protect the IA from transient overvoltages. According to *Analog Devices* (1994):

> [Negative] [Feedback through the Q1–A1–R1 loop and the Q2–A2–R2 loop maintains constant collector current of the input devices Q1, Q2 thereby impressing the input voltage across the external gain setting resistor R_{gain}. This creates a differential gain from the inputs to the A1/A2 outputs given by G = (R1 + R2)/RG + 1. The unity gain subtractor [DA] A3 removes any common-mode signal, yielding a single-ended output referred to as the REF [V_{REF}] pin potential.

> The value of RG also determines the transconductance of the preamp stage. As RG is reduced for larger gains, the transconductance increases

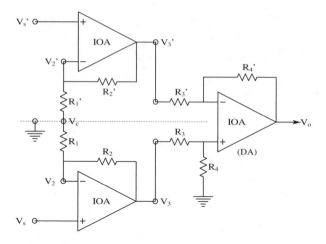

FIGURE 8.2
The three-op amp instrumentation amplifier.

asymptotically to that of the input transistors. This has three important advantages: (a) open-loop gain is boosted for increasing programmed gain, thus reducing gain-related errors. (b) The gain-bandwidth product (determined by C1, C2, and the preamp transconductance) increases with programmed gain, thus optimizing frequency response. (c) The input voltage noise is reduced to a value of 9 nV/√Hz, determined mainly by the collector current and base resistance of the input devices.

It is clear that the AD620 has many features that make it outperform the simple three-op amp IA shown in Figure 8.2. Given proper ohmic isolation, the AD620 can make an effective ECG amplifier. It can be run on batteries as low as ±2.3 V and its output can modulate a voltage-to-frequency converter (VFC), also battery powered, generating NBFM. The VFC's digital output can be coupled to the nonisolated world through a photo-optic coupler and thus be demodulated by conventional means, filtered, and further amplified.

8.3 Medical Isolation Amps

8.3.1 Introduction

All amplifiers used to record biopotential signals from humans (ECG, EEG, EMG, EOG, etc.) must meet certain safety standards for worst-case voltage breakdown and maximum leakage currents through their input leads attached to electrodes on the body, and maximum current through any driven output lead attached to the body. A variety of testing conditions or scenarios to ensure patient safety have been formulated by various regulatory agencies. The conservative leakage current and voltage breakdown criteria set by the National Fire Protection Association (NFPA; Quincy, MA) and the Association for the Advancement of Medical Instrumentation (AAMI) have generally been adopted by medical equipment manufacturers in the U.S. and by U.S. hospitals and other health care facilities. A number of other regulatory agencies also are involved in formulating and adopting electrical medical safety standards:

- International Electrotechnical Commission (IEC)
- Underwriters Laboratories (UL)
- Health Industries Manufacturers' Association (HEMA)
- National Electrical Manufacturers' Association (NEMA)
- U.S. Food and Drug Administration (FDA)

Most of the standards have been adopted to prevent patient electrocution, including burns, induction of fibrillation in the heart, pain, muscle spasms, etc.

Space does not permit detailing the effects of electroshock and the many scenarios by which it can occur. Nor can the technology of safe grounding practices and ground fault interruption be explored. The interested reader should consult Chapter 14 in Webster (1992) for comprehensive treatment of these details.

If the threshold ac heart surface current required to induce cardiac fibrillation in 50% of dogs tested is plotted vs. frequency, it is seen that the least current is required between 40 to 100 Hz. From 80 to 600 μA RMS of 60 Hz, current will induce cardiac fibrillation when applied directly to the heart, as through a catheter (Webster, 1992). Thus, the NFPA–ANSI/AAMI standard for ECG amplifier lead leakage is that isolated input lead current (at 60 Hz) must be <10 μA between any two leads shorted together and <10 μA for any input lead connected to the power plug ground (green wire) with and without the amplifier's case grounded. A more severe test is that isolation amplifier input lead leakage current must be <20 μA when any input lead is connected to the high side of the 120 Vac mains. The medical isolation amplifier has evolved to meet these severe tests for leakage.

Isolation is accomplished by electrically separating the input stage of the isolation amplifier (IsoA) from the output stage. That is, the input stage has a separate floating power supply and a "ground" that are connected to the output side of the IsoA by a resistance of over 1000 megohms, and a parallel capacitance in the low picofarad range. The signal input terminals of the input stage are isolated from the IsoA's output by a similar very high impedance, although the Thevenin output resistance of the IsoA can range from milliohms to several hundred ohms.

8.3.2   Common Types of Medical Isolation Amplifiers

Current practice uses *three* major means of effecting the Galvanic isolation of the input and output stages of IsoAs. The first means is to use a high-quality toroidal transformer to magnetically couple regulated, high-frequency ac power from the output side to the isolated input stage where it is rectified and filtered; it is also coupled to rectifiers and filters serving the output amplifiers. Frequencies in the range of 50 to 500 kHz are typically used with transformer isolation IsoAs. The output signal from the isolated headstage modulates an ac carrier magnetically coupled to a demodulator on the output side. Transformer coupling can provide 12- to 16-bit resolution and bandwidths up to 75 kHz. Galvanic isolation with transformers is excellent; their maximum breakdown voltage can be made as high as 10 kV, but is often much lower.

A second means of isolation is to use photo-optic coupling of the amplified signal; usually pulse-width or delta–sigma modulation of the optical signal is used, although direct linear analog photo-optic coupling can be used. In the optical type of IsoA, a separate isolated dc–dc converter must be used to power the input stage. Photo-optic couplers can be made to withstand voltages in the 4- to 7-kV range before breakdown.

A third means of isolation is to use a pair of small (e.g., 1 pF) capacitors to couple a pulse-modulated signal from the isolated input to the output stage. A separate isolated power supply must be used with the differential capacitor-coupled IsoA as well. Table 8.1 lists some of the critical specifications of five types of medical-grade IsoAs.

The Burr–Brown ISO121 differential capacitor-coupled IsoA is used with a separate isolated clock to run its duty cycle modulator. The clock frequency can be from 5 to 700 kHz, giving commensurate bandwidths, governed by the Nyquist criterion.

A simplified schematic of an Analog Devices AD289 magnetically coupled IsoA is shown in Figure 8.3. Note that this IsoA has a single-ended input. In this case, an AD620 IA is powered from the AD289's isolated power supply and provides true isolated differential input to the IsoA that rejects unwanted common-mode noise and interference. The clock power oscillator drives a toroidal core, T1, on which coils for the input and output isolated power supplies are wound and for the synchronizing signal for the double-side-band, suppressed-carrier (DSBSC) modulator and demodulator. A separate toroidal transformer, T2, couples the DSBSCM output signal to the output side of the IsoA. This is basically the architecture used in the Intronics 290 and the Burr–Brown BB3656 IsoAs.

An unmodulated feedback-type analog optical isolation system is used in the Burr–Brown BB3652 differential optically coupled linear IsoA. This IsoA still requires a transformer-isolated power supply for the input headstage and for the driver for the linear optocoupler. A feedback-type linear optocoupler, similar to that used in the BB3652, is shown in Figure 8.4. (In the B3652, OA1 is replaced with a high input impedance DA headstage.) The circuit works in the following manner.

TABLE 8.1

Comparison of Properties of Some Popular Isolation Amplifiers

Amplifier	IA294	BB3656	BB3652	BB ISO121	ISO-Z
Iso. type	Transformer	Transformer	Optical	Capacitor	Transformer?
Manufacturer	Intronics	Burr–Brown	Burr–Brown	Burr–Brown	Dataq
CMV isolation	±5000 V continuous; ±6500 V 10-MS pulse	±3500 V continuous; ±8000 V, 10 sec	±2000 V continuous; ±5000 V, 10 sec.	3500 RMS	1500 V continuous; 5000 V, 10 sec
CMRR @ 60 Hz	120 dB @ 60 Hz	108 dB	80 dB @ 60 Hz	115 dB IMR @ 60 Hz	>100 dB @ 60 Hz
Gain range	10 (fixed)	1 to 100	1 to >100, by formula	1 V/V (fixed)	10 (fixed)
Leakage to 120 Vac mains	10 μA max	0.5 μA	0.5 μA; 1.8 pF leakage capacitance	$I_{ac} = V2\pi fC; C \cong$ 2.21 pF	<5 μA, any input to ground
Noise	8 μV ppk; 0.05 to 100 Hz	5 μV pkpk; 0.05 to 100 Hz BW	8 μV pkpk 0.05 - 100 Hz BW	4 μVRMS/√Hz	<4 μVRMS, referred to input, "wideband"
Bandwidth	0 to 1 kHz	0 to 30 kHz; ±3 dB	0 - 15 kHz, ± 3 dB	0 to 60 kHz; (approx. 200 kHz clock)	0 to 8 kHz
Slew rate	?	+0.1, −0.04 V/μs	1.2 V/μs	2 V/μs	?

The summing junction of OA2 is at 0 V. DC bias current through R_{B1}, I_{B1}, drives the OA2 output negative, biasing the LED, D2, on at some I_{D20}. D2's light illuminates photodiodes D1 and D3 equally; the reverse photocurrent through D1 drives OA2's output positive, reducing I_{D2}. It thus provides a linearizing negative feedback around OA2, acting against the current produced by the input voltage, V_{in}/R_1. Because D1 and D3 are matched photo-diodes, the reverse photocurrent in D3 equals that in D1, i.e., $I_{D10} = I_{D30}$ and $V_o = R_3$ $(I_{D30} - I_{B3})$. The bias current I_{B3} makes $V_o \to 0$ when $V_{in} = 0$. Now when $V_{in} >$ 0, the input current, V_{in}/R_1, makes the LED D2 brighter, increasing $I_{D1} = I_{D3} >$ $I_{D10} = I_{D30}$, increasing V_o. Thus, $V_o = K_V V_{in}$. Note that analog opto-isolation eliminates the need for a high-frequency carrier, modulation, and demodulation, while giving a very high degree of Galvanic isolation. Unfortunately, the isolated headstage still must receive its power through a magnetically isolated power supply. It could use batteries, however, which would improve its isolation.

IsoAs using capacitor isolation use high-frequency duty-cycle modulation to transmit the signal across the isolation barrier using a differential 1-pF capacitor coupling circuit. This type of IsoA also needs an isolated power supply for the input stages, clock oscillator, and modulator. Figure 8.5 illustrates schematically a simplified version of how the Burr–Brown ISO121 capacitively isolated IsoA works.

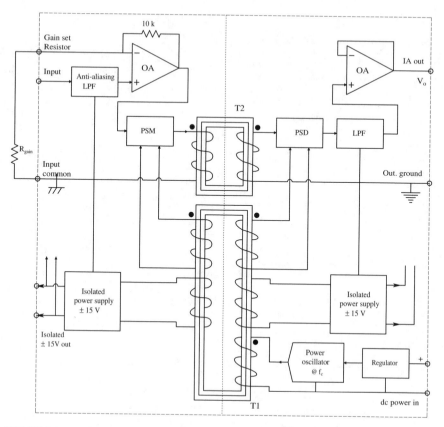

FIGURE 8.3

Simplified schematic of an Analog Device's AD289 magnetically isolated isolation amplifier (IsoA). An AD620 IA is used as a differential front end for the IsoA; it is powered from the AD289's isolated power supply.

The positive signal V_{in} is added to a high-frequency symmetrical triangle wave, V_T, with peak height, V_{pkT}. The sum of V_T and V_{in} is passed through a comparator, which generates a variable duty-cycle square wave, V_2. Note that the highest frequency in V_{in} is $\ll f_c$, the clock frequency, and $|V_{inmax}| < V_{pk}$. The state transitions in V_2 are coupled through the two 1-pF capacitors as spikes to a flip-flop on the output side of the IA. The flip-flop's transitions are triggered by the spikes. At the flip flop's output, a $\pm V_{3m}$-variable duty-cycle square wave, V_3, is then averaged by low-pass filtering to yield V_o.

The duty cycle of V_2 and V_3 can be shown to be:

$$\eta(V_{in}) \equiv T_+/T = \left(\frac{1}{2} + V_{in}/2V_{pkT}\right), \quad |V_{in}| < v_{pkT} \tag{8.1}$$

The average of the symmetrical flip-flop output is:

$$V_o = \overline{V}_3 = V_{in}\left(V_{3m}/V_{pkT}\right) \tag{8.2}$$

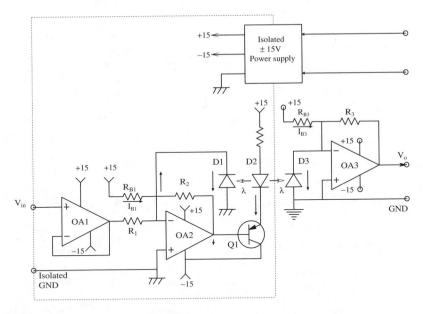

FIGURE 8.4
Simplified schematic of an analog feedback-type photo-optic coupler IsoA.

Thus, the output signal is proportional to V_{in}. The actual circuitry of the Burr–Brown ISO121 is more complex than described previously, but the basic operating principle remains the same.

Certified isolation amplifiers *must* be used in surgery and intensive-care hospital environments in which cardiac catheters are used. Although the scenarios for direct cardiac electroshock do not generally exist for outpatients, IsoAs are still used for ECG, EEG, and EMG applications to limit liability in the very unlikely event of an electroshock incident.

8.3.3 A Prototype Magnetic IsoA

All of the IsoAs described thus far use a carrier and can thus face problems of aliasing in the output signal when the input signal's highest frequency approaches one half the carrier frequency, as well as ripple in the output. One way to avoid the problems of carrier-based IsoAs is to use a technology that is dc coupled yet provides the required ohmic isolation. One approach is to use a transduction scheme that uses magnetic fields at signal rather than carrier frequencies. One such magnetic sensor is the Hall-effect device (Yang, 1988). Unfortunately, commercial Hall-effect sensors are not particularly sensitive and have low outputs that require amplification.

Fortunately, another relatively new technology was discovered in the late 1980s by Peter Gruenberg of the KFA Research Institute in Julich, Germany, and independently by Albert Fert at the University of Paris-Sud; this is the giant magnetoresistive (GMR) effect. Researchers at IBM extended the initial

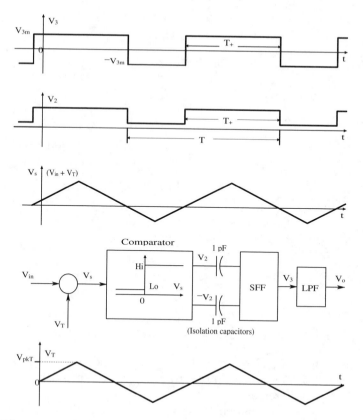

FIGURE 8.5

Waveforms relating to the operation of the Burr–Brown ISO121 capacitively coupled, duty cycle-modulated IsoA system. The low-frequency signal, V_{in}, is added to a symmetrical 0-mean triangle carrier wave; the sum is passed through a zero-crossing comparator that effectively performs duty-cycle modulation. If $V_{in} > 0$, $T_+/T > 0.5$; if $V_{in} < 0$, $T_+/T < 0.5$. The comparator output, V_2, and its complement, $\overline{V}_2$, are coupled to a flip-flop whose output square wave, V_3, has zero mean at 50% duty cycle. The text shows that the time average value of V_3, V_o, is proportional to V_{in}.

work on GMR devices; they developed sensitive GMR transducers based on sputtered thin film technology. IBM's interest in developing sensitive miniature GMR devices has been to improve the data density stored on computer floppy and hard-drive magnetic discs. IBM calls its GMR sensor the spin valve read-head.

GMR sensors have a resistance modulated by an imposed magnetic flux density; therefore, a Wheatsone bridge can be used to sense the $\Delta R/R_M$, and thus the ΔB. Unfortunately, GMRs are not particularly linear, which makes them acceptable for binary applications but presents problems for linear analog sensing.

A basic GMR sensor is a multiple-layer thin film device. In its simplest form, it has a nonmagnetic conductive spacing layer sandwiched between two ferromagnetic film layers. Usually, the magnetization in one ferromagnetic layer is fixed or pinned along a set direction. The magnetization of the free layer is allowed to rotate in response to an externally applied magnetic field. Low resistance occurs when the pinned and free layer are magnetically oriented in the same direction because electrons in the conductor layer with parallel spin directions move freely in both films. Higher resistance occurs when the magnetic orientations in the two films oppose each other because movement of electrons in the conductor of either spin direction is hampered by one or the other magnetic film. Depending on the strength and orientation of the applied external B field, the pinning direction, and the materials used and their thicknesses, the $R_M = f(B, \theta, \varphi)$ curve can have a variety of shapes (Wilson, 1996). In many cases, the GMR $R_M = f(B, \theta, \varphi)$ curve exhibits hysteresis and some dead zone as shown in Figure 8.6. This spin valve has the "crossed easy axis" configuration in which the applied **B** is perpendicular to the free layer easy axis and the pinning direction is parallel to **B**. The response is linear around Q and is relatively hysteresis free (Wilson, 1996). Because of its magnetic sensitivity, the GMR must be magnetically shielded from the Earth's field and stray magnetic fields from man-made power wiring and machinery. To be used as a linear device, such a sensor must be magnetically biased around the Q-point.

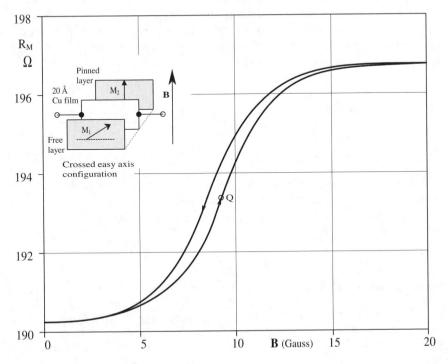

FIGURE 8.6
Resistance vs. flux density of a typical giant magnetoresistor (GMR). Note the hysteresis.

Much research is currently going on to improve the linearity and sensitivity of spin valves or GMR sensors. Attention is being paid to the use of multiple layered thin films of various compositions, including two pinned layers; 6 to 12 layers are being studied by Fujitsu (Kanai et al., 2001).

GMR sensors are available commercially. Infineon Technologies offers a four-element GMR IC package in which the four GMRs are connected in a bridge. Their GMR B6 is intended as a rotary position sensor in that the bridge output is a sinusoidal function of the input magnet's B field angle. The magnetic field-free value of each resistor is approximately 700 Ω. Rhopoint Components of Oxted, Surrey, U.K. offers a 12-sensor GMR device kit for experimenters and research and development use.

The author's version of a prototype IsoA design based on GM resistors is shown in Figure 8.7. Four GMR resistors are connected as a Wheatstone bridge (Wilson). The bridge can be powered with dc or ac; if ac is used, a phase-sensitive rectifier must be placed between the DA and the integrator. The quantity under isolated measurement is transduced to V_s, which is converted to a signal current, I_S, by a VCCS with transconductance, G_M. A dc bias current component, I_{so}, must be added to I_S to move the operating point of the GMR resistors to a linear region of its $R_M = f(B)$ curve. The current I_S through the coils on the opposite diagonals of the bridge creates equal **B** fields, which cause identical changes in the GMRs, ΔR_s, that, in turn, unbalance the bridge. The bridge output is amplified by the DA and serves as the input to an integrator. The integrator output causes a feedback current, I_F, to flow that forces $\Delta R_f = \Delta R_s$ in the other two diagonal R_Ms, which re-nulls the bridge output. Because of symmetry, the feedback current $I_F = I_S + I_{so}$ at null and the output voltage of the op amp transresistor is:

$$V_o = -I_F R_F = -V_s G_M R_F + I_{so} R_F \qquad (8.3)$$

Thus,

$$V_s = \left(I_{so} R_F - V_o\right)\big/\left(G_M R_F\right) \qquad (8.4)$$

Galvanic isolation of the GMR bridge IsoA depends on the insulation between the chip containing the four GMR resistors and the two input coils. The capacitance between the coils and R_Ms and the dielectric breakdown of this insulation are important.

8.4   Safety Standards in Medical Electronic Amplifiers

8.4.1   Introduction

The central rationale for safety standards for medical electronic equipment is based on the need to prevent harm to human patients and health-care

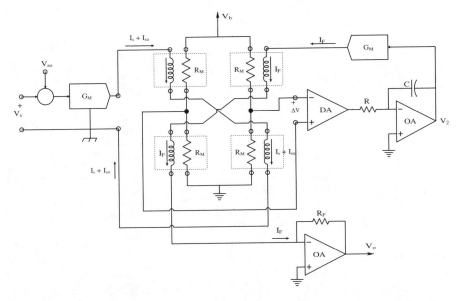

FIGURE 8.7

Architecture of an IsoA designed by the author using four GMR elements in a bridge. A type 1 feedback loop is used to autonull the bridge. Autonulling ensures linear operation of the GMRs. Note that the input circuit ground is separate from the signal conditioning and output ground. V_{so} is a bias voltage that causes the GMRs to operate in their linear ranges.

workers attached to or using such equipment. Besides user safety, having a biomedical electronic product certified by one or more of the qualified test agencies reduces the litigation risk for those persons who designed, sold, and used it in practice if any untoward incident should occur. (The U.S. is legendary for its medical malpractice litigation and the substantial awards that are made.) Product certification is also necessary in various jurisdictions in order to be able to sell a biomedical electronic product to hospitals, clinics, physicians, research labs, etc.

An excellent treatise on electrical safety and the physiological effects of electric currents on the body can be found in Chapter 14 of Webster (1992). A summary of the effects of injuries caused by electric current can also be found in the on-line Merck Manual, Section 20, Chapter 277 (2003). An excellent paper on safety standards and tests for medical electronic products can be found at the Eisner Safety Consultants Website (2003).

Electrical currents can enter the body in a variety of ways; probably the most common is through the skin on a hand, the head, or a foot. Note that for a circuit to exist, the current must leave the body, also through a hand, the head, or feet. Electric shock effects are usually described in terms of the current that flows through the body and if AC, the frequency of the current. Direct current can also have profound physiological effects, as can transient currents such as those from capacitor discharges, static electricity, and lightning. Table 8.2 summarizes typical physiological effects from dc, 60-Hz, and

TABLE 8.2

Physiological Effects in the Body of Electric Currents Introduced through the Hands

Current in mA			
60 Hz	10 kHz	DC	Effect
0 to 0.3	0 to 5	0 to 0.6	No sensation
2	8	3.5	Slight tingling on hand
1	11	6	"Shock"; not painful
10	51	58	Painful muscle spasms; recipient may let go
20	60	65	Painful; muscle tetanus; recipient cannot let go
>100		>500	Deep burns, edema, cardiac fibrillation, respiratory paralysis
>2000		>2000	All of the above; death

Note: A current × time product determines tissue damage once the power density in tissues reaches the level at which temperatures rise to a level at which "cooking" occurs. Values are "typical" and can vary widely among individuals due to fat, muscle mass, etc.

10-kHz electric currents in a macroshock scenario in which the current is applied between the hands. The data are based on several sources, including human and animal studies.

Figure 8.8 illustrates let-go current vs. frequency for the hand-to-hand current path in humans. Plotted is the current vs. frequency for the median of the test population; the bars show the 99.5 and 0.5 percentile limits. This curve and the preceding table teach that power line frequency (50 or 60 Hz) is the most physiologically effective in producing electric shock damage to the body and heart. Direct current and AC at 10 kHz are about one sixth as effective in doing damage. Consequently, impedance pneumographs and plethysmographs typically pass mA level currents with frequencies of approximately 75 kHz through the chest with no untoward effects.

When the heart is stimulated directly, as in open-heart surgery or cardiac pacemaker catheterization, the scenario is called *microshock.* The 60-Hz current required to induce ventricular fibrillation can be as low as 20 μA in dogs. In humans, microshock current causing fibrillation is on the order of 80 to 600 μA (Webster, 1990, Chapter 14).

8.4.2 Certification Criteria for Medical Electronic Systems

The data presented show that it is extremely important to prevent harmful currents from flowing into the body under macroshock conditions from any amplifier connected to the body by electrodes, such as in ECG, EEG, EMG, EOG, etc. measurements. The U.S. has a number of regulatory and certifying agencies that ensure medical electronic devices are safe, including :

- Food and Drug Administration (FDA)
- National Fire Protection Agency (NFPA) and its National Electrical Code (NEC)
- American National Standards Institute/Association for the Advancement of Medical Instrumentation (ANSI/AAMI ES1-1993)

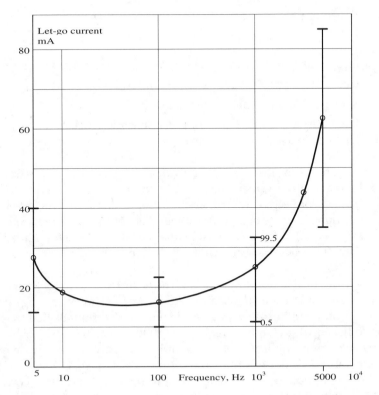

FIGURE 8.8

Let-go current vs. frequency for the hand-to-hand current path in humans. Note that the most dangerous frequency is around 50 to 60 Hz.

- Occupational Health and Safety Administration (OSHA)
- Underwriter's Laboratories (UL)

Europe has are two major organizations: (1) the European Committee for Electrotechnical Standardization (CENELEC) and (2) the International Electrotechnical Commission (IEC).

Gradually, the standards in the U.S. appear to be converging on those established by the IEC, which has developed a set of standards to certify medical instruments called the IEC60601-1 that covers all of the general requirements for all medical based products. (Some papers refer to IEC60601-1 as IEC601-1.) Many of the U.S. standards have been based on IEC requirements set in the past decade, but some, such as UL544, were phased out in January, 2003. The new UL2601-1 is largely based on the IEC regulations, with some exceptions (Mentelos, 2003).

The IEC60601-1 standards are subdivided into several IEC60601-X-YZ parts, which cover specific types of medical equipment. The interest here, however, is in medical isolation amplifiers used to record potentials from the body surface. Four classes of basic electrical safety tests are defined by the IEC. These include:

- Protective earth verification: ground continuity test; ground bond test
- Dielectric strength: AC hipot test; DC hipot test
- High resistance: insulation resistance test
- Leakage current: Earth leakage, touch/chassis (enclosure); patient leakage and patient auxiliary leakage

The *earth* (ground or green wire) *verification test* passes 25 amps from the line cord plug ground (green) terminal to the chassis, to ensure cord-to-chassis ground connection robustness, and measures the voltage between the current source and the chassis or cabinet. The resistance of the grounding system must be <0.1 Ω for a detachable line cord and <0.2 Ω for a fixed cord according to IEC60601-1 specifications. Resistance is calculated by Ohm's law: $R = V/25$ ohms.

The *dielectric strength test* applies a high ac or dc voltage to the line power input to ensure that no insulation breakdown or flashover (arcing) occurs between ground and the input power line with both terminals tied together. The basic IEC60601-1 standard requires the DUT to withstand 1250 VRMS at 60 Hz for 1 min. Medical isolation amplifiers easily exceed this requirement (see Table 8.1). For example, the Intronics IA175 IsoA is rated at 3000 V_{pk}, 60 Hz continuous from patient inputs to the outputs/power common. The IA175 runs on +15 VDC, so further isolation can be obtained by using a medical-grade power supply that meets IEC60601-1 standards.

The *insulation resistance test* is a voltmeter–ammeter test of the DUT's insulation using a high-voltage DC source. For example, a high DC potential is applied to the IsoA's power input common, e.g., 1000 V, and the steady-state current to ground is measured at the isolated power supply's neutral. Such current would be 1 nA DC if the resistance were 10^{12} Ω.

Finally, leakage currents are considered. The four types of leakage current defined by the IEC as described by Eisner (2001) are:

> Earth leakage: the most important and most common of the line leakage current tests, earth leakage current is basically the current flowing back through the ground conductor on the power cord [green wire]. It is measured by opening the ground conductor, inserting a circuit with the simulated impedance of the human body and measuring the voltage across part of the circuit with a true RMS voltmeter.
>
> Patient leakage: a line leakage current test that measures the current that would flow from or to applied parts such as sensor and patient leads.
>
> Patient auxiliary leakage: that line leakage current flowing in the patient in NORMAL use between applied parts of the DUT and not intended to produce a physiological effect.

Touch/chassis leakage: a line leakage current test [that] simulates the effect of a person touching exposed metal parts of a product and detects whether or not the leakage current that flows through the person's body remains below a safe level. Line leakage tests are conducted by applying power to the product being tested, then measuring the leakage current from any exposed metal on the chassis of the product under various fault conditions (such as "no ground"). A special circuit is used to simulate the impedance of the human body.

The circuit used to simulate the body's impedance as defined by IEC60601-1 is shown in Figure 8.9. At 60 Hz, this phantom presents an impedance of $999.7\angle-0.32°\ \Omega$, basically 1 k$\Omega$. The reactance of the 0.015 µF capacitor is $X_c = -1.768 \times 10^5\ \Omega$ at 60 Hz. (The author finds it curious that leakage currents are measured through this 1-kΩ body phantom, rather than using the short-circuit leakage current.) The Eisner (2001) Web paper on IEC60601-1 illustrates in detail the various circuits used to measure the four types of leakage current; space limitations prevent duplication of them here. Table 8.3 summarizes the leakage current limits from two U.S. standards and IEC60601-1 (Mentelos, 2003).

Modern medical isolation amplifiers such as the Intronics IA175 generally exceed specifications. For example, the maximum leakage currents, inputs to common @ 115 VAC, 60 Hz, are only 8 µA max. The actual input impedance of the IA175 is $10^8\ \Omega\ \|\ 3$ pF for DM in and $10^{11}\ \Omega\ \|\ 20$ pF for CM

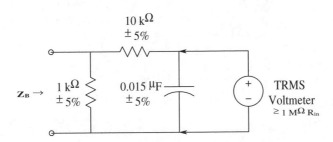

FIGURE 8.9
The IEC body phantom impedance model defined by the IEC60601-1 standard.

TABLE 8.3

Leakage Current Limits for Three Standards

Leakage Type	UL544	UL2601-1	IEC60601-1
Earth leakage	300 µA	300 µA	1 mA
Enclosure leakage	300 µA	300 µA	500 µA
Patient leakage (auxiliary)	10 µA input 20 µA at end of cable	50 µA	50 µA

Note: Units cannot be certified by UL544 after 1/1/03 ; UL certification expires after 1/1/05. UL2601-1 and IEC60601-1 should be used for all new designs of medical electronic equipment.

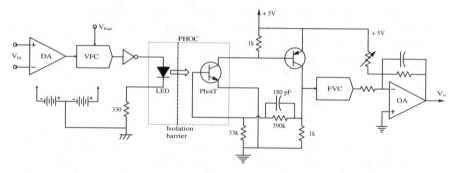

FIGURE 8.10

An IsoA architecture for ECG recording using a digital photo-optic coupler. Pulses from a voltage-to-frequency converter are sent to a frequency-to-voltage converter through the PhOC to recover a signal proportional to V_{in}.

inputs. The maximum CM voltage, inputs to outputs/input power common is 3000 Vpk, 60 Hz AC for 1 min. The peak continuous DC CM input voltage is ±5000 V. The CMRR with a balanced differential source is 126 dB at 60 Hz. The small-signal –3-dB frequency is 1 kHz, which is ideal for ECG, EEG, and EOG applications.

An inexpensive isolation amplifier to measure the ECG in an experimental setting can be made from a battery-operated AD620 IA connected to a battery-operated, low-current, voltage-to-frequency converter (VFC) such as the AD654. The VFC is given an FM center frequency with a bias voltage (not shown in Figure 8.10). The bipolar ECG signal output from the IA frequency modulates the VFC's digital output. To realize isolation, the VFC drives a photo-optic coupler with output that is the input to a frequency-to-voltage converter (FVC) such as the ADVFC32. The VFC carrier bias at the output of the FVC is subtracted out and the ECG signal is further amplified and filtered.

Figure 8.10 illustrates this system. The photo-optic coupler's phototransistor (PhotT) is given positive feedback to speed up its switching to a maximum of 500 kHz (Stapleton and O'Grady, 2001). Of course, if this design were to be used in a medical or clinical application, it would need to be tested and meet or exceed IEC60601-1 standards, etc. If the isolation and insulation on the PHOC were not adequate, one could use a fiber optic cable to couple the LED to the phototransistor.

Note that radiotelemetry is another means of providing extreme isolation between a battery-operated amplifier, modulator, and RF transmitter and a line-powered receiver, demodulator, and signal conditioner. In fisheries biology, fish are tracked underwater and data can be sent by battery-powered modulated ultrasonic "tags." Again, extreme isolation is inherent in ultrasonic telemetry.

8.5   Medical-Grade Power Supplies

The only practical way to achieve extreme galvanic isolation and still couple significant power from the mains to a low-voltage regulated dc supply that powers a medical amplifier is by toroidal transformer. The transformer can operate at line frequency or, for lighter weight and improved efficiency, can operate at frequencies in the 10- to 100-kHz range. A power oscillator must be used to drive the transformer's primary in the latter case. If a high-frequency oscillator is used, the transformer can be made smaller and lighter (a smaller core and fewer turns on the windings are required) and the output filter capacitor can be smaller and lighter.

A toroidal transformer is used for efficiency in magnetic coupling the primary to secondary windings; the toroidal core allows the primary and secondary to be separate physically on the core to minimize capacitive coupling between them. By physically separating the windings and insulating them from the core with special insulation, breakdown voltages between primary and secondary can be made 8 kV or greater and primary-to-secondary dc resistance can be on the order of 10^{12} Ω and greater. The secondary ac voltage is rectified by the usual means; the raw dc is low-pass filtered by a capacitor, and then regulated by a feedback regulator. The net result is a dc supply with guaranteed extreme galvanic isolation between the input power lines (high, low, and ground) and the output dc terminals (ground and V_{CC}).

Many power supply manufacturers make medical grade units; for example, GlobTek Inc. (www.globtek.com) offers a broad line of medical-grade, stand-alone power supplies including wall plug-in "bricks" and open-frame units. Their class II double insulated units withstand 4 kV ac or 5.65 kV dc input–output potential and have less than 100-μA leakage.

8.6   Chapter Summary

This chapter described the properties and uses of instrumentation amplifier ICs, including those that can be made from low-noise op amps. Requirements for and properties of medical isolation amplifiers were also examined. Galvanic isolation is required for patient safety in all settings (surgical, clinical, outpatient). Power supply isolation is achieved by batteries or special transformer-coupled power supplies. Isolation amplifier analog output must also be isolated. One way this can be done is by DSBSC modulation of a high-frequency ac carrier by the physiological signal, and coupling the modulated carrier to the output with a transformer, where the signal is recovered with a demodulator.

Another way of coupling the physiological signal to the output with isolation is to use a photo-optic coupler and transmit the signal directly in analog form (see Section 6.6.4 of Chapter 6). If the isolated physiological signal is sampled and converted by a serial output analog-to-digital converter, the digital output can also be transmitted through a digital photo-optic coupler to the output. Still another way of coupling an isolated signal to the output was by converting the signal to a pulse-width modulated (PWM) TTL square wave and coupling this wave to the output with two 1-pF capacitors. At the output, this wave is highly differentiated into a spike train. Flip-flops recover the PWM wave at the output and the signal is demodulated by averaging.

The physiological effects of electroshock were described, including induced cardiac fibrillation, apnea, and burns. Certification agencies for medical electronic devices worldwide were listed and some of their standards compared. The U.S. was seen to have five major certifying agencies; Europe had two. A trend in the U.S. is to converge on the IEC standards. To meet European marketing standards for medical electronic devices, U.S. manufacturers must meet IEC and CENELEC standards that, paradoxically in some areas, are less stringent than NFPA and other U.S. standards.

Finally, medical-grade power supplies that run off the mains were discussed.

9

Noise and the Design of Low-Noise Amplifiers for Biomedical Applications

9.1 Introduction

The noise considered in this chapter provides one limitation to the precision of biomedical measurements. Other factors that limit resolution are the distortion caused by signal conditioning system nonlinearity and quantization in the analog-to-digital conversion (ADC) of input signals. The degree to which a biosignal is resolvable can be determined by the signal-to-noise ratio at the output of the signal conditioning system. The noise in this chapter is considered to arise in a circuit, measurement system, or electrode from completely random processes. Although any physical quantity can be "noisy," this chapter will generally consider only completely random noise voltages and currents; these will be defined as being stationary (the physical process giving rise to the noise does not change with time) and having zero mean (zero additive dc components). An unwanted dc component accompanying a noise source in practice can be from an electrochemical EMF arising in a recording electrode or from amplifier dc offset voltage or bias current. The reduction of unwanted dc components will not be treated here.

Coherent interference (CI) can also be present at the output of biomedical signal conditioning systems. As its name suggests, CI generally has its origins in periodic, manmade phenomena, such as power line-frequency electric and magnetic fields; radio-frequency sources such as radio and television broadcast antennas; certain poorly shielded computer equipment; spark discharge phenomena such as automotive ignitions and electric motor brushes and commutators; and inductive switching transients generated by SCR motor speed controls, etc. It is well known that minimization of CI is often "arty" and may involve changing the grounding circuits for a system; shielding with magnetic and/or electric conducting materials; filtering; using isolation transformers, etc. (Northrop, 1997, Section 3.9). In this chapter, however, attention will be focused on purely random, stationary, incoherent noise.

Minimizing the impact of incoherent noise in a measurement system often involves a prudent choice of low-noise amplifiers and components, certain basic electronic design principles, and band-pass filtering. First, commonly used methods for describing stationary random noise will be examined.

9.2 Descriptors of Random Noise in Biomedical Measurement Systems

9.2.1 Introduction

When stationarity is assumed for a noise source, averages over time are equivalent to ensemble averages. An ensemble average is carried out at a given time on data from N separate records that are generated simultaneously from a stationary random process (SRP) (in the limit $N \rightarrow \infty$). If the stationary random process is ergodic, then only one record needs to be examined statistically because it is "typical" of all N records from the SRP.

An example of a nonstationary noise source is a resistor that, at time t = 0, begins to dissipate average power such that its temperature slowly rises above ambient, as does its resistance. (As demonstrated later, the mean-squared noise voltage from a resistor is proportional to its Kelvin temperature.)

Probability and statistics are used to describe random phenomena. Several statistical methods for describing random noise include but are not limited to the mean; the root-mean-square (RMS) value; the probability density function; the cross- and autocorrelation functions and their Fourier transforms; the cross- and autopower density spectra (PDS); and the root power density spectrum (RPS, which is simply the square root of the PDS). The PDS and RPS are, in general, functions of frequency. These descriptors are treated in detail next.

9.2.2 The Probability Density Function

The probability density function (PDF) is a mathematical model that describes the probability that any random sample of a noise function, $n(t)$, will lie in a certain range of values. The univariate PDF considers only the amplitude statistics of the noise waveform, not how it varies in time. The univariate PDF of the SRV, $n(t)$, is defined as:

$$p(x) \equiv \frac{\text{Probability that} \left[x < n \le (x + dx) \right]}{dx} \tag{9.1}$$

where x is a specific value of n taken at some time, t, and dx is a differential increment in x. The mathematical basis for many formal derivations and proofs in probability theory, the PDF has the properties:

$$\int_{-\infty}^{v} p(x)\,dx = \text{Prob}[x \le v] \tag{9.2}$$

$$\int_{v_2}^{v_1} p(x)\,dx = \text{Prob}[v_1 \le x \le v_2] \tag{9.3}$$

$$\int_{-\infty}^{\infty} p(x)\,dx = 1 = \text{Prob}[x \le \infty] \ (\text{a certainty}) \tag{9.4}$$

Several PDFs are widely used as mathematical models to describe the amplitude characteristics of electrical and electronic circuit noise. These include:

$$p(x) = \left(\frac{1}{\sigma_x \sqrt{2\pi}}\right) xp\left[-\frac{(x-\langle x\rangle)^2}{2\sigma_x^2}\right] \qquad \text{Gaussian or normal PDF} \tag{9.5}$$

$$p(x) = 1/2a, \quad \text{for } -a < x < a, \text{ and}$$
$$p(x) = 0, \qquad \text{for } x > a \qquad\qquad \text{Rectangular PDF} \tag{9.6}$$

$$p(x) = \left(\frac{x}{\alpha^2}\right) xp\left[\frac{-x^2}{2\alpha^2}\right] \qquad\qquad \text{Rayleigh PDF} \tag{9.7}$$

$$p(x) = \left(\frac{x^2}{\alpha^2}\right)\sqrt{(2/\pi)}\exp\left[\frac{-x^2}{2\alpha^2}\right] \qquad \text{Maxwell PDF, } x \ge 0 \tag{9.8}$$

In Equation 9.5, $\langle x\rangle$ is the true mean or expected value of the stationary random variable (SRV), x, and σ_x^2 is the variance of the stationary random variable (SRV), x, described next. The true mean of a stationary ergodic noisy voltage can be written as a time average over all time:

$$\langle x\rangle \equiv \lim_{T\to\infty}\frac{1}{T}\int_0^T x(t)\,dt \tag{9.9}$$

The mean of the SRV, x, can also be written as an expectation or probability average of x:

$$\mathbf{E}\{x\} \equiv \int_{-\infty}^{\infty} x\,p(x)\,dx = \langle x \rangle \tag{9.10}$$

Similarly, the mean squared value of x can be expressed by the expectation or probability average of x^2:

$$\mathbf{E}\{v^2\} = \int_{-\infty}^{\infty} v^2\,p(v)\,dv = \langle v^2 \rangle \tag{9.11}$$

The mean can be estimated by a finite average over time. For discrete data, this is called the sample mean, which is a statistical estimate of the true mean and as such has noise itself.

$$\bar{x} = \frac{1}{T}\int_0^T x(t)\,dt, \quad \text{or } \bar{x} = \frac{1}{N}\sum_{k=1}^{N} x_k \quad (\text{sample mean}) \tag{9.12}$$

The variance of the random noise, σ_x^2, is defined by:

$$\sigma_x^2 \equiv E\left\{\left[x - \langle x \rangle\right]^2\right\} = \int_{-\infty}^{\infty} \left[x - \langle x \rangle\right]^2 p(x)\,dx = \lim_{T\to\infty} \frac{1}{T}\int_0^T \left[x(t) - \langle x \rangle\right]^2 dt \tag{9.13}$$

It easy to show from this equation that $\langle x^2 \rangle = \sigma_x^2 + \langle x \rangle^2$, or $E\{x^2\} = \sigma_x^2 + E^2\{x\}$. Because the random noise to be considered has zero mean, the mean squared noise is also its variance.

Under most conditions, it is assumed that the random noise arising in a biomedical measurement system has a Gaussian PDF. Many mathematical benefits follow this assumption; for example, the output of a linear system is Gaussian with variance σ_y^2 given the input to be Gaussian with variance σ_x^2. If Gaussian noise passes through a nonlinear system, the output PDF generally will not be Gaussian; however, this chapter will show ways of describing the transformation of Gaussian input noise by a nonlinear system.

9.2.3   The Power Density Spectrum

A noise source can be thought of as the sum of a very large number of sine wave sources with different amplitudes, phases, and frequencies. Very heuristically, a power density spectrum (PDS) shows how the mean squared values of these sources is distributed in frequency.

One approach to illustrate the meaning of the PDS of the noise, $n(t)$, uses the autocorrelation function (ACF) of the noise. The ACF is defined in the following by the continuous time integral (Aseltine, 1958):

$$R_{nn}(\tau) = \lim_{T \to \infty} \frac{1}{2T} \int_{-T}^{T} n(t)n(t+\tau)dt = \lim_{T \to \infty} \frac{1}{2T} \int_{-T}^{T} n(t-\tau)n(t)dt \qquad (9.14)$$

The two-sided PDS is the continuous Fourier transform (CFT) of the autocorrelation function of the noise:

$$\Phi_{nn}(\omega) = \frac{1}{2\pi} \int_{-\infty}^{\infty} R_{nn}(\tau)e^{-j\omega\tau}d\tau \qquad (9.15)$$

Because $R_{nn}(\tau)$ is an even function, its Fourier transform, $\Phi_{nn}(\omega)$, is also an even function; stated mathematically, this means:

$$\Phi_{nn}(\omega) = \Phi_{nn}(-\omega) \qquad (9.16)$$

The following discussion will also consider the one-sided PDS, $S_n(f)$, which is related to the two-sided PDS by:

$$S_n(f) = 2 \Phi_{nn}(2\pi f) \text{ for } f \geq 0 \qquad (9.17)$$

and

$$S_n(f) = 0 \text{ for } f < 0. \qquad (9.18)$$

Note that the radian frequency, ω, is related to the Hertz frequency simply by $\omega = 2\pi f$.

To see how to find the one-sided PDS experimentally, examine the model system shown in Figure 9.1(A). Here, a noise voltage is the input to an *ideal* low-pass filter with an adjustable cut-off frequency, f_c. The output of the ideal low-pass filter is measured with a broadband, true RMS, AC voltmeter. Begin with $f_c = 0$ and systematically increase f_c, each time recording the square of the RMS meter reading, which is the mean squared output voltage, $\overline{v_{on}^2}$, of the filter. As f_c is increased, $\overline{v_{on}^2}$ increases monotonically, as shown in Figure 9.1(B). Because of the finite bandwidth of the noise source, $\overline{v_{on}^2}$ eventually reaches an upper limit, which is the total mean-squared noise voltage of the noise source. The plot of $\overline{v_{on}^2}(f_c)$ vs. f_c is called the cumulative mean-squared noise characteristic of the noise source. In this example, its units are mean-squared volts.

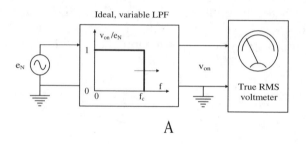

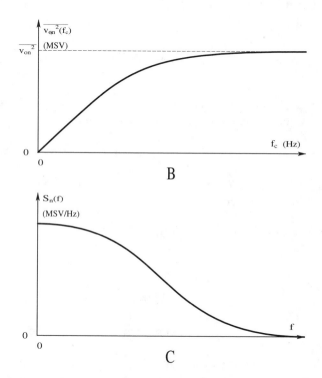

FIGURE 9.1
(A) System for measuring the integral power spectrum (cumulative mean-squared noise characteristic) of a noise voltage source, $e_N(f)$. (B) Plot of a typical integral power spectrum. (C) Plot
of a typical one-sided power density spectrum. See text for description.

A simple interpretation of the one-sided noise power density spectrum,
$S_n(f)$, is that it is the derivative, or slope, of the cumulative mean-squared
noise characteristic curve described previously. Stated mathematically, this
is:

$$S_n(f) \equiv \frac{d\overline{v_{on}^2(f)}}{df}, \quad 0 \leq f \leq \infty \quad \text{mean squared volts/hertz} \quad (9.19)$$

A plot of a typical noise PDS is shown in Figure 9.1(C). Note that a practical PDS drops off to zero as $f \to \infty$.

Those first encountering the PDS concept sometimes ask why it is called a power density spectrum. The power concept has its origin in the consideration of noise in communication systems and has little meaning in the context of noise in biomedical instrumentation systems. One way to rationalize the power term is to consider an ideal noise voltage source with a 1-ohm load. In this case, the average power dissipated in the resistor is simply the total mean-squared noise voltage ($P = \overline{v_{on}^2}/R$).

From the preceding heuristic definition of the PDS, it is possible to write the total mean-squared voltage in the noise voltage source as the integral of the one-sided PDS:

$$\overline{v_{on}^2} = \int_0^\infty S_n(f)\,df \tag{9.20}$$

The mean squared voltage in the frequency interval, (f_1, f_2), is found by:

$$\overline{v_{on}^2}(f_1, f_2) = \int_{f_1}^{f_2} S_n(f)\,df \quad \text{mean squared volts} \tag{9.21}$$

Often noise is specified or described using root power density spectra, which are simply plots of the square root of $S_n(f)$ vs. f, and have the units of RMS volts (or other units) per root Hertz.

Special (ideal) PDSs are used to model or approximate portions of real PDSs. These include the White noise PDS and the one-over-f PDS. A white noise PDS is shown in Figure 9.2(A). Note that this PDS is flat; this implies that

$$\int_0^\infty S_{nw}(f)\,df = \infty \tag{9.22}$$

which is clearly not realistic. A $1/f$ PDS is shown in Figure 9.2(B). The $1/f$ spectrum is often used to approximate the low-frequency behavior of real PDSs. Physical processes that generate $1/f$-like noise include ionic surface phenomena associated with electrochemical electrodes; carbon composition resistors carrying direct current (metallic resistors are substantially free of $1/f$ noise); and interface imperfections affecting diffusion and recombination phenomena in semiconductor devices. The presence of $1/f$ noise can present problems in the electronic signal conditioning systems used for low-level, low-frequency, and dc measurements.

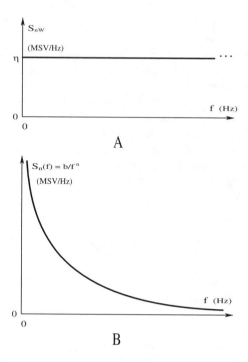

FIGURE 9.2

(A) A one-sided, white-noise power density spectrum. (B) A one-sided, one-over-f power density spectrum. Both of these spectra are idealized mathematical models. Their integrals are infinite.

9.2.4 Sources of Random Noise in Signal Conditioning Systems

Sources of random noise in signal conditioning systems can be separated into two major categories: noise from passive resistors and noise from semiconductor circuit elements such as bipolar junction transistors, field-effect transistors, and diodes. In most cases, the Gaussian assumption for noise amplitude PDFs is valid and the noise generated can generally be assumed to have a white (flat) power over a major portion of its spectrum.

9.2.4.1 Noise from Resistors

From statistical mechanics, it can be shown that any pure resistance at some temperature T Kelvins will have a zero-mean broadband noise voltage associated with it. This noise voltage appears in series with the (noiseless) resistor as a Thevenin equivalent voltage source. From dc to radio frequencies where the resistor's capacitance to ground and its lead inductance can no longer be neglected, the resistor's noise is well modeled by a Gaussian white noise source.

Noise from resistors is called thermal or Johnson noise; its one-sided white PDS is given by the well-known relation:

$$S_n(f) = 4kTR \text{ mean squared volts/Hertz} \tag{9.23}$$

where k is Boltzmann's constant (1.380×10^{-23} joule/Kelvin), T is in degrees Kelvin, and R is in ohms. In a given noise bandwidth, $B = f_2 - f_1$, the mean squared white noise from a resistor can be written:

$$\overline{v_{on}^2}(B) = \int_{f_1}^{f_2} S_n(f) df = 4kTR(f_2 - f_1) = 4kTRB \text{ MSV} \tag{9.24}$$

A Norton equivalent of the Thevenin Johnson noise source from a resistor can be formed by assuming an MS, white noise, short-circuit current source with PDS:

$$S_{ni}(f) = 4kTG \text{ MS amps/Hz} \tag{9.25}$$

This Norton noise current root spectrum, i_n RMS A/√Hz, is in parallel with a noiseless conductance, $G = 1/R$.

The Johnson noise from several resistors connected in a network may be combined into a single Thevenin noise voltage source in series with a single noiseless equivalent resistor. Figure 9.3 illustrates some of these reductions for two-terminal circuits.

It has been observed that when dc (or average) current is passed through a resistor, the basic Johnson noise PDS is modified by the addition of a low-frequency, $1/f$ spectral component, e.g.,

$$S_n(f) = 4kTR + A I^2/f \text{ MSV/Hz} \tag{9.26}$$

where I is the average or dc component of current through the resistor and A is a constant that depends on the material from which the resistor is constructed (e.g., carbon composition, resistance wire, metal film, etc.).

An important parameter for resistors carrying average current is the cross-over frequency, f_c, where the $1/f$ PDS equals the PDS of the Johnson noise. f_c is easily shown to be:

$$f_c = A I^2/4kTR \text{ Hz} \tag{9.27}$$

It is possible to show that the f_c of a noisy resistor can be reduced by using a resistor of the same type, but with a higher wattage or power dissipation rating. As an example of this principle, consider the circuit of Figure 9.4 in which a single resistor of R ohms, carrying a dc current I, is replaced by nine resistors of resistance R connected in a series-parallel circuit that also carries the current I. The nine-resistor circuit has a net resistance, R, which dissipates nine times the power of the single resistor R. The noise PDS in any one of the nine resistors is:

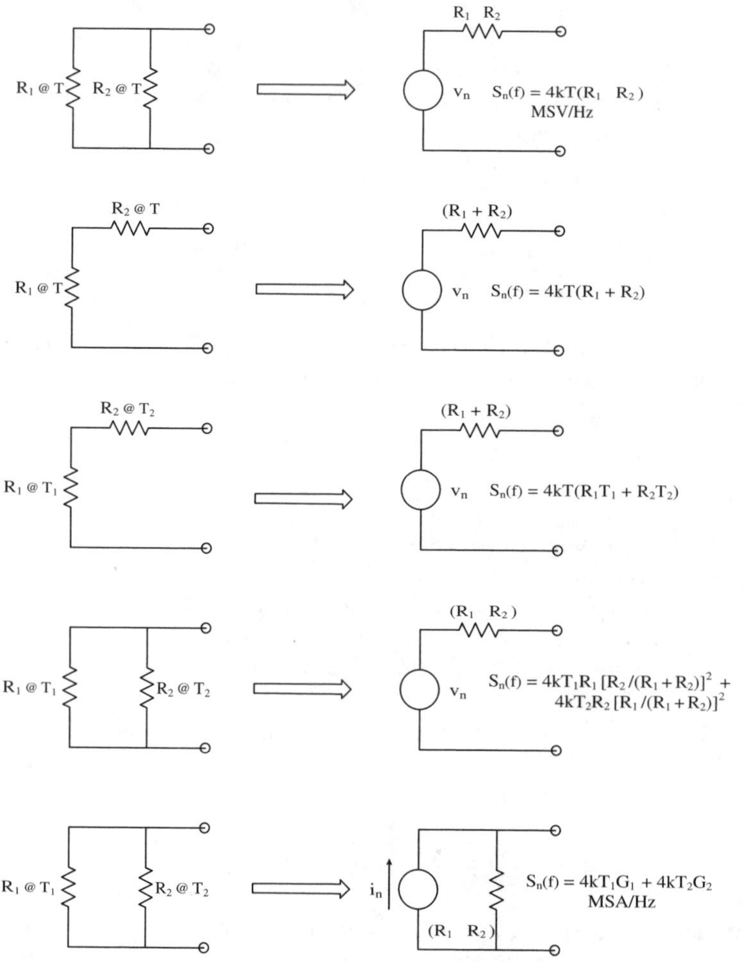

FIGURE 9.3
Examples of combining white Johnson noise power density spectra from pairs of resistors. In the resulting Thevenin models, the Thevenin resistors are noiseless.

$$S'_n(f) = 4kTR + A(1/3)^2/f \quad \text{MSV/Hz} \qquad (9.28)$$

Each of the nine PDSs given by the preceding equation contributes to the net PDS seen at the terminals of the composite 9-W resistor. Each resistor's equivalent noise voltage source "sees" a voltage divider formed by the other eight resistors in the composite resistor. The attenuation of each of the nine voltage dividers is given by

$$\frac{3R/2}{3R/2 + 3R} = 1/3 \qquad (9.29)$$

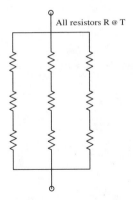

FIGURE 9.4
Nine identical resistors in series parallel have the same resistance as any one resistor, and nine times the wattage.

The net voltage PDS at the composite resistor's terminals may only be found by superposition of MS voltages or PDSs:

$$S_{n(9)}(f) = \sum_{j=1}^{9} \left[4kTR + A(I/3)^2 / f \right](1/3)^2 = 4kTR + AI^2/9f \quad \text{MSV/Hz} \quad (9.30)$$

Thus, the composite 9-W resistor enjoys a ninefold reduction in the $1/f$ spectral energy because the dc current density through each element is reduced by one third. The Johnson noise PDS remains the same, however. It is safe to generalize that the use of high wattage resistors of a given type and resistance will result in reduced $1/f$ noise generation when the resistor carries dc (average) current. The cost of this noise reduction is the extra volume required for a high-wattage resistor and its extra expense.

9.2.4.2 The Two-Source Noise Model for Active Devices

Noise arising in JFETs, BJTs, and complex IC amplifiers is generally described by the two-noise source input model. The total noise observed at the output of an amplifier, given that its input terminals are short-circuited, is accounted for by defining an equivalent short-circuited input noise voltage, e_{na}, which replaces the combined effect of all internal noise sources seen at the amplifier's output under short-circuited input conditions. The amplifier, shown in Figure 9.5, is now considered noiseless. e_{na} is specified by manufacturers for many low-noise discrete transistors and IC amplifiers. e_{na} is a root PDS, i.e., it is the square root of a one-sided PDS and is thus a function of frequency; e_{na} has the units of RMS volts per root Hertz. Figure 9.6 illustrates a plot of a typical $e_{na}(f)$ vs. f for a low-noise JFET. Also shown in Figure 9.6 is a plot of $i_{na}(f)$ vs. f for the same device.

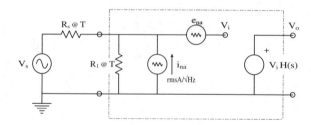

FIGURE 9.5
The two-noise source model for a noisy amplifier. e_{na} and i_{na} are root power density spectra. R_{out} is neglected.

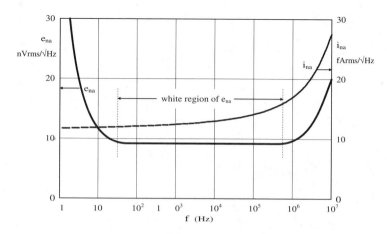

FIGURE 9.6
Plots of the e_{na} and i_{na} root power density spectra vs. f for a typical low-noise FET headstage amplifier. Note that e_{na} has a low frequency $1/\sqrt{f}$ component and i_{na} does not. i_{na} and e_{na} increase at very high frequencies.

In addition to the equivalent short-circuited input noise voltage, the modeling of the net noise characteristics of amplifiers requires the inclusion of an equivalent input noise current source, i_{na}, as shown in Figure 9.5. $i_{na}(f)$ is the root PDS of the input equivalent noise current; its units are RMS amps per $\sqrt{\text{Hertz}}$. Note that $e_{na}(f)$ and $i_{na}(f)$ have flat mid-frequency portions that invite approximation by white noise sources. At high frequencies, both equivalent noise root PDSs slope upward. For discrete JFETs and BJTs, and IC amplifiers, $e_{na}(f)$ shows a distinct $1/\sqrt{f}$ region at low frequencies.

9.2.4.3   Noise in JFETs

Certain selected discrete JFETs are sometimes used in the design of low-noise amplifier headstages for biomedical signal conditioning systems. Some JFETs give good low-noise performance in the audio and subaudio frequency regions of the spectrum; others excel in the video and radio-frequency end of the spectrum, giving them applications for RF oscillators, mixers, and tuned amplifiers used in ultrasound applications. Amplifiers using JFET headstages have relatively low input dc bias currents ($I_B \approx 10$ pA) and high input resistances ($>10^{10}$ Ω), both of which are desirable.

Van der Ziel (1974) showed that the theoretical thermal noise generated in the conducting channel of a JFET can be approximated by a white, equivalent short-circuited input noise with PDS given by:

$$e_{nn}^2 = 4kT/gm = 4kT/g_{m0}\sqrt{\frac{I_{DSS}}{I_{DQ}}} \text{ MSV/Hz} \tag{9.31}$$

where g_{m0} is the FET's small-signal transconductance measured when $V_{GS} = 0$ and $I_D = I_{DSS}$; I_{DSS} = the dc drain current measured for $V_{GS} = 0$ and $V_{DS} > V_P$; and I_{DQ} = the quiescent dc drain current at the FET's operating point where $V_{GS} = V_{GSQ}$. In reality, due to the presence of $1/f$ noise, the theoretical short-circuited input voltage PDS can be better modeled by:

$$e_{na}^2(f) = \left(4kT/g_m\right)\left(1 + f_c/f^n\right) \text{ MSV/Hz} \tag{9.32}$$

The exponent n has the range $1 < n < 1.5$ and is determined by device and lot. For algebraic simplicity, n is usually set equal to one. The origins of the $1/f^n$ effect in JFETs is poorly understood. Note that e_{na} given by Equation 9.32 is temperature dependent; heat sinking or actively cooling the JFET will reduce e_{na}. The parameter f_c used in Equation 9.32 is the corner frequency of the $1/f$ noise spectrum. Depending on the device, it can range from below 10 Hz to above 1 kHz. f_c is generally quite high in RF and video frequency JFETs because, in this type of transistor, $e_{na}(f)$ dips to around 2 nV/√Hz in the 10^5- to 10^7-Hz region, which is desirable.

JFET gates have a dc leakage or bias current, $I_{GL} = I_B$, which produces broadband shot noise that is superimposed on the leakage current. This noise component in I_{GL} is primarily due to the random occurrence of charge carriers that have enough energy to cross the reverse-biased gate–channel diode junction. The PDF of the gate current shot noise is generally assumed to be Gaussian and its PDS is approximated by:

$$i_{na}^2 = 2q\,I_{GL} \text{ MSA/Hz} \tag{9.33}$$

where $q = 1.602 \times 10^{-19}$ C (electron charge) and I_{GL} is the dc gate leakage current in amperes. I_{GL} is typically about 2 pA, so i_{na} is about 1.8 fA RMS/√Hz in the flat mid-range of $i_{na}(f)$. Like $e_{na}(f)$, $i_{na}(f)$ shows a $1/f$ characteristic at low frequencies, which can be modeled by:

$$i_{na}^2(f) = 2qI_{GL}\left(1 + f/f_{ic}\right) \text{ MSA/Hz} \tag{9.34}$$

where f_{ic} is the current noise corner frequency.

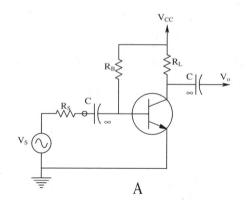

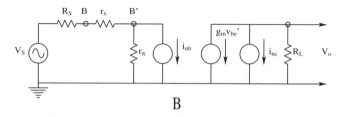

FIGURE 9.7
(A) A simple, grounded emitter BJT amplifier relevant to noise calculations. (B) The noise equivalent circuit for the BJT amplifier.

For some transistors, the measured $e_{na}(f)$ and $i_{na}(f)$ have been found to be greater than the predicted, theoretical values; in other cases, they have been found to be less. No doubt the causes for these discrepancies lie in the oversimplifications used in their derivations. Note that MOSFETs have no gate–drain diode and thus do not have a $1/f$ component in their i_{na}s.

9.2.4.4   Noise in BJTs

The values of e_{na} and i_{na} associated with bipolar junction transistor amplifiers depend strongly on the device's quiescent dc operating (Q) point because there are shot noise components superimposed on the quiescent base and collector currents. A mid-frequency, small-signal model of a simple grounded-emitter BJT amplifier is shown in Figure 9.7(B). In this circuit, negligible noise from R_L, the voltage-controlled current source, $g_m \, v_{be}$, and the small-signal base input resistance, r_π, is assumed. The shot noise PDSs are:

$$i_{nb}^2 = 2 \, q \, I_{BQ} \, \text{MSA/Hz} \qquad (9.35)$$

$$i_{nc}^2 = 2\,q\,\beta\,I_{BQ}\ \text{MSA/Hz} \tag{9.36}$$

where $\beta = h_{fe}$ is the BJT's small-signal forward current gain evaluated at the BJT's quiescent operating (Q) point. In this example, it is algebraically simpler not to find the equivalent input e_{na} and i_{na}, but to work directly with the two white shot noise sources in the mid-frequency, hybrid pi small-signal model. It can be shown (Northrop, 1990) that the total output noise voltage PDS is given by:

$$S_{NO}(f) = 4kTR_L + 2q(I_{BQ}/\beta)(\beta R_L)^2 + \frac{4kTR_s'(\beta R_L)^2 + 2q\,I_{BQ}\,R_s^2(\beta R_L)^2}{(V_T/I_{BQ} + r_x)^2}\ \text{MSV/Hz} \tag{9.37}$$

where it is clear that r_π is approximated by V_T/I_{BQ}, $R_s' = r_x + R_s$, and the Johnson noise from R_L is neglected because it is numerically small compared to the other terms.

It is easy to show (Northrop, 1990) that the mean squared output signal can be written as

$$\overline{v_{os}^2} = \overline{v_s^2}(\beta R_L)^2 \big/ \left(V_T/I_{BQ} + r_x\right)^2\ \text{MSV} \tag{9.38}$$

Thus, the MS signal-to-noise ratio at the amplifier output can be written:

$$\text{SNR}_O = \frac{v_s^2/B}{4kTR_s' + 2qI_{BQ}R_s'^2 + 2q(I_{BQ}/\beta)(V_T/I_{BQ} + R_s')^2} \tag{9.39}$$

where B is the specified equivalent (Hz) noise bandwidth for the system. The SNR_O given by the preceding equation has a maximum for some non-negative I_{BQMAX}. The I_{BQMAX} that will give this maximum can be found by differentiating the denominator of Equation 9.39 and setting the derivative equal to zero. This gives:

$$I_{BQMAX} = V_T \big/ \left(R_s'\sqrt{\beta + 1}\right)\ \text{DC amperes} \tag{9.40}$$

What should be remembered from the preceding exercise is that the best noise performance for BJT amplifiers is a function of quiescent biasing conditions (Q-point). Often these conditions must be found experimentally when working at high frequencies. Although individual BJT amplifiers may best be modeled for noise analysis with the two shot-noise current sources, it is more customary when describing complex BJT IC amplifier noise performance to use the more general and more easily used e_{na} and i_{na} two-source model parameterized for a given BJT Q-point.

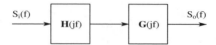

FIGURE 9.8
Two cascaded linear systems through which Gaussian noise is propagating.

9.3   Propagation of Noise through LTI Filters

In a formal rigorous treatment of noise in linear systems, it is possible to show that the PDF of the output of a linear system is Gaussian, given a Gaussian noise input. In addition, it can be shown rigorously (James et al., 1947) that the PDS of the system's output noise is given by

$$S_y(f) = S_x(f)\left|H(j2\pi f)\right|^2 \text{ MS units/Hz} \tag{9.41}$$

This is the scalar product of the positive-real input PDS and the magnitude squared of the LTI system's transfer function. This relation can be extended to include two or more cascaded systems, as shown in Figure 9.8.

$$S_y(f) = S_x(f)\left|H(j2\pi f)\right|^2 \left|G(j2\pi f)\right|^2 \text{ MSV/Hz} \tag{9.42}$$

or

$$S_y(f) = S_x(f)\left|H(j2\pi f)G(j2\pi f)\right|^2 \text{ MSV/Hz} \tag{9.43}$$

If white noise with a PDS, $S_x(f) = \eta$ MSV/Hz is the input to a linear system, then the output PDS is simply:

$$S_y(f) = \eta\left|H(j2\pi f)\right|^2 \text{ MSV/Hz} \tag{9.44}$$

The total mean-squared output noise of this system is given by:

$$\overline{v_{on}^2} = \int_0^\infty S_y(f)df = \eta \int_0^\infty \left|H(j2\pi f)\right|^2 df \text{ MSV} \tag{9.45}$$

For transfer functions with one more finite poles than zeros, the right-hand integral of Equation 9.45 may be shown to be the product of the transfer function's low-frequency or mid-band gain squared times the filter's equivalent

TABLE 9.1

Gain^2-Bandwidth Products for Some Common Filter Transfer Functions

Transfer Function[a]	Gain^2 Bandwidth[b]	Filter Type
1. $\dfrac{K_v}{s\tau+1}$	$K_v^2\left(\dfrac{1}{4\tau}\right)$	Low pass; one real-pole
2. $\dfrac{K_v}{(s\tau_1+1)(s\tau_2+1)}$	$K_v^2\left(\dfrac{1}{4(\tau_1+\tau_2)}\right)$	Low pass; two real poles
3. $\dfrac{K_v}{s^2/\omega_n^2+s2\xi/\omega_n+1}$	$K_v^2\left(\dfrac{\omega_n}{8\xi}\right)$	Low pass; underdamped quadratic
4. $\dfrac{sK_v(2\xi/\omega_n)}{s^2/\omega_n^2+s2\xi/\omega_n+1}$	$K_v^2(\xi\omega_n)$	Underdamped quadratic band pass
5. $\dfrac{s\tau_1K_v}{(s\tau_1+1)(s\tau_2+1)}$	$K_v^2\left(\dfrac{1}{4\tau_2(1+\tau_2/\tau_1)}\right)$	Overdamped quadratic band pass

[a] H(s)
[b] Hz

Hertz noise bandwidth. Thus, the filter's gain-squared bandwidth product is given by:

$$\text{GAIN}^2\text{BW} = \int_0^\infty \left|H(2\pi fj)\right|^2 df \tag{9.46}$$

Gain^2-bandwidth integrals have been evaluated for a number of transfer functions using complex variable theory (James et al., 1947). Table 9.1 gives the gain^2-bandwidth integrals for five common transfer functions. Note that the equivalent noise bandwidths (in brackets in each case) *are in Hertz*, not radians/second. Also note the absence of any 2π factors in these expressions. Gain^2-bandwidth integrals are used to estimate the total MS output noise from amplifiers with (approximate) white noise input sources and are thus useful in calculating output signal-to-noise ratios.

9.4 Noise Factor and Figure of Amplifiers

9.4.1 Broadband Noise Factor and Noise Figure of Amplifiers

An amplifier's noise factor, F, is defined as the ratio of the mean-squared signal-to-noise ratio at the amplifier's input to the MS signal-to-noise ratio at the amplifier's output. Because a real amplifier is noisy and adds noise to the signal as well as amplifying it, the output signal-to-noise ratio (SNR_o)

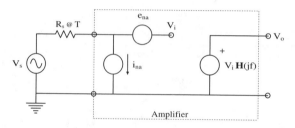

FIGURE 9.9
The simple two-noise source model for a noisy VCVS.

is always less than the input signal-to-noise ratio (SNR_i); thus, the noise factor is always greater than one for a noisy amplifier. F is a figure of merit for an amplifier — the closer to unity the better.

$$F \equiv \frac{\text{SNR}_i}{\text{SNR}_o} > 1 \tag{9.47}$$

The noise figure is defined as:

$$NF \equiv 10 \log_{10}(F) \text{ (decibels dB)} \tag{9.48}$$

when the SNRs are in terms of mean squared quantities. The closer NF is to zero, the quieter the amplifier is.

Figure 9.9 illustrates a simple two-noise source model for a noisy amplifier. Here it is assumed the spectrums of e_{na} and i_{na} are white and that $R_1 \gg R_s$. The MS input signal is $S_i = \overline{v_s^2}$, so the MS output signal is $S_o = K_V^2 \, \overline{v_s^2}$, where K_V^2 is the amplifier's mid-band gain squared. The MS input noise is simply that associated with v_s (here set to zero) plus the Johnson noise from the source resistance, R_s, in a specified Hertz noise bandwidth, B. It is:

$$N_i = 4kTR_s \, B \text{ MSV} \tag{9.49}$$

The mean-squared noise at the amplifier's output, N_o, is composed of three components: one from the R_s Johnson noise and two from the equivalent noise sources. N_o can be written as the sum of MS voltages:

$$N_o = \left(4kTR_s + e_{na}^2 + i_{na}^2 R_s^2\right) \int_0^\infty \left|\mathbf{H}(j\,2\pi f)\right|^2 df \tag{9.50}$$

$$= \left(4kTR_s + e_{na}^2 + i_{na}^2 R_s^2\right) K_v^2 B \text{ MSV}$$

Using the definition for F, the noise factor for the simple noisy amplifier model can be written as:

$$F = 1 + \frac{e_{na}^2 + i_{na}^2 R_s^2}{4kTR_s} \tag{9.51}$$

Note that this expression for F contains no bandwidth terms; they cancel out. When the NF is given for an amplifier, R_s must be specified, as well as the Hertz bandwidth, B, over which the noise is measured. The temperature should also be specified, although common practice usually sets T at 298 K (25°C).

For practical amplifiers, NF and F are functions of frequency because e_{na} and i_{na} are functions of frequency (see Figure 9.6). For a given R_s, F tends to rise at low frequencies due to the $1/f$ components in the equivalent input noise sources. F also increases at high frequencies — again, due to the high-frequency increases in e_{na} and i_{na}. Often, one is interested in the noise performance of an amplifier in low or high frequencies in which the NF and F are not minimum. To examine the detailed noise performance of an amplifier at low and high frequencies, use the spot noise figure (described next).

9.4.2 Spot Noise Factor and Figure

Spot noise measurements are made through a narrow band-pass filter in order to evaluate an amplifier's noise performance in a certain narrow frequency range, particularly where $e_{na}(f)$ and $i_{na}(f)$ are not constant, such as the $1/f$ range. Figure 9.10 illustrates a set of spot noise figure (SNF) contours for a commercial low-noise preamplifier with applications at audio frequencies. Note the area in $\{R_s, f\}$ space at which the spot noise figure is a minimum. For best noise performance, the Thevenin resistance of the source, R_s, should lie in the range of minimum SNF and the input signal's PDS should contain most of its energy in the range of frequencies at which the SNF is minimum.

A system for determining an amplifier's spot noise figure is shown in Figure 9.11. An adjustable white noise voltage source is used at the amplifier's input. Note that the output resistance of the white noise source plus some external resistance must add up to R_s, the specified Thevenin equivalent input resistance. The system is used as follows: first, the band-pass filter (BPF) is set to the desired center frequency, f_c, around which the amplifier's noise performance is to be characterized. Then the white noise generator is set to $e_N = 0$. Assume that the total mean squared noise at the system output under these conditions can be written as:

$$N_o(f_c) = \left[4kTR_s + e_{na}^2(f_c) + i_{na}^2(f_c)R_s^2 \right] K_V^2 B_F \text{ MSV} \tag{9.52}$$

where $e_{na}(f_c)$ is the value of e_{na} at the center frequency; f_c, B_F is the equivalent noise bandwidth of the BPF; and K_V is the combined gain of the amplifier under measurement at f_c, the BPF at f_c, and the postamplifier. K_V can be written:

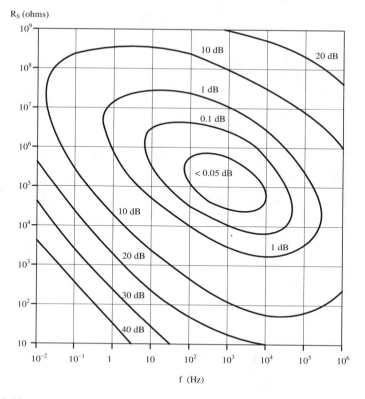

FIGURE 9.10
Curves of constant spot noise figure (SNF) for a typical commercial low-noise amplifier. Note the region in R_S-f space at which the SNF is minimum (optimum).

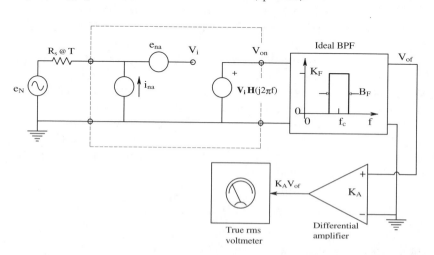

FIGURE 9.11
A test circuit for measuring an amplifier's SNF.

$$K_V = \left| \mathbf{H}(j\, 2\pi\, f_c) \right| K_F\, K_A \tag{9.53}$$

In the second step, the white noise source is made nonzero and adjusted so that the true RMS meter reads $\sqrt{2}$ higher than in the first case with $e_N = 0$. The MS output voltage can now be written:

$$N_o'(f_c) = 2N_o(f_c) = 2\left[4kTR_s + e_{na}^2(f_c) + i_{na}^2(f_c)R_s^2 \right] K_v^2 B_F$$

$$= \left[\overline{e_N^2} + 4kTR_s + e_{na}^2(f_c) + i_{na}^2(f_c)R_s^2 \right] K_v^2\, B_F \tag{9.54}$$

Under this condition, it is evident that

$$\overline{e_N^2} = 4kTR_s + e_{na}^2(f_c) + i_{na}^2(f_c) R_s^2 \tag{9.55}$$

so:

$$\left[e_{na}^2(f_c) + i_{na}^2(f_c) R_s^2 \right] = \left[\overline{e_N^2} - 4kTR_s \right] \tag{9.56}$$

If the left-hand side of this equation is substituted into Equation 9.51 for the noise factor, F,

$$F_{spot} = \overline{e_N^2} \big/ \left(4kTR_s \right) \tag{9.57}$$

Note that this simple expression for the SNF does not contain specific terms for the band-pass filter's center frequency, f_c, or its Hertz noise bandwidth, B_F. Note that these parameters must be specified when giving F_{spot} for an amplifier. F_{spot} is actually calculated by setting f_c and R_s, then determining the $\overline{e_N^2}$ value that doubles the mean squared output noise. This value of $\overline{e_N^2}$ is then divided by the calculated white noise spectrum from the resistor R_s.

It is also possible to measure F_{spot} using a sinusoidal source of frequency f_c, instead of the calibrated white noise source, e_N. See the home problems at the end of this chapter for a detailed treatment of this method.

9.4.3   Transformer Optimization of Amplifier NF and Output SNR

Figure 9.10 illustrates that, for a given set of internal biasing conditions, a given amplifier will have an optimum operating region in which NF_{spot} is a minimum in R_s, f_c-space. In some practical instances, the input transducer to which the amplifier is connected has an R_s far smaller than the R_s giving the lowest NF_{spot} on the amplifier's spot NF contours. Consequently, the signal conditioning system (i.e., transducer and amplifier) is not operating to give the lowest NF or the highest output SNR.

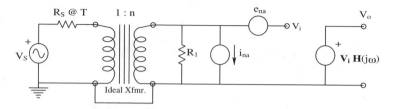

FIGURE 9.12
Use of an ideal transformer in an amplifier's input circuit to maximize the output MS signal-to-noise ratio, as well as minimize the SNF, given the optimum turns ratio.

One way of improving the output SNR is to couple the input transducer to the amplifier through a low-noise, low-loss transformer, as shown in Figure 9.12. Such coupling, of course, presumes that the signal coming from the transducer is ac and not dc, for obvious reasons. (A practical transformer is a band-pass device that loses efficiency at low and high frequencies, thus limiting the range of frequencies over which output SNR can be maximized.)

The output MS SNR can be calculated for the circuit of Figure 9.12 as follows: the MS input signal is simply $\overline{v_s^2}$. In the case of a sinusoidal input, it is well known that $\overline{v_s^2} = V_s^2/2$ MSV, where V_s is the peak value of the sinusoid. The MS signal at the output is:

$$S_o = \overline{v_s^2}\, n^2\, K_v^2 \tag{9.58}$$

where n is the transformer's secondary-to-primary turns ratio and K_V is the amplifier's mid-band gain.

The transformer is assumed to be ideal (and noiseless). In practice, transformer windings have finite resistance and thus make Johnson noise; their magnetic cores contribute Barkhausen noise to their outputs. (Barkhausen noise arises from the small transient voltages induced on the transformer winding when magnetic domains in the transformer's ferromagnetic core flip direction as the magnetizing field, **H**, varies in time. Domain flipping is effectively random at low $|\mathbf{H}|$ values.)

The ideal transformer, besides having infinite frequency response, is also lossless and noiseless. From this latter assumption, it is easy to show that the amplifier "sees" a transformed Thevenin equivalent circuit of the input transducer with an open-circuit voltage of $n\, v_s(t)$ and a Thevenin resistance of $n^2\, R_s$ (Northrop, 1990). Thus, the mean squared output noise of the transformer-input amplifier can be written

$$N_o = \left[n^2\, 4kTR_s + e_{na}^2 + i_{na}^2 \left(n^2 R_s \right)^2 \right] K_v^2\, B \text{ MSV} \tag{9.59}$$

and the output SNR is:

$$\text{SNR}_o = \frac{\overline{v_s^2}/B}{4kTR_s + e_{na}^2/n^2 + i_{na}^2 n^2 R_s^2} \tag{9.60}$$

The SNR$_o$ clearly has a maximum with respect to the turns ratio, n. (It can be shown that F is minimum when $n = n_o$, so SNR$_o$ is maximum (Northrop, 1997). If the denominator of Equation 9.60 is differentiated with respect to n^2 and set equal to zero, an optimum turns ratio, n_o, exists that will maximize SNR$_o$. n_o is given by:

$$n_o = \sqrt{e_{na}/(i_{na}R_s)} \tag{9.61}$$

If the noiseless (ideal) transformer is given the turns ratio of n_o, then it is easy to show that the maximum output SNR is given by:

$$\text{SNR}_{O\max} = \frac{\overline{v_s^2}/B}{4kTR_s + 2e_{na}i_{na}R_s} \tag{9.62}$$

The general effect of transformer SNR maximization on the system's noise figure contours is to shift the locus of minimum NF_{spot} to a lower range of R_s; no obvious shift occurs along the f_c axis. Also, the minimum NF_{spot} is higher with a real transformer because a practical transformer is noisy, as discussed earlier. As a rule of thumb, using a transformer to improve output SNR and reduce NF_{spot} is justified if $(e_{na}^2 + i_{na}^2 R_s^2) > 20\, e_{na}\, i_{na}\, R_s$ in the range of frequencies of interest (Northrop, 1990).

9.5   Cascaded Noisy Amplifiers

9.5.1   Introduction

To achieve the required high gain required for certain biomedical signal conditioning applications, it is often necessary to place several IC gain stages in series. A natural question to ask is whether *all* the component IC gain stages need to be low noise in the low-noise amplifier design. The good news is that as long as the headstage (input, or first stage) is low noise and has a gain magnitude of ≥10, the remaining gain stages *do not* need to be low noise in design. The headstage's noise sets the noise performance of the complete signal conditioning amplifier.

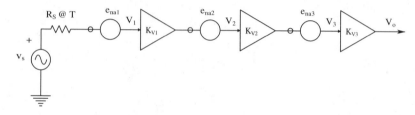

FIGURE 9.13
Three cascaded noisy amplifiers.

9.5.2 The SNR of Cascaded Noisy Amplifiers

Figure 9.13 illustrates three cascaded amplifier stages. The amplifier's overall gain is $K_V = K_{V1} K_{V2} K_{V3}$. The first stage has a white, short-circuit voltage, root power spectrum of e_{na1} RMSV/$\sqrt{\text{Hz}}$ and an input current noise root power spectrum of i_{na1} RMS V/$\sqrt{\text{Hz}}$. The other two stages have voltage noises of e_{na2} and e_{na3}, respectively, and zero current noises. (It can be assumed that the current noises are zero because the output resistance of the previous stages is assumed to be very low, so that $i_{na2} R_{o1} \ll e_{na2}$, and $i_{na3} R_{o2} \ll e_{na3}$.) Assume a sinusoidal input signal, $v_s(t) = V_s \sin(2\pi ft)$; thus, the MS input voltage is $V_s^2/2$. The MS output voltage is simply $\overline{v_{os}^2} = (V_s^2/2)(K_{V1}K_{V2}K_{V3})^2$. The total MS noise output voltage is the sum of the MS noise components from the noise sources: $v_{on}^2 = [e_{na1}^2 + i_{na1}^2 R_s^2](K_{V1}K_{V2}K_{V3})^2 + e_{na2}^2 (K_{V2}K_{V3})^2 + e_{na3}^2 (K_{V3})^2$. The output MS signal-to-noise ratio can now be examined for the three-stage amplifier:

$$\text{SNR}_o = \frac{\left(V_s^2/2\right)\left(K_{V1}K_{V2}K_{V3}\right)^2}{\left\{\left[e_{na1}^2 + i_{na1}^2 R_s^2\right]\left(K_{V1}K_{V2}K_{V3}\right)^2 + e_{na2}^2\left(K_{V2}K_{V3}\right)^2 + e_{na3}^2\left(K_{V3}\right)^2\right\}B}$$

$$\downarrow$$

$$\text{SNR}_o = \frac{\left(V_s^2/2\right)/B}{\left[e_{na1}^2 + i_{na1}^2 R_s^2\right] + e_{na2}^2/K_{V1}^2 + e_{na3}^2/\left(K_{V1}K_{V2}\right)^2} \cong \frac{\left(V_s^2/2\right)/B}{\left[e_{na1}^2 + i_{na1}^2 R_s^2\right]} \quad (9.63)$$

Thus, the SNR_o of the three-stage cascaded amplifier is set by the headstage alone, as long as the headstage gain $|K_{V1}| > 10$.

What if the headstage is of necessity a source or emitter follower with near-unity gain? If the preceding equation is examined, it can be seen that it reduces to a lower value for $K_{V1} \to 1$, e.g.,

$$\text{SNR}_o \cong \frac{\left(V_s^2/2\right)/B}{\left[e_{na1}^2 + i_{na1}^2 R_s^2\right] + e_{na2}^2 + e_{na3}^2/\left(K_{V2}\right)^2} \quad (9.64)$$

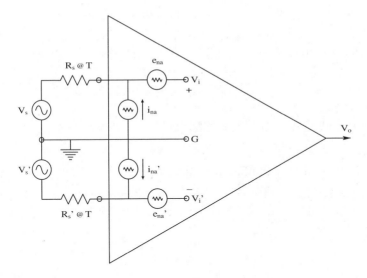

FIGURE 9.14
Equivalent input circuit for a noisy differential amplifier. In this model, both input transistors make noise.

Now the second stage's voltage noise, e_{na2}, becomes important and K_{V2} that should be >10; the first and the second stages must use low-noise amplifiers.

9.6 Noise in Differential Amplifiers

9.6.1 Introduction

As Chapter 3 discussed, the headstage of a differential amplifier contains two active elements (BJTs, JFETs, or MOSFETs) and thus two, *independent*, *uncorrelated* sources of e_{na} and i_{na}. The equivalent input circuit of a DA is shown in Figure 9.14. To simplify analysis, the two amplifier input resistances that appear in parallel with the i_{na}s have been set to infinity (i.e., omitted) because $R_s \ll R_{in}$. All the noise sources are assumed to be white, $e_{na} = e_{na}'$ RMSV/√Hz, and $i_{na} = i_{na}'$ RMSA/√Hz, although certainly $e_{na}(t) \neq e_{na}'(t)$ and $i_{na}(t) \neq i_{na}'(t)$, except very rarely. Recall that, for a DA,

$$v_o = \mathbf{A_D}v_{id} + \mathbf{A_C}v_{ic} \tag{9.65}$$

where A_D is the scalar difference-mode gain; A_C is the scalar common-mode gain; v_{id} is the difference-mode input signal; and v_{ic} is the common-mode input signal. By definition:

$$v_{id} \equiv (v_i - v_i')/2 \tag{9.66A}$$

$$v_{ic} \equiv (v_i + v_i')/2 \tag{9.66B}$$

Also recall that the common-mode rejection ratio for the simple DA could be expressed as:

$$\text{CMRR} \equiv A_D/A_C \tag{9.67}$$

Under normal operating conditions, $|A_D| \gg |A_C|$ and CMRR $\gg 1$.

9.6.2 Calculation of the SNR$_o$ of the DA

Referring to Figure 9.14, the DA noise model circuit has *six* independent, uncorrelated noise sources. Thus the total noise PDS at the v_i node can be written:

$$S_{ni} = e_{na}{}^2 + i_{na}{}^2 R_s{}^2 + 4kTR_s \text{ MSV/Hz} \tag{9.68}$$

Similarly, the total noise PDS at the v_i' node is:

$$S_{ni}' = e_{na}'^2 + i_{na}'^2 R_s{}^2 + 4kTR_s \text{ MSV/Hz} \tag{9.69}$$

To find the MS SNR$_o$ of the noisy DA, assume that the input signal is pure DM. Thus $v_{ic} = 0$, $v_{id} = v_s$, and $\overline{v_{os}^2} = A_D{}^2\, \overline{v_s^2}$ MSV. To find the MS noise output, set $v_s = v_s' = 0$ and consider that the six noise sources add in quadrature (in an MS sense). First, note that in the time domain:

$$v_i(t) = e_{na}(t) + i_{na}(t)R_s + e_{nrs}(t) \text{ V} \tag{9.70}$$

and

$$v_i'(t) = e_{na}'(t) + i_{na}'(t)R_s' + e_{nrs}'(t) \text{ V} \tag{9.71}$$

Now expand and square Equation 9.65 for the amplifier output:

$$v_{on}^2(t) = A_D^2\left[\frac{v_i^2 - 2v_i v_i' + v_i'^2}{4}\right] + 2A_D A_C\left[\frac{v_i - v_i'}{2}\right]\left[\frac{v_i + v_i'}{2}\right] + A_C^2\left[\frac{v_i^2 + 2v_i v_i'}{4} + v_i'^2\right] \tag{9.72}$$

When the expressions for $v_i(t)$ and $v_i'(t)$ from Equation 9.70 and Equation 9.71 are substituted into Equation 9.72 and the expectation or mean is taken, cross terms between v_i and v_i' vanish because of statistical independence and no correlation. Also, the means of self-cross terms such as $e_{na}'(i_{na}'R_s')$ also vanish for the same reasons. Recall that because the DA is symmetrical, $e_{na} = e_{na}'$ RMSV/$\sqrt{\text{Hz}}$, $i_{na} = i_{na}'$ RMSA/$\sqrt{\text{Hz}}$ and $R_s = R_s'$. After some algebra that will not be reproduced here, the MS output noise is given by:

$$\overline{v_{on}^2} = \frac{A_D^2 + A_C^2}{2}\left(e_{na}^2 + i_{na}^2 R_s^2 + 4kTR\right)B \text{ MSV} \tag{9.73}$$

B is the Hertz noise bandwidth of the DA acting on the white PDSs. Now the MS output SNR of the DA for a pure DM input is easily found to be:

$$SNR_o = \frac{2\overline{v_{sd}^2}/B}{\left(1 + CMRR^{-2}\right)\left(e_{na}^2 + i_{na}^2 R_s^2 + 4kTR_s\right)} \tag{9.74}$$

Note that $CMRR^{-2} \ll 1$ and is negligible. The 2 in the numerator is real, however, and illustrates the advantage of using a DA with pure DM signals.

9.7 Effect of Feedback on Noise

9.7.1 Introduction

Chapter 4 and Chapter 5 showed that negative voltage feedback (NVFB), correctly applied, has many important beneficial effects in signal conditioning. These include but are not limited to reduction of harmonic distortion, extension of bandwidth, and reduction of output impedance. A common misconception is that negative voltage feedback also acts to improve output SNR and reduce the NF. It will be shown next that NVFB has quite the opposite effect: it reduces the output SNR and increases the NF.

9.7.2 Calculation of SNR$_0$ of an Amplifier with NVFB

Figure 9.15 illustrates a noisy differential amplifier with NVFB applied through a voltage divider to the inverting input. To simplify calculations, assume that the DA has a finite difference-mode gain, A_D, and an infinite CMRR, i.e., $A_C \to 0$. Also, neglect the input voltages produced by the current noise sources. The DA's output is given by:

$$v_o = A_D'(v_i - v_i') \tag{9.75}$$

The noninverting input node signal voltage is $v_i = v_s$. The inverting input node voltage is:

$$v_i' = v_o\left(\frac{R_1}{R_1 + R_F}\right) = v_o\beta \tag{9.76}$$

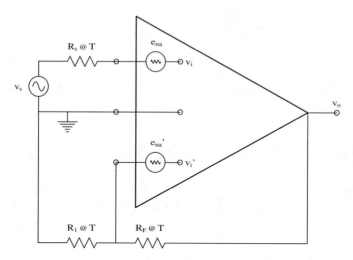

FIGURE 9.15
Circuit model for a DA with negative voltage feedback. The i_{na}s are neglected.

When the expressions for v_i and v_i' are substituted into Equation 9.75, v_o is found to be:

$$v_o = \frac{v_s A_D'}{1+\beta A_D'}$$
(9.77)

The mean-squared output signal voltage is thus:

$$\overline{v_{os}^2} = \overline{v_s^2}\,\frac{A_D'^2}{\left(1+\beta A_D'\right)^2}$$
(9.78)

When considering the noises, v_s is set to zero and, for the time signals:

$$v_o = A_D'\Big[e_{na} + e_{ns} - \big\{e_{na}' + \beta v_o + \beta e_{nf} + (1-\beta)e_{n1}\big\}\Big]$$
(9.79)

The preceding equation is solved for $v_o(t)$:

$$v_o\big(1+\beta A_D'\big) = A_D'\Big[e_{nn} + e_{ns} - e_{na}' - \beta e_{nf} - (1-\beta)e_{n1}\Big]$$
(9.80)

Note that $\beta \equiv R_1/(R_1 + R_F)$ and $e_{na} = e_{na}'$ statistically but not necessarily in the time domain; e_{ns}, e_{n1}, and e_{nf} = the thermal noise voltages from R_s, R_1, and R_F, respectively — all at Kelvin temperature T. One can now write the expression for the mean squared v_o over the noise Hertz bandwidth B:

$$\overline{v_{on}^2} = \frac{A_D'^2}{\left(1+\beta A_D'\right)^2}\left[2e_{na}^2 + 4kTR_s + \beta^2\, 4kTR_F + \left(1-\beta\right)^2 4kTR_1\right]B \qquad (9.81)$$

The MS signal-to-noise ratio of the feedback amplifier is found by taking the ratio of Equation 9.78 to Equation 9.81:

$$\text{SNR}_o = \frac{\overline{v_s^2}/B}{2e_{na}^2 + 4kT\left[R_s + \beta^2\, R_F + \left(1-\beta\right)^2 R_1\right]} \qquad (9.82)$$

It is left as an exercise for the reader to show that, in the absence of feedback (no feedback resistors at all), the output SNR is:

$$\text{SNR}_o = \frac{\overline{v_s^2}/B}{2e_{na}^2 + 4kTR_s} \qquad (9.83)$$

Note that the presence of the feedback voltage divider resistors adds noise to the output and gives a lower SNR_o. Contemplate the effect of applying feedback through a purely capacitive voltage divider. Capacitors do not generate thermal noise.

9.8 Examples of Noise-Limited Resolution of Certain Signal Conditioning Systems

9.8.1 Introduction

In following examples, assume that the stationary sources of noise (resistor thermal noise, amplifier e_{na} and i_{na}) are statistically independent, are uncorrelated, have white spectra in the range of frequencies of interest, and are added in the MS sense as PDSs are. Aside from their short-circuit input voltage noise, e_{na}, the op amps are assumed to be ideal.

9.8.2 Calculation of the Minimum Resolvable AC Input Voltage to a Noisy Op Amp

Figure 9.16 illustrates a simple inverting op amp circuit with a sinusoidal input. Assume that $i_{na}\, R_F \ll e_{na}$ and thus i_{na} produces negligible noise at the amplifier output and is deleted from the model. Only amplifier e_{na} and resistor Johnson noise contribute to the amplifier's noise output. The mean-squared signal output is given by:

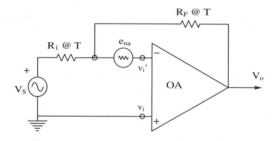

FIGURE 9.16
A simple inverting op amp circuit with a sinusoidal voltage input. White thermal noise is assumed to come from the two resistors and also from the op amp's e_{na}.

$$\overline{v_{os}^2} = \left(V_S^2/2\right)\left(-R_F/R_1\right)^2 \tag{9.84}$$

The noise voltages in this circuit are all conditioned by different gains: e_{n1} is the thermal noise from R_1; it is conditioned by the same gain as v_s, i.e., $(-R_F/R_1)$. Because the summing junction is at 0 V due to the ideal op amp assumption, the thermal noise in R_F, e_{nf}, is seen at the output as simply e_{nf} (a gain of unity). Again, the gain for e_{na} is found by assuming $v_i' = 0$. The voltage at the R_1–R_F node thus must be e_{na}; therefore, the voltage divider ratio gives $v_o = e_{na}(1 + R_F/R_1)$. Note that these three gains are derived assuming e_{na}, e_{nf}, and e_{n1} are voltages varying in time. When the MS noise at the output is examined, the gains must be squared.

Using the principles described previously, the total MS noise at the op amp output is:

$$\overline{v_{on}^2} = \left\{ 4kTR_1\left(-R_F/R_1\right)^2 + 4kTR_F + e_{na}^2\left(1+R_F/R_1\right)_2 \right\} B$$

Note that the equivalent noise bandwidth, B, must be used to effectively integrate the white output PDS, giving MSV. The MS SNR_o of the amplifier is thus:

$$SNR_o = \frac{\left(V_S^2/2\right)\left(-R_F/R_1\right)^2}{\left\{ 4kTR_1\left(-R_F/R_1\right)^2 + 4kTR_F + e_{na}^2\left[1+2R_F/R_1+\left(R_F/R_1\right)^2\right] \right\} B} \tag{9.86}$$

$$\downarrow$$

$$SNR_o = \frac{\left(V_S^2/2\right)/B}{\left\{ 4kTR_1 + 4kTR_F\left(R_1/R_F\right)^2 + e_{na}^2\left[1+2R_F/R_1+\left(R_F/R_1\right)^2\right]\left(R_1/R_F\right)^2 \right\}} \tag{9.87}$$

$$\downarrow$$

$$\text{SNR}_o = \frac{\left(V_S^2/2\right)\!/B}{\left\{4kTR_1 + 4kT\left(R_1^2/R_F\right) + e_{na}^2\left[\left(R_1/R_F\right)^2 + 2R_1/R_F + 1\right]\right\}} \tag{9.88}$$

↓

$$\text{SNR}_o = \frac{\left(V_S^2/2\right)\!/B}{\left\{4kTR_1\left(1 + R_1/R_F\right) + e_{na}^2\left[1 + \left(R_1/R_F\right)\right]^2\right\}} \tag{9.89}$$

To maximize Equation 9.89 for SNR_o, it is clear that R_1/R_F must be small or, equivalently, that the amplifier's signal gain magnitude, R_F/R_1, must be large. This is an unusual result because it says the SNR_o is gain dependent. Most SNR_os to be calculated are independent of gain.

Equation 9.89 can be solved for the minimum V_S to give a specified SNR_o. For example, let the required MS SNR_o be set to 3; $4kT \equiv 1.656 \times 10^{-20}$; $R_1 = 1k$; $R_F = 10k$; $e_{na} = 10$ nVRMS/$\sqrt{\text{Hz}}$; and $B = 1000$ Hz. The source frequency is 10 kHz and lies in the center of B. The minimum peak sinusoidal voltage, V_S, is found to be 0.914 µV.

9.8.3 Calculation of the Minimum Resolvable AC Input Signal to Obtain a Specified SNR_0 in a Transformer-Coupled Amplifier

Figure 9.17 illustrates an op amp circuit used to condition an extremely small AC signal from a low impedance source. An impedance-matching transformer is used because R_S is much less than $R_{Sopt} = e_{na}/i_{na}$ ohms. Assume that the op amp is ideal except for e_{na} and i_{na}. The summing junction of the op amp, looking into the transformer's secondary winding, can be shown to

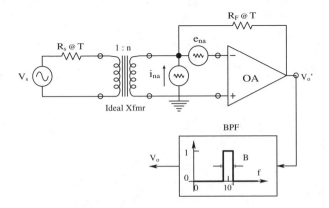

FIGURE 9.17
Circuit showing the use of an ideal impedance-matching transformer to maximize the output SNR. R_s and R_F are assumed to make thermal white noise; e_{na} and i_{na} are assumed to have white spectra. An ideal unity gain BPF is used to limit output noise msv.

"see" an input Thevenin equivalent circuit with an open-circuit voltage of $n\,v_s$ and a Thevenin resistance of $n^2\,R_S$ (Northrop, 1990). Thus, the output voltage due to the signal is $v_{os} = n\,v_s\,[-R_F/n^2\,R_S]$ and the MS signal is:

$$\overline{v_{os}^{\,2}} = \overline{v_s^{\,2}}\left[R_F/n\,R_S\right]^2 \text{ MSV} \tag{9.90}$$

The op amp's output is filtered by an (ideal) band-pass filter with peak gain = 1 and noise bandwidth, B, Hertz centered at f_s, the signal frequency. The filter is used to restrict the noise power at the output while passing the signal.

Finding the output noise is somewhat more complicated. The gain for e_{ns}, the thermal noise from R_S, is the same as for v_s, i.e., $[R_F/n^2R_S]$. The gain for i_{nf}, the thermal noise from R_F, is 1. The gain (transresistance) for i_{na} is R_F. The gain for e_{na} can be shown to be $[1 + R_F/(n^2R_S)]$ (Northrop, 1990). By using the superposition of mean-squared voltages, the total noise MS output voltage can be written:

$$\overline{v_{on}^{\,2}} = \left\{ e_{na}^2\left[1 + R_F/\left(n^2R_S\right)\right]^2 + i_{na}^2\,R_F^2 + 4kTR_F + 4kTR_S\left[R_F/n\,R_S\right]^2 \right\} B \text{ MSV} \tag{9.91}$$

The output SNR is easily written:

$$\text{SNR}_o = \frac{\overline{v_s^{\,2}}/B}{4kTR_S + e_{na}^2\left[n\,R_S/R_F + 1/n\right]^2 + i_{na}^2\,R_S^2\,n^2 + 4kTR_F\left[n\,R_S/R_F\right]^2} \tag{9.92}$$

The denominator of Equation 9.92 has a *minimum* for some non-negative transformer turns ratio, n_o; thus, SNR$_o$ is *maximum* for $n = n_o$. To find n_o, differentiate the denominator with respect to n^2 and set the derivative equal to zero, then solve for n_o.

$$0 = \frac{d}{dn^2}\left\{ 4kTR_S + e_{na}^2\left[n\,R_S/R_F + 1/n\right]^2 + i_{na}^2R_S^2n^2 + 4kTR_F\left[n\,R_S/R_F\right]^2 \right\} \tag{9.93}$$

$$\downarrow$$

$$0 = e_{na}^2\left[R_S/R_F\right]^2 + e_{na}^2\left[-1/n_o^4\right] + i_{na}^2\,R_S^2 + 4kTR_F\left[R_S/R_F\right]^2 \tag{9.94}$$

$$\downarrow$$

$$n_o = \frac{\sqrt{e_{na}/R_S}}{\left\{\left(e_{na}^2/R_F\right)^2 + 4kTR_F + i_{na}^2\right\}^{1/4}} \tag{9.95}$$

Now calculate the turns ratio, n_o, that will maximize SNR_o. Define the parameters: e_{na} = 3 nVRMS/√Hz (white); i_{na} = 0.4 pARMS/√Hz (white); R_F = 10^4 ohms; R_S = 10 ohms; $4kT$ = 1.656×10^{-20}; and B = 10^3 Hz. Using Equation 9.95, n_o = 14.73 (the secondary-to-primary ratio does not need to be an integer). Using n_o = 14.73, the desirable MS SNR_o = 3; substitute the preceding numerical values into Equation 9.92 and solve for the v_s RMS required: v_s = 28.3 nVRMS. If no transformer is used (equivalent to n = 1 in Equation 9.92), v_s = 166 nVRMS is needed for the MS SNR_o = 3.

9.8.4 The Effect of Capacitance Neutralization on the SNR_0 of an Electrometer Amplifier Used for Glass Micropipette Intracellular Recording

Measurement of the transmembrane potential of neurons, muscle cells, and other cells is generally done with hollow glass micropipettes filled with a conductive electrolyte solution such as 3M KCl (Lavallée et al., 1969). In order for the glass micropipette electrode to penetrate the cell membrane, the tips are drawn down to diameters of the order of 0.5 μm; the small diameter tips give micropipettes their high series resistance, R_μ. Figure 9.18 illustrates a simplified lumped-parameter model for a glass microelectrode with its tip in a cell. R_μ is on the order of 50 to 500 megohms. C_T is the equivalent lumped shunt capacitance across the electrode's tip glass; it is on the order of single picofarads.

The electrometer amplifier (EA) used to condition signals recorded intracellularly with a glass micropipette microelectrode is direct-coupled, has a low noninverting gain between 2 and 5, and is characterized by its extremely high input impedance (approximately 10^{15} Ω) and very low dc bias current (approximately 100 fA). The latter two properties are necessary because the

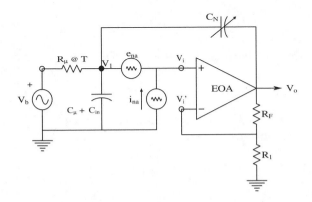

FIGURE 9.18
Circuit used to model noise in a capacity-neutralized electrometer amplifier supplied by a glass micropipette electrode. Only white thermal noise from the microelectrode's internal resistance is considered along with the white noises, e_{na} and i_{na}.

Thevenin source resistance of the microelectrode is so high and, for practical reasons, negligible dc bias current should flow through it to prevent ion drift at the tip. For all practical purposes, the EA can be treated as a noisy but otherwise ideal voltage amplifier. The so-called capacitive neutralization is accomplished by positive feedback applied though the variable capacitor, C_N.

The transfer functions for the biosignal, V_b, and the amplifier noises, e_{na} and i_{na}, will now be found. Assume the EA's gain is +3. To do this, first write the node equation for the v_1 node in terms of the Laplace variable, s:

$$V_1 [G_\mu + sC_T + sC_N] - 3V_1 \, sC_N = V_b \, G_\mu \tag{9.96}$$

Equation 9.96 can be solved for V_1:

$$V_1 = \frac{V_b}{1 + sR_\mu(C_T - 2C_N)} \tag{9.97}$$

Thus,

$$V_o = \frac{3V_b}{1 + sR_\mu(C_T - 2C_N)} \tag{9.98}$$

Note that, in this simple case, when C_N is made $C_T/2$, the amplifier's time constant $\to 0$, thus the break frequency $f_b = 1/2\pi\tau \to \infty$ and $V_o = 3V_b$.

Now consider the transfer function for the EA's current noise, i_{na}:

$$V_1 [G_\mu + s \, (C_T + C_N)] - 3V_1 C_N = i_{na} \tag{9.99}$$

This node equation leads to the transfer impedance:

$$\frac{V_o}{i_{na}} = \frac{3R_\mu}{1 + sR_\mu(C_T - 2C_N)} \tag{9.100}$$

Now find the transfer function for e_{na}. Again, write a node equation:

$$V_1'[G_\mu + s \, (C_T + C_N)] - 3V_1 C_N = 0 \tag{9.101}$$

Note that when $V_1' = V_1 - e_{na}$ is substituted into Equation 9.101, it is possible to solve for the transfer function:

$$\frac{V_o}{e_{na}} = \frac{3\left[1 + sR_\mu(C_T + C_N)\right]}{1 + sR_\mu(C_T - 2C_N)} \tag{9.102}$$

In summary, when $C_N = C_T/2$, the amplifier is neutralized and the noise gains are:

$$V_o = 3\, e_{n\mu} \ (e_{n\mu} \text{ is the thermal noise from } R_\mu.) \tag{9.103A}$$

$$V_o = 3R_\mu\, i_{na} \tag{9.103B}$$

$$V_o = e_{na}\, 3[1 + sR_\mu(3C_T/2)] \tag{9.103C}$$

The total MS noise output of the C-neut. amp is found by superposition of the three mean-squared noise components:

$$N_o = \left\{9\left(4kTR_\mu\right) + 9R_\mu^2 i_{na}^2\right\} B + \int_0^B 9e_{na}^2 \left|1 + j2\pi f R_\mu\left(3C_T/2\right)\right|^2 df \ \text{MSV} \tag{9.104A}$$

$$\downarrow$$

$$N_o = \left\{\left(4kTR_\mu\right) + R_\mu^2 i_{na}^2 + e_{na}^2\right\} 9B + 9e_{na}^2\left(B^3/3\right)\left[2\pi R_\mu\left(3C_T/2\right)\right]^2 \ \text{MSV} \tag{9.104B}$$

The fourth term in Equation 9.104B represents excess noise introduced by the positive feedback through the neutralizing capacitor. B is the Hertz noise bandwidth of the unity-gain ideal low-pass filter used to limit the output noise. Calculating the RMS output noise of the neutralized amplifier: the parameters are amplifier gain = 3; e_{na} = 35 nV RMS/$\sqrt{\text{Hz}}$ (white); i_{na} = 1.1 × 10^{-16} A RMS/$\sqrt{\text{Hz}}$ (white); R_μ = 10^8 Ω; C_T = 5 pF; $4kT$ = 1.656 × 10^{-20}; and B = 5E3 Hz. When substituted into Equation 9.104B, v_{on} = 2.915 × 10^{-4} V RMS, or about 0.3 mV RMS. The corner frequency for the output noise due to e_{na} under conditions of neutralization is:

$$f_c = 1\Big/\left[2\pi R_\mu\left(3C_T/2\right)\right] \ \text{Hz} \tag{9.105}$$

Numerically, this is 212 Hz.

Finally, the SNR$_o$ of the neutralized amplifier can be written:

$$\text{SNR}_o = \frac{\overline{V_b^2}}{\left\{\left(4kTR_\mu\right) + R_\mu^2 i_{na}^2 + e_{na}^2\right\} B + e_{na}^2\left(B^3/3\right)\left[2\pi R_\mu\left(3C_T/2\right)\right]^2} \tag{9.106}$$

As a final exercise, find the RMS V_b required to give an MS SNR$_o$ = 9. Substituting the preceding numerical values, V_b = 8.75 × 10^{-4} V RMS.

9.8.5 Calculation of the Smallest Resolvable ΔR/R in a Wheatstone Bridge Determined by Noise

9.8.5.1 Introduction

The Wheatstone bridge is typically associated with the precision measurement of resistance. However, this simple ubiquitous circuit is used as an

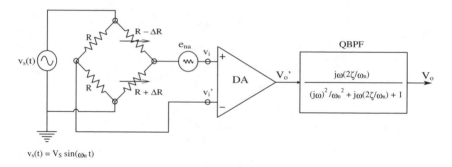

$v_s(t) = V_S \sin(\omega_n t)$

FIGURE 9.19
Schematic of a DA and BPF used to condition the ac output of a two-active arm Wheatstone bridge. The thermal noise from the bridge resistors is assumed white, as is the DA's e_{na}. The quadratic BPF is used to limit the output noise far from ω_n.

output transducer in many biomedical measurement systems in which the quantity under measurement (QUM) causes a sensor to change resistance. Some examples of variable resistance sensors include: thermistors; platinum resistance thermometers; photoconductors; strain gauges; hot-wire anemometers; and direct resistance change by mechanical motion (potentiometers). Bridges used with ΔR sensors generally have ac sources for increased sensitivity. The bridge output under ac excitation can be shown to be double-sideband, suppressed-carrier (DSBSC) modulated ac (Northrop, 1997). DSBSC operation allows enhanced detection sensitivity and noise reduction by band-pass filtering.

9.8.5.2   Bridge Sensitivity Calculations

Figure 9.19 illustrates a Wheatstone bridge with an output conditioned by a noisy but otherwise ideal DA. The ac output of the bridge is then passed through a simple quadratic band-pass filter to reduce noise and demodulated by a phase-sensitive rectifier/low-pass filter to give an analog voltage proportional to the QUM causing the sensor's ΔR. The system appears complex, but in reality is exquisitely sensitive.

In the bridge, two arms are fixed with resistance R and two vary with the QUM — one increasing $(R + \Delta R)$ and the other decreasing $(R - \Delta R)$, a situation often found in strain gauge systems used in blood pressure sensors. Five sources of white noise are in the circuit: the amplifier's e_{na} and the thermal noise from the four bridge resistors. It is assumed that the DA has ∞ CMRR. The voltage at the left-hand corner of the bridge is: $v_1' = v_s/2$. The voltage at the right-hand corner is $v_1 = (v_s/2)(1 + \Delta R/R)$. The voltage at the DA output is thus:

$$v_0' = K_d\,(v_1 - v_1') = K_d\,(v_s/2)(\Delta R/R) \tag{9.107}$$

$$v_s(t) = V_s\,\sin(2\pi f_s\,t) \tag{9.108}$$

v_o' passes through the BPF with unity gain, so the MS output due to $\Delta R/R$ is:

$$\overline{v_{os}^2} = \left(V_s^2/2\right)\left(1/4\right)\left[K_d\left(\Delta R/R\right)\right]^2 \text{ MSV} \qquad (9.109)$$

9.8.5.3 Bridge SNR$_o$

The noise power density spectrum at the DA output is found by superposition of PDSs:

$$S_{no}'(f) = [4kTR/2 + 4kTR/2 + e_{na}^2]\, K_d^2 \text{ MSV/Hz (white)} \qquad (9.110)$$

The gain^2-bandwith integral for the unity-gain quadratic BPF with $Q = 1/2\xi$ has been shown to be $(2\pi f s/2Q)$ Hz. Thus, the MS noise at the filter output is:

$$\overline{v_{on}^2} = \left[4kTR + e_{na}^2\right] K_d^2 \left(2\pi f s/2Q\right) \text{ MSV} \qquad (9.111)$$

and the SNR$_o$ is:

$$\text{SNR}_o = \frac{\left(V_s^2/2\right)\left(1/4\right)\left[K_d\left(\Delta R/R\right)\right]^2}{\left[4kTR + e_{na}^2\right] K_d^2 \left(2\pi f s/2Q\right)} \qquad (9.112)$$

Equation 9.112 can be used to find the numerical $\Delta R/R$ required to give a SNR$_o = 1$. Let $f_s = 1$ kHz; $4kT = 1.656 \times 10^{-20}$; $Q = 2$; $e_{na} = 10$ nVRMS/$\sqrt{\text{Hz}}$; $R = 400$ Ω; $K_d = 10^3$; and $V_s = 5$ Vpk. From these values, $\Delta R/R$ is found to be 2.315×10^{-7} and $\Delta R = 0.2315$ mΩ. Also, the DA output is 0.579 mVpk.

If a sensor's sensitivity (e.g., for a blood pressure sensor), and how many mmHg cause a given $\Delta R/R$ are known, it is easy to find the noise-limited ΔP from Equation 9.112.

9.8.6 Calculation of the SNR Improvement Using a Lock-In Amplifier

A lock-in amplifier (LIA) is used to measure coherent signals, generally at audio frequencies, that are "buried in noise." More precisely, the input signal-to-noise ratio is very low, often as low as –60 dB. There are two basic architectures used for LIAs. One uses an analog multiplier for signal detection followed by a low-pass filter; this system is shown in Figure 9.20(A). A second LIA architecture, shown in Figure 9.20(B), uses a synchronous rectifier followed by a low-pass filter to measure the amplitude of a coherent signal of constant frequency that is present in an overwhelming amount of noise.

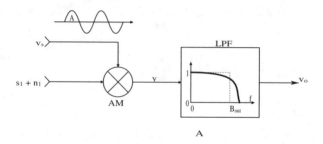

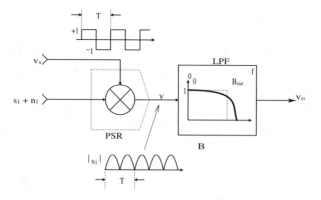

FIGURE 9.20
(A) Basic model for synchronous detection by a lock-in amplifier. A sinusoidal sync. signal is used with an ideal analog multiplier and a low-pass filter. (B) Lock-in operation when the sinusoidal signal to be detected, s_1, is effectively multiplied by a ±1 sync signal with the same frequency and phase as s_1. Note that s_1 is effectively full-wave rectified by the multiplication, but n_1 is not.

Assume the input to the LIA is

$$x(t) = n_i(t) + V_s \cos(\omega_o t) \qquad (9.113)$$

and that the noise is zero-mean Gaussian white noise with one-sided power density spectrum, $S_n(f) = \eta$ MSV/Hz. The MS input SNR is:

$$\text{SNR}_{in} = \frac{V_s^2/2}{\eta B_{in}} \qquad (9.114)$$

where B_{in} is the Hertz bandwidth over which the input noise is measured.

In the analog multiplier form of the LIA, $x(t)$ is multiplied by an in-phase sync signal, $v_s(t) = A \cos(\omega_o t)$. The multiplier output is thus:

$$y = v_s(n_i + s_i) = A\cos(\omega_o t)[n_i(t) + V_s\cos(\omega_o t)]$$

$$= An(t)\cos(\omega_o t) + AV_s\cos^2(\omega_o t) \tag{9.115}$$

$$y(t) = An_i(t)\cos(\omega_o t) + (AV_s/2)[1 + \cos(2\omega_o t)]$$

Note that the one-sided power spectrum of the first term in Equation 9.115 is the noise PDS shifted up to be centered at $\omega = \omega_o$. Because $S_n(f)$ is white, shifting the center of $S_n(f)$ from 0 to $f_o = \omega_o/2\pi$ does not change the noise output of the LIA's output band-pass filter. Thus, the MS output noise voltage from the LIA is $v_{on}^2 = A^2 \eta(1/4\tau)$ MSV, where $(1/4\tau)$ can be shown to be the equivalent noise Hertz bandwidth of the simple output R–C low-pass filter, and τ is the output LPF's time constant. The output LPF removes the $2\omega_o$ frequency term in the right-hand term of Equation 9.115, leaving a dc output proportional to the peak value of the sinusoidal signal. Clearly, $v_{os} = AV_s/2$. Thus, the MS SNR at the LIA output is:

$$\text{SNR}_{out} = \frac{A^2 V_s^2/4}{A^2\eta(1/4\tau)} = V_s^2 \tau/\eta \tag{9.116}$$

The noise figure, F, is defined as the ratio of SNR_{in} to SNR_{out}. For an amplifier, F should be as small as possible. In a noise-free amplifier (the limiting case), $F = 1$. It is easy to show that F for this kind of LIA is:

$$F_{LIA} = B_{out}/B_{in} \tag{9.117}$$

where $B_{out} = 1/4\tau$ is the Hertz noise bandwidth of the LIA's output LPF and B_{in} is the Hertz noise bandwidth over which the input noise is measured. Because the LIA's desired output is a dc signal proportional to the peak sinusoidal input signal, B_{out} can be on the order of single Hertz and F_{LIA} can be $\ll 1$.

In the second model for LIA noise, consider the synchronous rectifier LIA architecture of Figure 9.20(B). Now the sinusoidal signal is full-wave rectified by passing it through an absolute value function that models the synchronous rectifier. The full-wave rectified sinusoidal input signal can be shown to have the Fourier series (Aseltine, 1958):

$$y(t) = |v_s(t)| = V_s(2/\pi)[1 - (2/3)\cos(2\omega_o t) - (2/15)\cos(4\omega_o t) - \ldots] \tag{9.118}$$

Clearly, the average or dc value of y is $V_s(2/\pi)$.

Curiously, the zero-mean white noise *is not* conditioned by the absval function of the synchronous rectifier. This is because the synchronous rectifier is really created by effectively multiplying $x(t) = n_i(t) + V_s \cos(\omega_o t)$ by an even ± 1 square wave having the same frequency as, and in phase with, $V_s \cos(\omega_o t)$. This square wave can be represented by the Fourier series:

$$SQWV(t) = \sum_{n=1}^{\infty} a_n \cos(n\omega_o t) \tag{9.119}$$

where $\omega_o = 2\pi/T$ and

$$a_n = (2/T) \int_{-T/2}^{T/2} f(t)\cos(n\omega_o t)dt = (4/n\pi)\sin(n\pi/2) \ [\text{nonzero for n odd}] \tag{9.120}$$

For a unit cosine (even) square wave that can be written in expanded form,

$$SQWV(t) =$$
$$(4/\pi)\left[\cos(\omega_o t)-(1/3)\cos(3\omega_o t)+(1/5)\cos(5\omega_o t)-(1/7)\cos(7\omega_o t)+...\right] \tag{9.121}$$

The input Gaussian noise is multiplied by $SQWV(t)$:

$$y_n(t) = n(t) \times (4/\pi)$$
$$\left[\cos(\omega_o t)-(1/3)\cos(3\omega_o t)+(1/5)\cos(5\omega_o t)-(1/7)\cos(7\omega_o t)+...\right] \tag{9.122}$$

Before passing through the LIA's output LPF, the white one-sided noise power density spectrum can be shown to be:

$$S_n(f) = \eta(4/\pi)^2\left[1-(1/3)+(1/5)-(1/7)+(1/9)-(1/11)+(1/13)-...\right]^2 \tag{9.123}$$
$$= \eta \ \text{MSV/Hz}$$

This white noise is conditioned by the output LPF, so the output MS SNR is:

$$SNR_{out} = \frac{V_s^2(2/\pi)^2}{\eta B_{out}} \tag{9.124}$$

The MS SNR at the input to the LIA is:

$$SNR_{in} = \frac{V_s^2/2}{\eta B_{in}} \tag{9.125}$$

Thus, F for this LIA architecture is found to be:

$$F = \frac{SNR_{in}}{SNR_{out}} = \frac{\pi}{2^3} \frac{B_{out}}{B_{in}} = 1.23 \frac{B_{out}}{B_{in}} \tag{9.126}$$

which can be made quite small by adjusting the ratio of B_{out} to B_{in}.

As an example of signal recovery by an LIA, consider an LIA of the analog multiplier architecture. Let the signal to be measured be $v_s(t) = 20 \times 10^{-9} \cos(2\pi\, 50 \times 10^3\, t)$. The Gaussian white noise present with the signal has a root power spectrum of $\sqrt{\eta} = 4$ nVRMS/$\sqrt{Hz}$. The input amplifier has a voltage gain of $K_v = 10^4$ with a 100-kHz noise and signal bandwidth. Thus, the raw input MS SNR is:

$$SNR_{in1} = \frac{(20 \times 10^{-9})^2 / 2}{(4 \times 10^{-9}) \times 10^5} = \frac{2 \times 10^{-16}\ MSV}{1.6 \times 10^{-12}\ MSV} = 1.25 \times 10^{-4}, \text{ or } -39 \text{ dB} \tag{9.127}$$

If the sinusoidal signal is conditioned by an (ideal) unity-gain LPF with a $Q = 50 =$ center freq./bandwidth, the noise bandwidth $B = 50 \times 10^3/50 = 1$ kHz. The MS SNR at the output of the ideal BPF is still poor:

$$SNR_{filt} = \frac{2 \times 10^{-16}\ MSV}{(4 \times 10^{-9})^2 \times 10^3} = 1.25 \times 10^{-2}, \text{ or } -19 \text{ dB} \tag{9.128}$$

Now the signal plus noise is amplified and passed directly into the LIA and the LIA's output LPF has a noise bandwidth of 0.125 Hz. The output dc component of the signal is $K_v V_s/2$ V. Thus, the MS dc output signal is $\overline{v_{so}^2} = K_v^2 V_s^2/4 = K_v^2 \times 1 \times 10^{-16}$ MSV. The MS noise output is $\overline{v_{no}^2} = K_v^2 (4 \times 10^{-9})^2 \times 0.125$ MSV; the MS $SNR_{out} = 50$, or +17 dB.

The costs for using an LIA are that the ac signal is reduced to a proportional dc level and that the output LPF means that the LIA does not reach a new steady-state output, given a change in V_s, until about three time constants of the LPF (about 3 sec in the preceding example). The benefit of using an LIA is that coherent signals buried in up to 60-dB noise can be measured.

9.8.7 Signal Averaging of Evoked Signals for Signal-to-Noise Ratio Improvement

9.8.7.1 *Introduction*

The signal-to-noise ratio (SNR) of a periodic signal recorded with additive noise is an important figure of merit that characterizes the expected resolution of the signal. SNRs are typically given at the input to a signal conditioning system, as well as at its output. SNR can be expressed as a positive real number or in decibels (dB). The SNR can be calculated from the MS, RMS, or peak signal voltage divided by the MS or RMS noise voltage in a defined noise bandwidth. If the MS SNR is computed, the SNR(dB) $= 10 \log_{10}$ (msSNR); otherwise it is SNR(dB) $= 20 \log_{10}$(RMSSNR)

Signal averaging is widely used in experimental and clinical electrophysiology in order to extract a repetitive, quasi-deterministic, electrophysiological transient response buried in broadband noise. One example of the type of signal extracted is the evoked cortical response recorded directly from the surface of the brain (or from the scalp) by an electrode pair while the subject is given a repetitive periodic sensory stimulus, such as a tone burst, flash of light, or tachistoscopically presented picture. Every time the stimulus is given, a "hard-wired" electrophysiological transient voltage, $s_j(t)$, lasting several hundred MS is produced in the brain by the massed activity of cortical and deeper neurons. When viewed directly on an oscilloscope or recorder, each individual evoked cortical response is invisible to the eye because of the accompanying noise.

Signal averaging is generally used to extract the evoked potential, $s(t)$, from the noise accompanying it. Signal averaging is also used to extract evoked cortical magnetic field transients recorded with SQUID sensors (Northrop, 2002) and to extract multifocal electroretinogram (ERG) signals obtained when testing the competence of macular cones in the retina of the eye. A small spot of light illuminating only a few cones is repetitively flashed on the macular retina. ERG averaging is done over N flashes for a given spot position in order to extract the local ERG flash response, then the spot is moved to a new, known position on the macula and the process is repeated until a 2-D macular ERG response of one eye is mapped (Northrop, 2002).

Signal averaging is ensemble averaging; following each identical periodic stimulus, the response can be written for the jth stimulus:

$$x_j(t) = s_j(t) + n_j(t), \, 0 \leq j \leq N \qquad (9.129)$$

where $s_j(t)$ is the jth evoked transient response and $n_j(t)$ is the jth noise following the stimulus. t is the local time origin taken as 0 when the jth stimulus is given.

The noise is assumed to be generally nonstationary, i.e., its statistics are affected by the stimulus. Assume that the noise has zero mean, however, regardless of time following any stimulus, i.e., $E\{n(t)\} = 0$, $0 \leq t < T_i$. T_i is the interstimulus interval. Also, to be general, assume that the evoked response varies from stimulus to stimulus; that is, $s_j(t)$ is not exactly the same as $s_{j+1}(t)$, etc.

Each $x_j(t)$ is assumed to be sampled and digitized beginning with each stimulus; the sampling period is T_s and M samples are taken following each stimulus. Thus, there are N sets of sampled $x_j(k)$, $0 \leq k \leq (M - 1)$; also, $(M - 1)T_s = T_D < T_i$. T_D is the total length of analog $x_j(t)$ digitized following each input stimulus (epoch length).

When the jth stimulus is given, the $x(k)^{th}$ value is summed in the kth data register with the preceding $x(k)$ values. At the end of an experimental run, $[x_1(k) + x_2(k) + x_3(k) + \ldots + x_N(k)]$ in the kth data register. Figure 9.21 illustrates the organization of a signal averager. Early signal averagers were stand-alone dedicated instruments. Modern signal averagers typically use a PC or

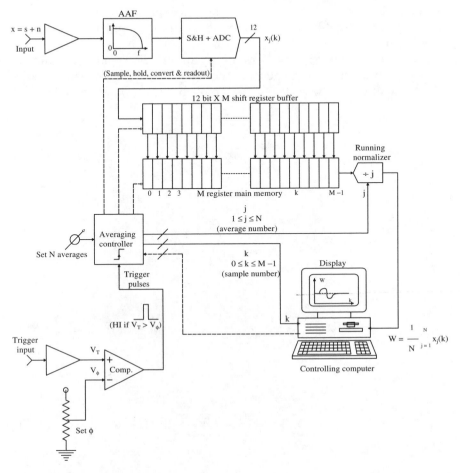

FIGURE 9.21
Block diagram of a signal averager. The memory and averaging controller are actually in the computer and are drawn outside for clarity.

laptop computer with a dual-channel A/D interface to handle the trigger event that initiates sampling the evoked transient plus noise, $x_j(t) = s_j(t) + n_j(t)$. Modern averagers give a running display in which the main register contents are continually divided by the running j value as j goes from 1 to N.

9.8.7.2 Analysis of SNR Improvement by Averaging

The average contents of the kth register after N epochs are sampled can be written formally

$$\overline{x(k)}_N = \frac{1}{N}\sum_{j=1}^{N} s_j(k) + \frac{1}{N}\sum_{j=1}^{N} n_j(k), \ 0 \le k \le (M-1) \qquad (9.130)$$

where the left-hand summation is the signal sample mean at t = kT_s after N stimuli and the right-hand summation is the noise sample mean at t = kT_s after N stimuli.

It has been shown that the variance of the sample mean is a statistical measure of its noisiness. In general, the larger N is, the smaller the noise variance will be. The variance of the sample mean of $x(k)$ is written as:

$$Var\{x(k)_N\} = E\left\{\left[\frac{1}{N}\sum_{j=1}^{N}x_j(k)\right]^2\right\} - \langle x(k)\rangle^2$$

$$\downarrow$$

$$Var\{x(k)_N\} = E\left\{\left[\frac{1}{N}\sum_{j=1}^{N}x_j(k)\right]\left[\frac{1}{N}\sum_{i=1}^{N}x_i(k)\right]\right\} - \langle x(k)\rangle^2$$

$$\downarrow$$

$$Var\{x(k)_N\} = \frac{1}{N^2}\sum_{j=1}^{N}\sum_{i=1}^{N}E\{x_j(k)x_i(k)\} - \langle x(k)\rangle^2$$

$$\downarrow$$

$$Var\{x(k)_N\} = \frac{1}{N^2}\overset{(N\ terms,\ j=1)}{\sum_{j=1}^{N}}E\{x_j^2(k)\} + \frac{1}{N^2}\overset{(N^2=N\ terms)}{\underset{j\neq1}{\sum_{j=1}^{N}\sum_{i=1}^{N}}}E\{x_j(k)x_i(k)\} - \langle x(k)\rangle^2 \quad (9.131)$$

Now for the N squared terms:

$$E\{x_j^2(k)\} = E\left\{\left[s_j(k)+n_j(k)\right]^2\right\} = E\{s_j^2(k)\} + 2E\{s_j(k)\}E\{n_j(k)\} + e\{n_j^2(k)\}$$
(9.132)
$$= \sigma_s^2(k) + \langle s(k)\rangle^2 + \sigma_n^2(k)$$

and, for the ($N^2 - N$) terms with unlike indices:

$$E\{x_j(k)x_i(k)\} = E\left\{\left[s_j(k)+n_j(k)\right]\left[s_i(k)+n_i(k)\right]\right\}$$
(9.133)
$$= E\{s_j(k)s_i(k)\} + E\{n_j(k)n_i(k)\} + E\{s_j(k)n_i(k) + s_i(k)n_j(k)\}$$

Several important assumptions are generally applied to the preceding equation. First, noise and signal are uncorrelated and statistically independent, which means that E{s n} = E{s} E{n} = E{s} 0 = 0. Also, assuming that noise samples taken at or more than $t = T$ seconds apart will be uncorrelated leads to $E\{n_j(k)\,n_i(k)\} = E\{n_j(k)\}\,E\{n_i(k)\} \to 0$. So, $E\{x_j(k)\,x_i(k)\} = E\{[s_j(k)\,s_i(k)]\}$. It is also assumed that $s_j(k)$ and $s_i(k)$ taken at or more than T seconds apart are independent. So finally:

$$E\{x_j(k)x_i(k)\} = E\{[s_j(k)s_i(k)]\} = E\{s_j(k)\}E\{s_i(k)\} = \overline{s(k)}^2 \qquad (9.134)$$

Now, putting all the terms together:

$$Var\{\overline{x(k)}_N\} = \frac{1}{N^2}\left\{N\left[\sigma_s^2(k) + \overline{s(k)}^2 + \sigma_n^2(k)\right] + \left(N^2 - N\right)\overline{s(k)}^2\right\} - \overline{s(k)}^2 \qquad (9.135A)$$

$$\downarrow$$

$$Var\{\overline{x(k)}_N\} = \frac{\sigma_s^2(k) + \sigma_n^2(k)}{N} \qquad (9.135B)$$

The variance of the sample mean for the kth sample following a stimulus is a measure of the noisiness of the averaging process. The variance of the averaged signal, x, is seen to decrease as $1/N$, where N is the total number of stimuli given and of responses averaged.

Another measure of the effectiveness of signal averaging is the noise factor, $F \equiv \dfrac{S_{in}/N_{in}}{S_o/N_o}$, where S_{in} is the mean-squared input signal to the averaging process; N_{in} is the MS input noise; S_o is the MS output signal; and N_o is the MS output noise. The noise factor is normally used as a figure of merit for amplifiers. Because amplifiers generally add noise to the input signal and noise, the output signal-to-noise ratio (SNR) is less than the input SNR; thus, for a nonideal amplifier, $F > 1$. For an ideal noiseless amplifier, $F = 1$. The exception to this behavior is in signal averaging, in which the averaging process generally produces an output SNR greater than the input SNR, making $F < 1$. Note that the noise figure of a signal conditioning system is defined as:

$$NF \equiv 10 \log_{10}(F) \text{ dB} \qquad (9.136)$$

From the preceding calculations on the averaging process:

$$S_{in}(k) = E\{s_j^2(k)\} = \sigma_s^2(k) + \overline{s(k)}^2 \qquad (9.137)$$

$$N_{in}(k) = E\{n_j^2(k)\} = \sigma_n^2(k) \qquad (9.138)$$

$$S_o(k) = E\{s_o^2(k)\} = \frac{\sigma_s^2(k)}{N} + \overline{s(k)}^2 \qquad (9.139)$$

$$N_o(k) = \frac{\sigma_n^2(k) + \sigma_s^2(k)}{N} \tag{9.140}$$

These terms can be put together to calculate the noise factor of the averaging process:

$$F = \frac{\left[\sigma_s^2(k) + \overline{s(k)}^2\right]\left[1 + \sigma_s^2(k)/\sigma_n^2(k)\right]}{\left[\sigma_s^2(k) + N\overline{s(k)}\right]^2} \tag{9.141}$$

Note that if the evoked transient is exactly the same for each stimulus, $\sigma_s^2(k) \to 0$ and $F = 1/N$.

The reader should appreciate that this is an idealized situation; in practice, a constant level of noise, σ_a^2, is present on the output of the signal averager. This noise comes from signal conditioning amplifiers, quantization accompanying analog-to-digital conversion, and arithmetic round-off. The averager MS output noise can thus be written:

$$N_o = \frac{\sigma_n^2(k) + \sigma_s^2(k)}{N} + \sigma_a^2 \quad \text{mean-squared volts} \tag{9.142}$$

and, as before, the MS signal is:

$$S_o(k) = \frac{\sigma_s^2(k)}{N} + \overline{s(k)}^2 \tag{9.143}$$

The averaged MS output SNR is just:

$$\text{SNR}_o = \frac{\sigma_s^2(k) + N\overline{s(k)}^2}{\sigma_s^2(k) + \sigma_n^2(k) + N\sigma_a^2} \tag{9.144}$$

and, if the evoked response is deterministic, $\sigma_s^2(k) \to 0$, then:

$$\text{SNR}_o = \frac{N\overline{s(k)}^2}{\sigma_n^2(k) + N\sigma_a^2} \tag{9.145}$$

Note that if the number, N, of stimuli and responses averaged becomes very large, then

$$\text{SNR}_o \to \frac{\overline{s(k)}^2}{\sigma_a^2} \tag{9.146}$$

and also in the limit,

$$F \to \frac{\sigma_a^2}{\sigma_n^2(k)} .$$ (9.147)

Signal averaging can recover a good estimate of $s(k)$ even when $\sigma_n(k)$ is 60 dB larger than $s(k)$. From Equation 9.145, it is possible to find the N required to give a specified SNR_o, given $\sigma_n^2(k)$, σ_a^2 and $\overline{s(k)^2}$.

9.8.7.3   Discussion

Signal averaging is widely used in biomedical research and diagnosis. A periodic stimulus (e.g., noise, flash, electric shock, pin prick, etc.) is given to a subject. The response is generally electrophysiological, i.e., an evoked cortical potential (ECP), an electrocochleogram (ECoG), or an electroretinogram (ERG) — all richly contaminated with noise. By averaging, the noise is reduced (its sample mean tends to zero) as the number of averaging cycles, N, increases, while the signal remains the same. Thus, signal averaging increases the SNR in the averaged signal. However, as demonstrated, there are practical limits to the extent of SNR improvement.

9.9   Some Low-Noise Amplifiers

TABLE 9.2

Partial Listing of Commercially Available Low-Noise Op Amps and Instrumentation Amplifiers with Low-Noise Characteristics Suitable for Biomedical Signal Conditioning Applications

Amp. Model	Type[a]	e_{na}[b]	i_{na}[c]	Low freq V_n[d]	R_{in}[e]	f_T[f]	A_{v0}[g]
PMI OP-27	OP/BJT	3	0.4 pA	0.08 µVppk	6 M	5	10^6
PMI OP-61A	OP/BJT	3.4	0.8 pA	—	—	200	4×10^5
HA 5147A	OP/BJT	3	0.4 pA	0.08 µVppk	6M	140	10^6
BB OPA111BM	OP/FET	6	0.4 fA	1.6 µVppk	10^{13} (DM); 10^{14} (CM)	2	125 dB
LT1028	OP/BJT	0.85	1 pA	35 nVppk	20M (DM); 300M (CM)	75	7×10^6
AM-427	OP/BJT	3	0.4 pA	0.18 µVppk	1.5M (DM)	5	120 dB
NE5532	OP/BJT	5	0.7 pA	—	300K	10	10^5
MAX 4106/7	OP/BJT	0.75	2.5 pA	—	1 MΩ (CM)	300 (−3)	10^5
PMI AMP-011	IA/BJT	5	0.15 pA	0.12 µVppk	10G (DM); 20G (CM)	26	$1 - 10^3$
PMI AMP-021	IA/FET	9	0.4 fA	0.4 µVppk	10G (DM); 16.5G (CM)	5	$1 - 10^3$
AD624	IA/BJT	4	60 pAppk; 0.1–10 Hz	10 nVppk	1G ǀ 10 pF (CM & DM)	1	$1 - 10^3$

TABLE 9.2 (continued)

Partial Listing of Commercially Available Low-Noise Op Amps and Instrumentation Amplifiers with Low-Noise Characteristics Suitable for Biomedical Signal Conditioning Applications

Amp. Model	Type[a]	e_{na}[b]	i_{na}[c]	Low freq V_n[d]	R_{in}[e]	f_T[f]	A_{V0}[g]
AD6251	IA/BJ	4	0.3 pA	0.2 µV	1G (DMandCM)	25	$1 - 10^3$
BB INA1102	IA/FET	10	1.8 fA	1 µVppk	2×10^{12} (DM); 5×10^{12} (CM)	12	$1 - 500$
PMI AMP-052	IA/FET	16	10 fA	4 µVpp	10^{12} (DM & CM)	3	$1 - 10^3$
ZN459CP	IA/BJT	0.8	1 pA	—	7k (Single ended)	15(–3)	60 dB
ZN424	IA/BJT	5.5	0.3 pA	— 200k	4	2×10^4	

[a] Type refers to whether the amplifier is an op amp (OP) or an instrumentation amplifier (IA), and whether it has a BJT or FET headstage.
[b] e_{na} is given in nV RMS/√Hz measured at 1 kHz.
[c] i_{na} is given in picoamps (pA) or femtoamps (fA) RMS/√Hz measured at 1 kHz.
[d] Low freq. V_n is the equivalent peak-to-peak, short-circuit input noise measured over a standard 0.1- to 10-Hz bandwidth.
[e] R_{in} is the input resistance.
[f] f_T is the unity gain bandwidth in MHz, unless followed by (–3), in which case it is the high-frequency –3-dB frequency.
[g] A_{V0} for op amps is their open-loop dc gain; the useful gain range is given for IAs.

9.10 The Art of Low-Noise Signal Conditioning System Design

9.10.1 Introduction

Consider the scenario in which a physiological signal such as nerve action potentials (spikes) is to be recorded extracellularly from the brain with a metal microelectrode embedded in the cortex. The signal has a peak amplitude, v_{spk}, generally in the tens of microvolts. The input signal is assumed to be accompanied by additive white noise and to be resolved above the total broadband noise at the preamplifier's input. It has been shown previously that the MS input noise is:

$$N_i = [e_{na}^2 + i_{na}^2 R_s^2 + 4kTR_s + e_{ns}^2] \, B \text{ MSV.} \tag{9.148}$$

where e_{na} and i_{na} are white root noise spectra that are properties of the amplifier used and e_{ns} is a white noise root power spectrum added to the recorded signal in the brain.

It is also assumed that the thermal noise in the source resistance, R_s, is white and B is the Hertz bandwidth over which the signal and input noises are considered. Low-noise amplifier design is particularly desired when v_{spk}

$$< 3\sqrt{[e_{na}^2 + i_{na}^2 R_s^2 + 4kTR_s]B} \ V.$$

The first step in designing a low-noise signal conditioning system is to choose a low-noise headstage amplifier that also meets other design criteria for parameters such as bandwidth, slew rate, input dc offset voltage (V_{OS}) and bias current (I_B), and V_{OS} and I_B tempcos. Modern low-noise IC amplifiers typically have e_{na}s < 7 nV/$\sqrt{\text{Hz}}$ in the white region. Such amplifiers may use super beta BJT headstages that, unlike FET headstages, have higher values of I_B and i_{na} and a relatively lower R_{in}. See Table 9.2 for examples.

Because the noise performance of a multistage amplifier used for signal conditioning is set by the noise characteristics of the (input) headstage, it is necessary to give the low-noise headstage at least a gain of 5, preferably 10. Having done this, following amplifier stages need not be expensive low-noise types. Any resistance used in an input high-pass filter coupling the electrode to the headstage should be a low-noise metal film type, not carbon composition.

Finally, a band-pass filter with noise bandwidth B should follow the amplifier stages. The filter's corner frequencies to pass nerve spikes and to exclude high- and low-frequency noise should be at 30 Hz and 3 kHz. The noise Hertz BW, B, is generally close to but greater than the signal passband. For a simple two-real-pole BPF with low break frequency at $f_{lo} = 1/(2\pi\tau_1)$ Hz and a high break frequency at $f_{hi} = 1/(2\pi\tau_2)$ Hz, the noise BW from Table 9.1 is:

$$B = \frac{1}{4\tau_2\left(1+\tau_2/\tau_1\right)} \text{ Hz} . \tag{9.149}$$

The signal's -3-dB Hz bandwidth is easily seen to be:

$$\text{SBW} = \frac{\left(\tau_1 - \tau_2\right)}{2\pi\,\tau_1\,\tau_2} \text{ Hz} \tag{9.150}$$

For example, if $\tau_2 = 10^{-4}$ sec and $\tau_1 = 10^{-2}$ sec then $B = 2.475 \times 10^3$ Hz for noise and the signal BW is SBW $= 1.576 \times 10^3$ Hz.

Section 9.4.3 described the use of an input transformer to maximize the SNR at the output of the analog signal conditioning system. It may be worthwhile to consider transformer coupling of the source to the headstage if the Thevenin source resistance of the electrode, R_s, is less than $1/10$ of $R_{sopt} = e_{na}/i_{na}$ Ω. Transformer coupling carries a price tag, however. Special expensive, low-loss, low-noise transformers are used that generally have extensive magnetic shielding to prevent the pick-up of unwanted, time-varying magnetic fields, such as those from power lines, etc. The author has never heard of SNR_o-maximizing coupling transformers being used with metal microelectrodes. The R_s of a typical metal microelectrode is on the order of 15 kΩ with its tip platinized (Northrop and Guignon, 1970). If an instrumentation amplifier such as the AD624 is used as the headstage, its $e_{na} = 4$ nV/$\sqrt{\text{Hz}}$ and its $i_{na} = 0.4$ pA/$\sqrt{\text{Hz}}$, so its $R_{sopt} = e_{na}/i_{na} = 10^5$ Ω. If a transformer were to be used, its turns ratio to maximize SNR_{out} would be 2.58.

Experience indicates that, although SNR_{out} improvement would occur, it would be too small to justify the expense of the transformer. (It would be only 1.08 times the SNR of the amplifier with no transformer.) On the other hand, if the same amplifier were to be used with a transducer having $R_s = 10$ Ω, the transformer turns ration would be $n_o = 100$ and the improvement in SNR_{out} over an amplifier with no transformer would be:

$$
\rho = \frac{4kTR_s + e_{na}^2 + i_{na}^2 R_s^2}{4kTR_s + 2e_{na}i_{na}R_s}
$$

$$
= \frac{1.656 \times 10^{-19} + 16 \times 10^{-18} + 16 \times 10^{-26} \times 100}{1.656 \times 10^{-19} + 2 \times 4 \times 10^{-9} \times 4 \times 10^{-13} \times 10} = 81.81
$$

(9.151)

Thus, the use of the transformer under the preceding conditions would lead to a significant improvement in the output MS SNR.

Section 9.7 and Section 9.8.2 examined the effect of negative feedback applied around an amplifier through a resistive voltage divider. A surprising result was found for a sinusoidal voltage source connected to a standard inverting, ideal op amp circuit with short-circuit equivalent input noise root power spectrum, e_{na} ($i_{na} = 0$ in this case) and noisy resistors. Namely, the amplifier's SNR_{out} increases monotonically with amplifier gain magnitude, R_F/R_1, to a best asymptotic value of:

$$
\text{SNR}_{outmax} = \frac{\left(V_s^2/2\right)/B}{4kTR_1 + e_{na}^2}
$$

(9.152)

Thus the output MS SNR depends on the absolute value of the input resistor and the amplifier's overall closed-loop gain.

As a design example, examine the SNR_{out} for an op amp used in the noninverting mode. Although both op amp inputs are properly characterized with their own e_{na} and i_{na}, it is common practice to assume infinite CMRR and combine the noises as one net e_{na} and i_{na} at the amplifier's summing junction, as shown in Figure 9.22. Assume that the three resistors make thermal white noise and that the signal is sinusoidal. The MS output signal is:

$$
S_o = \left(V_s^2/2\right)\left(1 + R_F/R_1\right)^2 \text{ MSV}
$$

(9.153)

The MS output noise has five independent components:

$$
N_o = \left\{\left(4kTR_s + e_{na}^2\right)\left(1 + R_F/R_1\right)^2 + \left(i_{na}^2 + 4kTG_1 + 4kTG_F\right)G_F^2\right\}B \text{ MSV}
$$

(9.154)

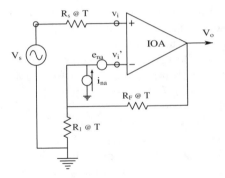

FIGURE 9.22
Noisy noninverting op amp amplifier relevant to the design example in Section 9.10.

Now the output MS SNR can be written:

$$\text{SNR}_{out} = \frac{\left(V_s^2/2\right)/B}{4kTR_s + e_{na}^2 + i_{na}^2\left(R_F\|R_1\right)^2 + 4kT\left(R_F\|R_1\right)} \tag{9.155}$$

where $(R_F\|R_1) = R_F R_1/(R_F + R_1)$.

SNR_{out} is maximized by (1) choosing an op amp with low i_{na} and e_{na}; and (2) making $(R_F\|R_1)$ small. The latter condition says nothing about the amplifier's voltage gain, $(1 + R_F/R_1)$, only that $R_F R_1/(R_F + R_1)$ must be small. For example, for small-signal operation, let $R_1 = 100\ \Omega$, and $R_F = 99.9\ k\Omega$, for a gain of 10^3. R_F and R_1 should be low XS noise types, i.e., wire-wound or metal film.

Low noise amplifier design also includes strategies to minimize the pick-up of coherent interference. These strategies are not covered here; the interested reader can find descriptions of shielding, guarding, and ground loop elimination in Section 3.9 in Northrop (1997), and also in Barnes (1987) and Ott (1976).

9.11 Chapter Summary

This chapter introduced key mathematical ways of describing the random noise accompanying recorded signals and also originating in resistors and amplifiers. Concepts, properties, and significance of the probability density function, auto- and cross-correlation functions and their Fourier transforms, and auto- and cross-power density spectrums were examined.

Random noise was shown to arise in all resistors, the real parts of impedances or admittances, diodes, and active devices including BJTs, FETs, and

IC amplifiers. To find the total noise from a circuit, it is necessary to add the mean squared noise voltages rather than the RMS noises; then the square root is taken to find the total RMS noise. The same superposition of mean squared noises can also be applied to noise power density spectra (PDS).

After showing that the output noise PDS from a linear system can be expressed as the product of the input power density spectrum and the magnitude squared of the system's frequency response function as shown in Equation 9.41, concepts of noise factor, noise figure, and signal-to-noise ratio as figures of merit for low-noise amplifiers and signal conditioning systems were introduced. Clearly, it is desirable to maximize the output SNR and minimize F and NF. Broadband and spot noise factor were treated, as well as the use of an input transformer to minimize F and maximize the output SNR when the Thevenin source resistance is significantly lower than e_{na}/i_{na}.

Also considered was the behavior of noise in cascaded amplifier stages, in differential amplifiers, and in feedback amplifiers. Section 9.8 gave many examples of the calculation of the minimum input signal to get a specified output SNR, including signal averaging. This chapter concluded by listing some low-noise op amps and IAs currently available and discussing the general principles of low-noise signal conditioning system design.

Home Problems

9.1   Assume the circuit in Figure P9.1 is at T Kelvins.

    a. Derive an expression for the one-sided noise voltage power density spectrum, $S_n(f)$, in MSV/Hz at the v_o node.

    b. Integrate $S_n(f)$ over $0 \leq f \leq \infty$ to find the total mean-squared noise voltage at v_o.

    c. Let $i_s(t) = I_s \sin(2\pi f_o t)$. Find an expression for the MS output voltage signal-to-noise ratio. Sketch and dimension SNR_{out} vs. C.

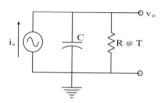

FIGURE P9.1

9.2   Repeat problem 9.1 for the circuit of Figure P9.2. Let $f_o = 1/(2\pi\sqrt{LC})$.

9.3   A white noise voltage with one-sided PDS of $S_n(f) = \eta$ MSV/Hz is added to the sinusoidal signal, $v_s(t) = V_s \sin(2\pi f_o t)$. Signal plus noise are conditioned by a simple low-pass filter with transfer function: $H(s) = 1/(\tau s + 1)$.

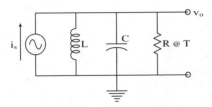

FIGURE P9.2

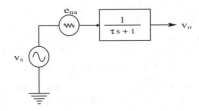

FIGURE P9.3

a. Find an expression for the mean-squared output signal voltage, $\overline{v_{os}^2}$.

b. Find an expression for the mean-squared output noise voltage, $\overline{v_{on}^2}$.

c. Find an expression for the optimum filter break frequency, $f_{opt} = 1/(2\pi\tau_{opt})$, that will maximize the mean-squared output signal-to-noise ratio. Give an expression for the MS optimum output SNR.

9.4 See Figure P9.4. A noisy but otherwise ideal op amp is used to condition a small ac current, $i_s(t) = I_s \sin(2\pi f_o t)$. It is followed by a noiseless, ideal band-pass filter with center frequency, f_o, and Hertz bandwidth B. Let $I_s = 10^{-11}$ A; $f_o = 10^4$ Hz; $4kT = 1.66 \times 10^{-20}$; $e_{na} = 100$ nVRMS/$\sqrt{\text{Hz}}$; and $i_{na} = 1$ pARMS/$\sqrt{\text{Hz}}$. Assume all noise sources are white.

a. Find an expression for and the numerical value of the MS output signal voltage.

b. Find an expression for and the numerical value of the MS output noise voltage.

c. Find B in Hertz required to give an MS output SNR = 10.

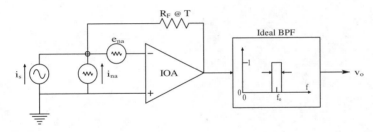

FIGURE P9.4

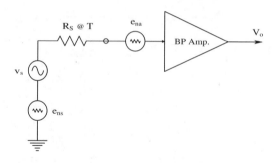

FIGURE P9.5

9.5 A tuned (band-pass) video amplifier, shown in Figure P9.5, is used to condition a 900-kHz Doppler ultrasound signal to which various uncorrelated noise signals are added. The amplifier's peak gain is 10^4 and its noise bandwidth B is 10 kHz centered on 900 kHz. Let $e_{na} = 10$ nVRMS/$\sqrt{\text{Hz}}$ (white); $e_{ns} = 25$ nVRMS/$\sqrt{\text{Hz}}$ (white); $R_s = 1200$ Ω; $4kT = 1.66 \times 10^{-20}$; and $v_s(t) = V_s \sin(2\pi\, 9.01 \times 10^5\, t)$.

a. Find the RMS output noise voltage.

b. Find the peak signal voltage, V_s, to give an RMS $\text{SNR}_{out} = 10$.

9.6 A noisy but otherwise ideal op amp is used to condition the signal from a silicon photoconductor (PC) light sensor as shown in Figure P9.6. Resistor R_c is used to compensate for the PC's dark current so that $V_{os} = 0$ in the dark. $i_{na} = 0.4$ pARMS/$\sqrt{\text{Hz}}$ (white); $e_{na} = 3$ nVRMS/$\sqrt{\text{Hz}}$ (white); $R_c = 2.3 \times 10^5$ Ω; $R_F = 10^6$ Ω; and $4kT = 1.66 \times 10^{-20}$. The photoconductor can be modeled by a fixed dark conductance, $G_D = 1/R_D$, in parallel with a light-sensitive conductance given by $G_P = I_P/V_C = P_L \times 742.27$ S. P_L is the incident optical power in watts and the photoconductance parameter is computed from various physical constants (see Section 2.6.5 in Chapter 2). The amplifier is followed by a noiseless LPF with $\tau = 0.01$ sec.

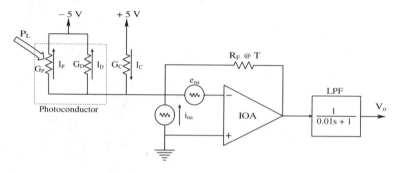

FIGURE P9.6

a. Derive an expression for and calculate the numerical value of the RMS output noise voltage, v_{on}, in the dark. Assume all the resistors make thermal white noise and are at the same temperature. (Note that there are five uncorrelated noise sources in the dark.)

b. Give an expression for the dc V_{os} as a function of I_p. What is the PC's dark current, I_D?

c. What photon power in watts, P_L, must be absorbed by the PC in order that the dc V_{os} be equal to three times the RMS noise voltage, v_{on}, found in part a?

9.7 In an attempt to increase the output SNR of a signal conditioning system, the circuit architecture of Figure P9.7 is proposed. N low-noise preamplifiers, each with the same value of short-circuit input voltage noise, e_{na}, are connected as shown. The ideal op amp and resistors R and R/N are assumed to be noiseless. R_S, however, is at temperature T Kelvins and makes Johnson noise. Find an expression for the MS output SNR.

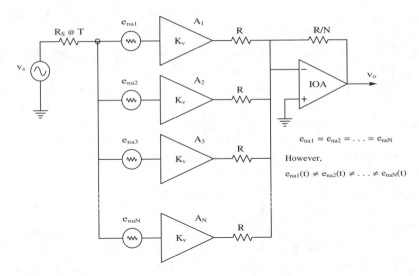

FIGURE P9.7

9.8 A four-arm, unbonded strain gauge bridge is used in a physiological pressure sensor. The bridge is excited by a 400-Hz ac signal. A PMI AMP-01 IA is used to condition the bridge's output. The IA is followed by a noiseless, unity-gain ideal band-pass filter with center frequency at 400 Hz, and signal and noise bandwidth, B Hertz. Assume $e_{na} = 5$ nVRMS/$\sqrt{Hz}$; $V_B = 5$ V peak; $B = 100$ Hz; $K_v = 10^3$; $R = 600\ \Omega$; and $\Delta R(t)$ contains no frequencies above 50 Hz. $4kT = 1.656 \times 10^{-20}$. $v_b(t) = V_B \sin(2\pi 400 t)$.

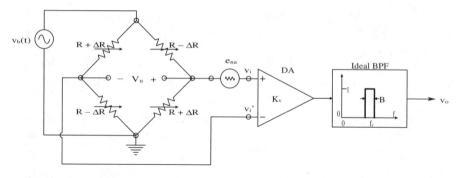

FIGURE P9.8

  a. Give an expression for $V_u(t)$ in terms of R, $\Delta R(t)$, and $v_b(t)$.

  b. Assume $\Delta R \equiv 0$ in computing system Johnson noise. Give an algebraic expression for the output MS SNR. Consider the input signal to be $\Delta R/R$.

  c. Find a numerical value for $\Delta R/R$ to get an output SNR = 10. Calculate the RMS output signal for this $\Delta R/R$.

9.9 A PIN photodiode is used in the biased (fast) mode, as shown in Figure P9.9. The op amp used has $e_{na} = 3$ nV/$\sqrt{Hz}$; $i_{na} = 0.4$ pA/$\sqrt{Hz}$; $R_F = 1$ MΩ; and $4kT = 1.656 \times 10^{-20}$. The PD is biased so that its dc dark current is $I_{DK} = 10$ nA, $[\eta q/(h\nu)] = 0.34210$ A/W @ 850 nm. Assume that the PD makes only shot noise MS current given by $i_{sh}^2 = 2q(I_{DK} + I_P)B$ mean square amperes. Let $B = 10^6$ Hz, $T = 300$ K, and $I_{rs} = 0.1$ nA, and assume the biased PD presents an infinite dynamic resistance to e_{na}. Also, assume that all noises are white and that the feedback resistor makes thermal noise.

  a. Derive an algebraic expression for the MS voltage SNR at the output of the amplifier.

  b. Find the input photon power, P_i, that will give a MS output voltage exactly equal to the total MS noise output voltage.

  c. Examine $\overline{v_{on}^2}$ numerically. Use the P_i value above. Which noise source in the circuit contributes the most and which contributes the least to $\overline{v_{on}^2}$?

9.10 Gaussian white noise is added to a sinusoidal signal of frequency, f_o. Their sum, $x(t)$, is: $x(t) = n(t) + V_s \sin(2\pi f_o\ t)$. The noise one-sided power density spectrum is: $S_n(f) = \eta$ MSV/Hz. $x(t)$ is passed through a linear filter described by the ODE:

$$\dot{v}_o = -1v_o + K x(t).$$

  a. Find an expression for the steady-state output, MS, and SNR.

  b. Find the value of "a" that will maximize the output SNR.

  c. Give an expression for the maximized output SNR.

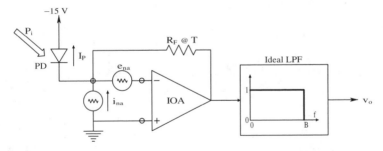

FIGURE P9.9

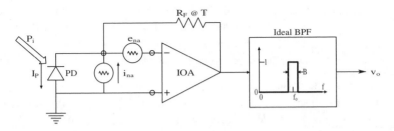

FIGURE P9.11

9.11 The current output of a PIN photodiode operating in the zero voltage mode is conditioned by an OP37 op amp. The input signal is sinusoidally modulated light power at 640 nm wave-length: $P_i(t) = 0.5 \, P_{pk} \, [1 + \sin(\omega_o t)]$. Assume the PD's $I_{rs} = 0.1$ nA; $V_T = 0.0259$ V; the photocurrent $I_P = [\eta q/(h\nu)] \, P_i$ A; and the PD makes shot noise *and* white thermal noise currents with the one-sided power density spectrum: $S_{Dn}(f) = [2q \, I_{Pave} + 4kTg_d]$ MSA/Hz. g_d is the PD's small-signal conductance at zero bias, easily shown to be: $g_d = I_{rs}/V_T$, where $V_T \equiv kT/q$. q is the electron charge magnitude, T is the Kelvin temperature, and k is Boltzmann's constant (1.38×10^{-23} J/Kelvin). The op amp has $e_{na} = 3$ nV/√Hz (white) and $i_{na} = 0.4$ pA/√Hz. R_F makes thermal white noise. Use $4kT = 1.656 \times 10^{-20}$. The noise bandwidth is $B = 1$ kHz around $f_o = \omega_o/2\pi = 10$ kHz.

  a. Write an expression for the MS output voltage SNR.

  b. Find a numerical value for P_{pk} that will make the output MS SNR = 1.0.

  c. What P_{pk} will saturate v_o at 12.5 V?

9.12 Calculate the RMS thermal noise voltage from a 0.1-MΩ resistor at 300 K in a 100- to 10-kHz bandwidth. Boltzmann's constant is 1.38×10^{-23}.

9.13 A certain amplifier has an equivalent short-circuit, white input noise root power spectrum, $e_{na} = 10$ nVRMS/√Hz. What value equivalent series input resistor at 300 K will give the same noise spectrum?

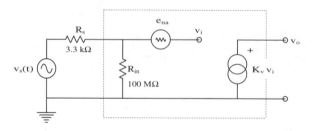

FIGURE P9.14

9.14 An amplifier shown in Figure P9.14 has a 100-MΩ input resistance, e_{na} = 12 nVRMS/$\sqrt{Hz}$, and a sinusoidal (Thevenin) source $v_s(t)$ in series with a 3.3-kΩ resistor. Both resistors are at 300 K. Amplifier bandwidth is 100 Hz to 20 kHz. Assume the resistors make white noise and that e_{na} is white. The sinusoidal source's frequency is 1 kHz and the amplifier's gain is 10^3. Find the RMS value of $v_s(t)$ so that the output mean-squared SNR = 1.

9.15 An OP-27 low-noise op amp is connected to a Thevenin source [v_s, R_s @ T] through an ideal, noiseless transformer to maximize the MS output SNR. Consider the op amp ideal except for its noises. R_F makes thermal noise. See Figure P9.15.

   a. Give an expression for the mean-squared output signal voltage, $\overline{v_{os}^2}$. Hint: What is the Thevenin equivalent circuit looking back from the summing junction toward the transformer?

   b. Give an expression for the MS output noise, $\overline{v_{on}^2}$.

   c. Find a numerical value for the transformer's turns ratio, n_o, will maximize SNR$_{out}$. Let $4kT$ = 1.66 × 10^{-20}; R_F = 10^5 Ω; e_{na} = 3 nVRMS/$\sqrt{Hz}$ (white); i_{na} = 0.4 pARMS/$\sqrt{Hz}$ (white); R_s = 50 Ω; and the noise bandwidth B = 10^4 Hz.

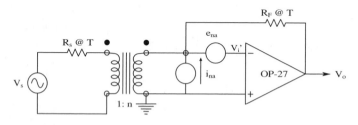

FIGURE P9.15

9.16 Signal averaging: a periodically evoked transient signal, which can be modeled by $s(t) = (V_{so}/2)[1 + \sin(2\pi t/T)]$ for $3T/4 \leq t \leq 7T/4$, 0 elsewhere, is added to Gaussian broad-band noise having zero mean and variance, σ_n^2. Assume the averager is noiseless (σ_a^2 = 0) and the signal is deterministic so its variance, σ_s^2 = 0.

a. Find an algebraic expression for the number of averages, N, required to get a specified MS $SNR_{out} > 1$ at the peak of the signal.
b. Evaluate N numerically so that when $(V_{so}/2) = 1 \ \mu V$ and $\sigma_n = 10 \ \mu VRMS$, the MS SNR_{out} at peak $s(t)$ will be 10.

10

Digital Interfaces

10.1 Introduction

Digital interfaces enable us to convert analog signals to a digital format that can be an input to a computer or a digital data storage system and, conversely, take digital data from a computer and convert it to an analog signal (voltage, current, light intensity, etc.). An analog-to-digital converter (ADC) performs the former task, while a digital-to-analog converter (DAC) undertakes the latter operation. There are many types of ADCs and DACs.

The majority of ADC and DAC operations involve sampling, i.e., the periodic conversion of signals to digital or analog format. Because sampling occurs in the time domain, it can also be described in the frequency domain by appropriate transformation. Two major sources of error in periodic data conversion will be discussed in this chapter: (1) a phenomenon known as *aliasing*, in which an analog signal is effectively sampled too slowly for its bandwidth; and (2) a finite number of binary digits used to characterize an analog signal; the finite-size binary words produce quantization errors, effectively introducing noise into the sampled signal. The problem of aliasing in sampled data will be discussed first

10.2 Aliasing and the Sampling Theorem

10.2.1 Introduction

As shown in Figure 10.1, a modern biomedical instrumentation system generally includes a digital computer that is used to supervise, coordinate, and control the measurements, and which often is used to store (data logging), condition, and display data in a meaningful summary form on a monitor. In describing signal conversion interfaces, it is expedient first to consider digital-to-analog converters (DACs) because these systems are also used in the designs of several analog-to-digital converters (ADCs). Data conversion

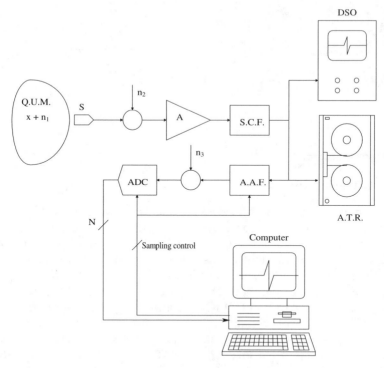

FIGURE 10.1
A typical instrumentation system. DSO = digital storage oscilloscope; ATR = analog tape recorder; SCF = signal conditioning filter (analog); AAF = anti-aliasing low-pass filter (analog); ADC = N-bit analog-to-digital converter under computer control; QUM = quantity under measurement.

from analog to digital form or digital to analog form is generally done periodically. Periodic data conversion has a great effect on the information content of the converted data, as will be shown next.

10.2.2 The Sampling Theorem

The sampling theorem describes the analog filter required to recover an analog signal, $x(t)$, from its impulse-modulated (sampled) form, $x^*(t)$. The theorem states that if the highest frequency present in the CFT of $y(t)$ is f_{max}, then when $x(t)$ is sampled at a rate $f_s = 2 f_{max}$, $x(t)$ can be exactly recovered from $x^*(t)$ by passing $x^*(t)$ through an ideal low-pass filter, $H_{IL}(j2\pi f)$.

The weighting function (impulse response) of $H_{IL}(j2\pi f)$ is (Proakis and Manolakis, 1989):

$$h_{IL} = \frac{\sin(2\pi f_{max}t)}{(2\pi f_{max}t)}$$

(10.1)

Thus, in the time domain, $x(t)$ is given by the real convolution:

$$x(t) = x^*(t) \otimes h_{IL}(t) \tag{10.2}$$

The sampling rate, $f_s = 2 f_{max}$, must be at least twice the highest frequency of the signal, $x(t)$ to prevent aliasing. Note that many practical $x(t)$s can have spectra in which their RMS values approach zero asymptotically as $f \to \infty$. In this case, the Nyquist frequency can be chosen to be the value at which the RMS value of $x(t)$ is some fraction of its maximum value, e.g., $1/10^3$ or -60 dB.

Note that $H_{IL}(j2\pi f)$ is an ideal LPF and is not physically realizable. In practice, the sampling rate is made three to five times f_{max} in order to compensate for the finite attenuation characteristics of the real anti-aliasing low-pass filter and for any "long tail" on the spectrum of $x(t)$. Even so, some small degree of aliasing is often present in $X^*(j2\pi f)$.

The sampling theorem is important because it establishes a criterion for the minimum sampling rate to be used to digitize a signal with a given low-pass power density spectrum. The relation between the highest significant frequency component in the signal's power density spectrum and the sampling frequency is called the *Nyquist criterion*; the implications of this criterion and aliasing are discussed later.

Because analog-to-digital data conversion is generally a periodic process, it is necessary first to analyze what happens when an analog signal, $x(t)$, is periodically and ideally sampled. The ideal sampling process generates a data sequence from $x(t)$ defined only and exactly at the sampling instants, when $t = nT_S$, where n is an integer ranging from $-\infty$ to $+\infty$ and T_S is the sampling period.

It is easy to show that an ideal sampling process is mathematically equivalent to impulse modulation, as shown in Figure 10.2. Here the continuous analog time signal, $x(t)$, is multiplied by an infinite train of unit impulses or delta functions that occur only at the sampling instants. This multiplication process produces a periodic number sequence, $x^*(t)$, at the sampler output. In the frequency domain, $X^*(j\omega)$ is given by the complex convolution of $X(j\omega)$ with the Fourier transform of the pulse train, $P_T(j\omega)$. In the time domain, the pulse train can be written as:

$$P_T(t) = \sum_{n=-\infty}^{\infty} \delta(t - nT_S) \tag{10.3}$$

The periodic function, P_T, can also be represented in the time domain by a Fourier series in complex form:

$$P_T(t) = \sum_{n=-\infty}^{\infty} C_n \exp(+j\omega_s t) \tag{10.4}$$

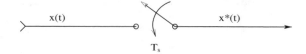

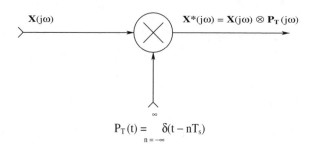

$$P_T(t) = \sum_{n=-\infty}^{\infty} \delta(t - nT_s)$$

FIGURE 10.2
(A) A sampler equivalent of periodic analog-to-digital conversion. (B) An impulse modulator equivalent to a sampler.

where

$$\omega_s = \frac{2\pi}{T_S} \ \text{r/s} \tag{10.5}$$

and the complex-form Fourier series coefficients are given by the well-known integral:

$$C_n = \frac{1}{T_S} \int_{-T_s/2}^{T_s/2} P_T(t) \exp(-j\omega_s t)\, dt = \frac{1}{T_S} \tag{10.6}$$

Thus, the complex Fourier series for the pulse train is found to be:

$$P_T(t) = \frac{1}{T_S} \sum_{n=-\infty}^{\infty} \exp(+jn\omega_s t) \tag{10.7}$$

The sampler output in the time-domain is the product of $P_T(t)$ and $x(t)$:

$$x^*(t) = x(t)\frac{1}{T_S} \sum_{n=-\infty}^{\infty} \exp(+jn\omega_s t) \tag{10.8}$$

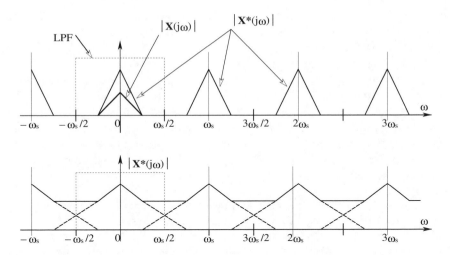

FIGURE 10.3
(A) The spectrum of a signal and spectrum of an ideally sampled signal that is not aliased.
(B) Spectrum of an aliased, sampled signal.

$$= \frac{1}{T_S} \sum_{n=-\infty}^{\infty} x(t) \exp(+jn\omega_s t)$$

The Fourier theorem for complex exponentiation is:

$$F\{y(t)\exp(+jat)\} \equiv Y(j\omega - ja) \qquad (10.9)$$

Using this theorem, the Fourier transform for the sampler output can be written:

$$X^*(j\omega) = \frac{1}{T_S} \sum_{n=-\infty}^{\infty} X(j\omega - jn\omega_s) \qquad (10.10)$$

Equation 10.10 for $X^*(j\omega)$ is the result of the complex convolution of $X(j\omega)$ and $P_T(j\omega)$; it is in the Poisson sum form, which helps to visualize the effects of (ideal) sampling in the frequency domain, as well as to understand the phenomenon of aliasing. In Figure 10.3(A), the magnitude of $X(j\omega)$ is plotted; note that $X(j\omega)$ is assumed to have negligible power above the Nyquist frequency, $\omega_s/2$. When $x(t)$ is sampled, a periodic spectrum for $X^*(j\omega)$ is seen.

As stressed earlier, $x(t)$ can be recovered from the sampler output by passing $x^*(t)$ through an ideal low-pass filter, as shown in Figure 10.3(A). Figure 10.3(B) assumes that the base-band spectrum of $x(t)$ extends beyond $\omega_s/2$. When such an $x(t)$ is sampled, the resultant $X^*(j\omega)$ is also periodic, but the high frequency corners of the component spectra overlap. An ideal low-pass filter thus cannot uniquely recover the base-band spectrum, so $x(t)$. This condition of overlapping spectral components in $X^*(j\omega)$ is called *aliasing*; it can lead to serious errors in subsequent digital signal processing.

Because of the problem of aliasing, all properly designed analog-to-digital conversion systems used in FFT spectrum analyzers, time-frequency analyzers, and related equipment must operate on input signals that obey the Nyquist criterion, i.e., the power density spectrum of $x(t)$, $S_{XX}(f)$, must have no significant power at frequencies above one half the sampling frequency. One way to ensure that this criterion is met is to use a properly designed analog low-pass anti-aliasing filter immediately preceding the sampler. According to Northrop (1990, Chapter 14):

> Anti-aliasing filters are generally high-order linear phase LPFs that attenuate the input signal at least by 40 dB at the Nyquist frequency. Many designs are possible for high-order anti-aliasing filters. For example, Chebychev filters maximize the attenuation cut-off rate at the cost of some passband ripple. Chebychev filters can achieve a given attenuation cut-off slope with a lower order (fewer poles) than other filter designs. It should be noted that in the limit as passband ripple approaches zero, the Chebychev design approaches the Butterworth form of the same order, which has no ripple in the passband. Chebychev filters are designed in terms of their order, n, their cut-off frequency, and the maximum allowable peak-to-peak ripple (in decibels) of their passband.
>
> If ripples in the frequency response stopband of an anti-aliasing filter are permissible, then elliptical or Cauer filter designs may be considered. With stopband ripple allowed, even sharper attenuation in the transition band than obtainable with Chebychev filters of a given order can be obtained. Elliptic LPFs are specified in terms of their order, their cutoff frequency, the maximum peak-to-peak passband ripple, and their minimum stopband attenuation.
>
> Bessel or Thomson filters are designed to have linear phase in the passband. They generally have a "cleaner" transient response, that is, less ringing and overshoot at their outputs, given transient inputs.

One problem in the design of analog anti-aliasing filters to be used with instruments having several different sampling rates concerns adjusting the filters to several different Nyquist frequencies. One way of handling this problem is to have a fixed filter for each separate sampling frequency. Another way is to make the filters easily tunable by digital or analog voltage means. Some approaches to the tunable filter problem are discussed in Section 7.3 in Chapter 7 and in Chapter 10 of the text by Northrop (1990).

Anti-aliasing LPFs are generally not used at the inputs of digital oscilloscopes because one can see directly on the display if the sampled waveform is sampled too slowly for resolution. An optional analog LPF is often used to cut high-frequency interference on digital oscilloscope inputs; this, however, is not an anti-aliasing filter.

10.3 Digital-to-Analog Converters (DACs)

10.3.1 Introduction

A digital-to-analog converter accepts as inputs an N-bit digital word (0s and 1s) representing a numerical value of an analog output signal and a convert enable (CE) command. A DAC's output is a voltage or current determined by the digital word input. The output is held until the next word is presented (as parallel or serial data) and the next CE command is given. DACs (voltage or current output) are used in many applications that include but are not limited to: high-fidelity sound systems; analog CRT display systems used in computers and TV; generation of analog signals used in test and measurement systems, etc.

10.3.2 DAC Designs

DACs can be classified by whether they use bipolar junction transistor switches or MOS transistor technology. The following DAC architectures are found with MOS technology:

- Binary-weighted resistor DAC
- R–2R ladder
- Inverted R–2R ladder
- Inherent monolithic ladder
- Switched-capacitor DAC

The following DAC designs use BJT technology:

- Binary-weighted current sources
- R–2R ladder using current sources

Figure 10.4 illustrates four common DAC architectures. Figure 10.4(A) shows the binary weighted resistor DAC. This is an impractical design for IC fabrication; one needs accurate resistor ratios over a wide range of resistor values. Also, the op amp is presented with varying input impedances, depending on the input word, thus making the DAC subject to op amp DC bias current errors. The SPDT switches used in this design are generally MOS transistors designed to have very low ON resistance and high OFF resistance. The output voltage of this DAC is given by:

$$V_o = \frac{-V_R}{2^N} \sum_{k=1}^{N} b_k 2^k \qquad (10.11)$$

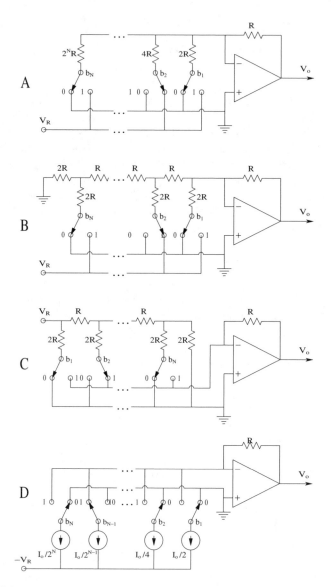

FIGURE 10.4
Four kinds of DAC circuits using op amps: (A) a binary-weighted resistor DAC (not practical for $N > 8$); (B) the R–$2R$ ladder DAC; (C) the inverted R–$2R$ ladder DAC; and (D) a binary-weighted current source DAC (not practical for $N > 8$).

where N is the bit length of the binary "word" being converted and b_k is "0" or "1," depending on the word.

Figure 10.4(B) illustrates the popular R–$2R$ ladder DAC. Here only two resistor values are used; their exact values are not critical, but the ratio must be exactly 2 between all $2R$ and R valued resistors. Switches with low ON resistance and zero offset voltage are required. The output can be shown to be:

$$V_o = \frac{-V_R}{2^{N+1}} \sum_{2^{N+1}}^{-V_R} b_k 2^k \qquad (10.12)$$

Full-scale output voltage occurs when all the switches are set to V_R. This is:

$$V_{oFS} = -V_R \frac{2^N - 1}{2^N} \qquad (10.13)$$

The inverted R–$2R$ DAC architecture is shown in Figure 10.4(C). This is a relatively switching glitch-free DAC, well suited for CMOS switches. Note that the ladder resistors' currents are constant and independent of the switch positions because the op amp's summing junction is at virtual ground. Bit b_1 is the most significant bit (MSB). With $b_1 = 1$ and all others $= 0$, $V_o = -V_R/2$.

Figure 10.4(D) illustrates the overall architecture of the binary-weighted current source DAC. This circuit is easily implemented with BJT current sources and switches. There are a number of approaches to realizing the switches and current sources for this type of DAC (Franco, 1988). The output voltage of this DAC is given by:

$$V_o = \left(I_o R\right) \sum_{k=1}^{N} b_k 2^{-k} \qquad (10.14)$$

When the MSB is HI ($b_1 = 1$) and all other $b_k = 0$, $V_o = I_o R/2$; when the LSB is HI ($b_N = 1$) and all other $b_k = 0$, then $V_o = I_o R/2^N$.

Figure 10.5 illustrates a simplified schematic of a low-power DAC using switched weighted capacitors (SWC). The MSB output of the SWC DAC can be found by observing that when $b_1 \to 1$, all other $b_k = 0$, and the charge in C_1 is also the charge in C_F. Also, the summing junction is assumed to be at virtual ground. Thus:

$$Q_1 = 2^{N-1} C V_R = Q_F = V_o 2^N C \qquad (10.15)$$

$$\downarrow$$

$$V_o = V_R/2 \qquad (10.16)$$

The LSB output of the SWC DAC is found the same way: by assuming $b_N \to 1$, all other $b_k = 0$.

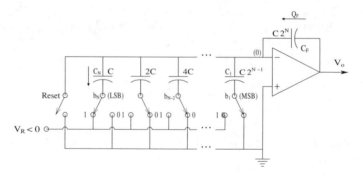

FIGURE 10.5
A switched, weighted capacitor DAC (not practical for $N > 8$).

$$Q_N = V_R 2^0 C = Q_F = V_o 2^N C \tag{10.17}$$

$$\downarrow$$

$$V_o = \frac{V_R}{2^{N-1}} \tag{10.18}$$

The general output can be written:

$$V_o = \frac{V_R C}{2^N} \sum_{k=1}^{N} b_k 2^{k-1} \tag{10.19}$$

Some practical problems emerge in considering the SWC DAC: (1) C_1 must have 2^{N-1} times the area of C_N on the substrate. This limits N practically to 8. (2) The op amp must have a MOS transistor front end to obtain ultra-low bias current so that V_o will not significantly drift over a sampling period.

In Figure 10.6, a design strategy enables the use of a 1:8 capacitor area ratio, rather than a 1:128 area ratio required for the 8-bit DAC shown in Figure 10.5. The MSB output is found from the capacitive voltage divider made from the input array. The input capacitor is $C_1 = C$. It can be shown that the series-parallel combination of the rest of the capacitors having $b_k = 0$, so they are grounded is C. Thus, $V_{o(MSB)}$ is simply $V_R/2$. The LSB output is found the same way by considering the capacitor voltage divider; it can be shown to be $V_{o(LSB)} = V_R/256$. The complete charge-scaling DAC output is given by:

$$V_o = V_r \sum_{k=1}^{N} b_k 2^{-k} \tag{10.20}$$

Multiplying DACs (MDACs) are a special class of DAC in which the reference signal is made variable and the DAC output is the product of the analog value of $v_R(t)$ and the digital scaling input. Thus two-quadrant multiplication can be realized for a straight unipolar binary input:

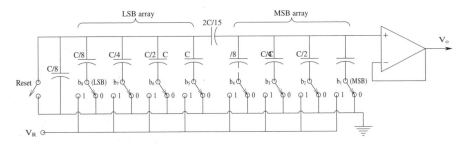

FIGURE 10.6
A charge-scaling switched-capacitor DAC.

$$v_o(t) = v_R(t) \left[2^{-N} \sum_{k=1}^{N} 2^k \right] \qquad (10.21)$$

If the DAC is set up for bipolar offset binary (BOB) operation, true four-quadrant multiplication occurs. The output of a DAC configured for BOB, such as the AD7845 12-bit MDAC, is given by:

$$v_o(t) = v_R(t) \left[-1 + \frac{1}{2^{N-1}} \sum_{k=1}^{N} b_k 2^{k-1} \right] \qquad (10.22)$$

For $N = 12$:

$$\{b_k\} = 1111\ 1111\ 1111,\ V_o = v_R(t)\frac{2047}{2048} \qquad (10.23A)$$

$$\{b_k\} = 1000\ 0000\ 0001,\ V_o = v_R(t)\frac{1}{2048} \qquad (10.23B)$$

$$\{b_k\} = 1000\ 0000\ 0001,\ V_o = v_R(t)\frac{0}{2048} = 0 \qquad (10.23C)$$

$$\{b_k\} = 0111\ 1111\ 1111,\ V_o = -v_R(t)\frac{1}{2048} \qquad (10.23D)$$

$$\{b_k\} = 0000\ 0000\ 0000,\ V_o = -v_R(t)\frac{2048}{2048} = -v_R(t) \qquad (10.23E)$$

MDACs find application in waveform generation; digitally controlled attenuators; programmable power supplies; programmable gain amplifiers;

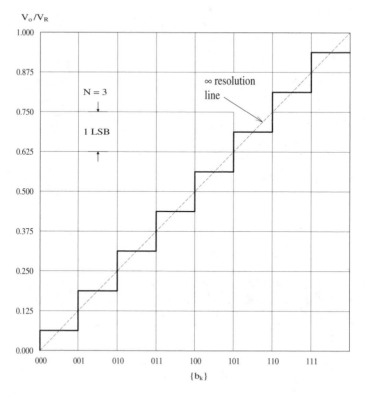

FIGURE 10.7
I/O characteristic of an ideal 3-bit DAC.

and self-nulling systems. The unity gain small-signal bandwidth (f_T) of the AD7845 is 600 kHz; its full-power bandwidth is 250 kHz.

10.3.3   Static and Dynamic Characteristics of DACs

Figure 10.7 illustrates the input/output characteristic of an ideal binary, $N = 3$-bit DAC (in practice the smallest N is typically 8 bits). Note that the analog output has one half LSB of output added to it to minimize conversion error. In general, the LSB and full-scale output of the 3-bit binary input DAC are given by:

$$LSB = V_R/2^N \tag{10.24}$$

$$V_{oFS} = V_R - LSB/2 = V_R\,[1 - 2^{-(N+1)}] \tag{10.25}$$

For the N = 3 DAC, $V_{oFS} = V_R \times 0.9375$.

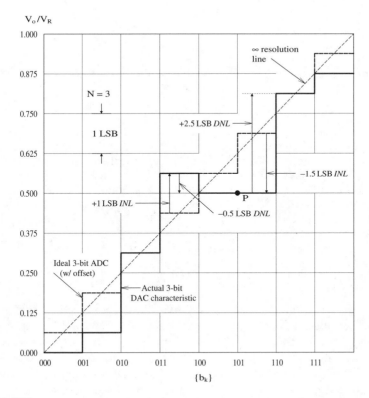

FIGURE 10.8

I/O characteristic of a nonideal, 3-bit DAC, showing types of errors. (Adapted from Allen, P.E. and D.R. Holberg, 2002, *CMOS Analog Circuit Design*, Oxford University Press, New York.)

DAC static errors can be described by the integral nonlinearity (INL) and the differential nonlinearity (DNL). According to Allen and Holberg (2002):

> [The] INL is the maximum difference between the actual finite resolution characteristics and the ideal finite resolution characteristic measured vertically. Integral nonlinearity can be expressed as a percentage of the full scale range or in terms of the least significant bit. Integral nonlinearity has several subcategories, which include absolute, best-straight-line, and end-point nonlinearity. The INL of a 3-bit [DAC] characteristic is illustrated in Figure [10.8]. The INL of an N-bit DAC can be expressed as a positive INL and a negative INL. The positive INL is the maximum positive INL. The negative INL is the maximum negative INL. In Figure [10.8], the maximum +INL is 1.0LSB and the maximum −INL is −1.5LSB.

> [The] DNL is a measure of the separation between adjacent levels measured at each vertical jump. Differential nonlinearity measures bit-to-bit deviations from ideal output steps, rather than along the entire output range. If V_{cx} is the actual voltage change on a bit-to-bit basis and V_s is the ideal change, then the differential nonlinearity can be expressed as

$$\mathrm{DNL} = \frac{V_{cx} - V_s}{V_s} \times 100\% = \left(V_{cx}/V_s - 1\right)\mathrm{LSBs} \qquad [10.26]$$

For an *N*-bit DAC and a full-scale voltage range of VFSR,

$$V_s = V_{FSR}/2^N \qquad [10.27]$$

Figure [10.8] also illustrates differential nonlinearity. Note that DNL is a measure of the step size and is totally independent of how far the actual step change may be from the infinite resolution characteristic at the jump. The change from 101 to 110 results in a maximum +DNL of 2.5LSBs (V_{cx}/V_s = 2.5LSBs). The maximum negative DNL is found when the digital input code changes from 011 to 100. The change is –0.5 LSB (V_{cx}/V_s = –0.5LSB), which gives a DNL of –0.5LSB. It is of interest to note that as the digital input code changes from 100 to 101, no change occurs (point *P*). Because we know that a change should have occurred, we can say that the DNL at point *P* is –0.5LSB.

Dynamic DAC characteristics of DACs limit the speed at which they can convert digital words to analog signals. If a DAC IC has an on-chip op amp for current-to-voltage conversion, the op amp's f_T and slew rate, η, provide one factor that limits conversion speed. Another factor comes from on-chip parasitic capacitances that shunt all resistors and transistors to substrate ground. Conversion speed is also limited by the rate at which MOS and/or BJT switches can turn on and off. Glitches — unwanted (artifactual) transients on the DAC output immediately following a digital word input — are another problem with high-speed DACs. Franco (1988) describes their origin and a cure:

> … these are due to the internal circuitry's nonuniform response to input bit changes and to poor synchronization of the bit changes themselves. For instance, if during the center-scale transition from 011…1 to 100…0 the MSB is perceived as going on before (after) all other bits go off, the output will momentarily [try to] swing to full-scale (to zero), thus causing an output glitch.

> Glitches are of particular concern in CRT display applications. Filtering doesn't solve the problem since the area under the glitch is integrated and carried over subsequent steps [i.e., as the filter's impulse response], which will therefore also be in error. Glitches can be minimized either by synchronizing the input bit changes with a high-speed parallel latch register, or by processing the DAC output with a[n] S/H [sample and hold] deglitcher circuit. The circuit is switched to hold mode just prior to the input code change and is returned to the track mode only after the DAC gas settle[s] to its new level, thus preventing any glitches from reaching the output.

The fast video DACs available in 2003 can convert at approximately 200 MSPS. For example the 10-bit, Analog Devices AD9732 DAC is rated at 200 MSPS and takes 5 ns to settle to one half LSB. The Faraday 8-bit DAC8001 also is rated at 200 MSPS and claims a 4-ns analog settling time.

10.4 Hold Circuits

Just as the sampling process can be interpreted in the frequency domain, so can the process of sample (or track) and hold of analog signals from a DAC. Note that the digital input to a DAC is generally periodic with period T_s. The DAC's analog output from the nth digital input is generally held constant until the $(n + 1)^{th}$ input updates it. This process generates a stepwise output waveform if $\{b_k\}$ is changing and can be viewed as linear filtering operation. The impulse response of the zero-order hold (ZOH) filter to a unit input word at t = 0, and zero inputs at sampling instants thereafter is:

$$h_o(t) = U(t) - U(t - T_s) \tag{10.28}$$

where $U(t)$ is the unit step function, defined as zero for all negative argument, and 1 for all positive argument. $h_o(t)$ is thus a pulse of unit height and duration $(0, T_s)$, else zero. The Laplace transform of $h_o(t)$ is:

$$H_o(s) = \frac{1}{s} - \frac{1}{s}e^{-sT_s} = \frac{1 - e^{-sT_s}}{s} \tag{10.29}$$

To find the frequency response of the ZOH, let $s \to j\omega$ and use the Euler relation for $e^{j\theta}$. The ZOH's frequency response is easily shown to be:

$$H_o(j\omega) = T_s \frac{\sin(\omega T_s/2)}{(\omega T_s/2)} e^{-j\omega T_s/2} \tag{10.30}$$

Note that the zeros in $H_o(j\omega)$ occur at $\omega = n2\pi/T_s$ r/s, where n = 1, 2, 3, ..., and $2\pi/T_s$ is the radian sampling frequency of the system. Thus, the overall process of sampling an analog signal, $x(t)$, and reconverting to (held) analog form by a DAC can be written in the frequency domain (neglecting quantization) as (Northrop, 1990):

$$X(j\omega) = \sum_{n=0}^{\infty} \frac{\sin(\omega T_s/2)}{(\omega T_s/2)} X(j\omega - jn\omega_s) e^{j\omega T_s/2} \tag{10.31}$$

Note that other more sophisticated holds exist; their realization is at the expense of some circuit complexity, however. For example, the first-difference extrapolator hold that generates linear slope transitions between sampling instants (instead of steps) can be realized with three DACs, a resettable analog integrator, and an analog adder (Northrop, 1990). Its transfer function can be shown to be:

$$H_e(s) = \frac{1-e^{-sT}}{s} + \frac{1-2e^{-sT}+e^{-2sT}}{s^2} - \frac{\left(1-e^{-sT}\right)e^{-sT}}{s} \qquad (10.32)$$

10.5 Analog-to-Digital Converters (ADCs)

10.5.1 Introduction

Although the technology for DACs is relatively simple, there are many diverse kinds of ADCs and ADC algorithms. The five major categories of ADC are:

1. Tracking (servo) converters
2. Successive approximation converters
3. Integrating converters
4. Flash (parallel) converters
5. Oversampled (sigma–delta) converters

Next, each category will be examined and a description of how it works given.

Figure 10.9 shows the transfer characteristic of a 3-bit binary-output ADC. Note that an infinite-resolution analog signal, $x(t)$, is quantized into eight 3-bit binary words, depending on its value. Figure 10.10 illustrates the normalized quantization error, $(NQE) \equiv v_e/LSB$, of this converter; the quantization error voltage is given by:

$$v_c = v_x - V_{FS}\sum_{k=1}^{N}b_k 2^{-k} = v_x - V_{FS}\left(b_1 2^{-1}+b_2 2^{-2}+b_3 2^{-3}\right), \text{ for } N = 3. \quad (10.33)$$

Note that the NQE is bounded by plus or minus one half LSB except for $v_x/V_{FS} \geq 7/8$, where it reaches +1 LSB at $v_x/V_{FS} = 1$. 1 LSB $= V_{FS}/2^3 = V_{FS}/8$ for this 3-bit ADC.

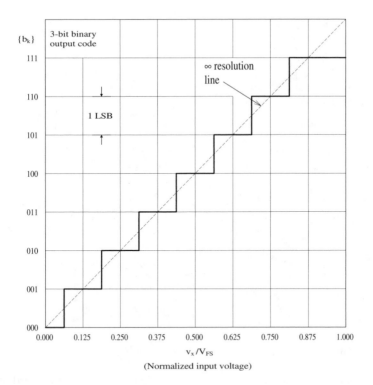

FIGURE 10.9
Transfer characteristic of an ideal 3-bit binary-output ADC.

10.5.2 The Tracking (Servo) ADC

The first ADC considered is the tracking (servo) ADC, aka the counting ADC. A block diagram for this ADC is shown in Figure 10.11. When conversion is initiated, the up/down counter is reset and then counts up. The up/down counter's digital output goes to a DAC. The DAC's voltage output ramps up at a rate easily shown to be:

$$\eta = V_{oFS}/\left(2^{N}T_{c}\right) \ V/\text{sec} \qquad (10.34)$$

where N is the number of bits of the DAC and U/D counter and T_c is the clock period.

V_{oFS} is generally made equal to V_{xmax}. If $N = 10$ bits, $T_c = 5 \times 10^{-7}$ sec ($f_c = 2$ MHz), and $V_{omax} = 10$ V, then the V_o slew rate is $\eta = 1.953 \times 10^{4}$ V/sec. By resetting the counter following each 10-V conversion, approximately 1,950 10-V conversions can be made per second. If conversion is not stopped when the comparator output goes LO ($V_o > V_x$) and the counter is not reset, then the counter will increment down by 1 LSB at the next clock cycle,

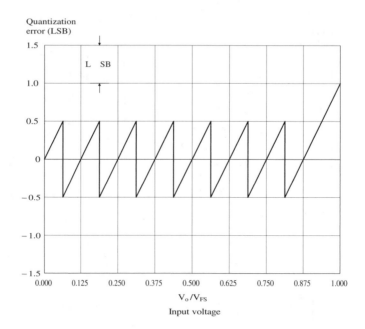

FIGURE 10.10
Normalized quantization error vs. input voltage for an ideal 3-bit binary ADC.

causing V_o to decrease by 1 LSB, thus bringing $V_o < V_x$; the comparator then goes HI and the next clock pulse increments the counter up, so V_o then exceeds V_x. The process repeats cyclically, generating a steady-state 1-LSB dither in the digital output.

When this ADC is used in the tracking mode to improve conversion speed, the LSB output is not used in order to avoid the steady-state dither. If the ADC is reset after each conversion, the end of conversion (EOC) signal occurs when $V_o > V_x$ by 1 LSB the first time after conversion is initiated. Although this mode of operation avoids dither, it is slower and still has a conversion error between 0 and +1 LSB.

The servo counting ADC is well suited for data conversion of DC or low-frequency AC signals. It is also easy to implement in hardware (ICs). One disadvantage is that conversion time depends on the value of v_x/V_{xmax}, i.e., it is variable. Another disadvantage is the LSB dither seen in the steady-state tracking mode.

10.5.3   The Successive Approximation ADC

Like the servo counting ADC, the successive approximation ADC (SAADC) uses a comparator and a DAC in a closed-loop architecture, as shown in Figure 10.12. The conversion cycle for a 10-bit SAADC begins with a start signal from the controlling computer's I/O interface at $t = nT$. Start causes the analog input signal, V_x, to be held at $[V_x(nT)]$ and the counter's

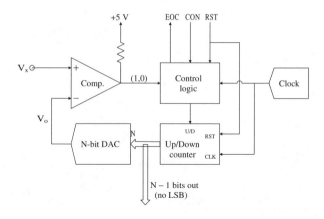

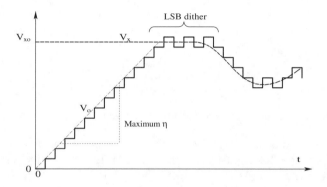

FIGURE 10.11
Top: block diagram of a tracking or servo ADC. Bottom: DAC output of the servo ADC showing numerical slew-rate limiting and dither.

output register is cleared (all $b_k \rightarrow 0$ except for $b_1 = 0$ (MSB)). This action causes the DAC output, V_o, to go to $512V_R/1024 = V_R/2$. The comparator subtracts this V_o from $[V_x(nT)]$ and performs the operation,

$$Q = \text{sgn}\left([V_x(nT)] - V_R/2\right) \tag{10.35}$$

If $Q = 1$, then b_1 is kept 1 (HI); if $Q = -1$, then b_1 is set to 0 (LO). Next, b_2 is set to 1 (b_1 retains the value determined in the first cycle). Now the DAC output is $V_o = V_R (b_1/2 + 1/2^2)$. The comparator tests to see if $\text{sgn}\{[V_x((n + 1)T] - V_o\} = 1$. If yes, b_2 stays at 1, if no, $b_2 \rightarrow 0$, completing the second bit's conversion cycle. Now $b_3 \rightarrow 1$ and $V_o = V_R (b_1/2 + b_2/4 + 1/2^3)$ and the process continues. $Q = \text{sgn}\{V_x((n + 2)T] - V_o\}$ is tested, etc. until all 10 bits have been tested. Figure 10.13, adapted from Northrop (1990), illustrates a logical flowchart for the operation of a 10-bit SAADC; note $b_1 = $ MSB and $b_{10} = $ LSB.

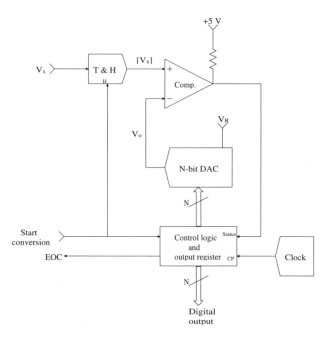

FIGURE 10.12
Block diagram of the popular successive-approximation ADC.

The conversion time of an SAADC is $T_c = NT$, i.e., about N clock periods. For example, the Texas Instruments TLC1225 12-bit SAADC can convert in 12 μs, given a 2-MHz clock input. The TI TLC1550I 10-bit SAADC can convert in 6 μs, given a 7.8-MHz clock, which is about 166 kSa/sec.

10.5.4 Integrating Converters

Integrating converters are also called serial analog DACs. Two basic architectures will be considered in this section: (1) single-slope and (2) dual-slope integrating DACs (IDACs). Figure 10.14 illustrates the block diagram of one version of a single-slope IDAC (SSIDAC). An op amp integrator that can be reset is used as a ramp generator; it integrates the DC $V_R < 0$ to produce a positive ramp with slope V_R/RC. The ramp, V_2, is the negative input to a comparator, the positive input to which is the held signal being converted, $[V_x] > 0$.

At the start of conversion $[V_x] > V_2$, so the comparator output, Q, is HI, enabling the AND gate to pass clock pulses to the binary counter. When $V_2 > [V_x]$, Q goes LO. This event stops the counting and, through the control logic, causes the integrator to be reset to $V_2 \to 0$ and the track and hold circuit to again track $v_x(t)$. $Q \to 0$ also causes the counter to present the total count at its parallel output and the control logic to signal end of conversion (EOC). The SSIDAC is now in standby mode waiting

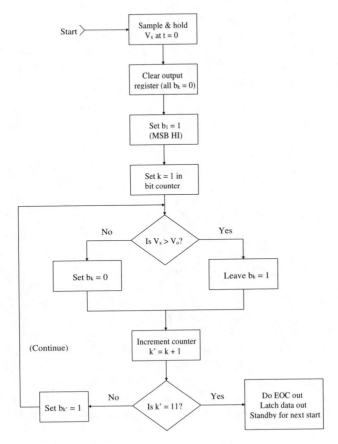

FIGURE 10.13
Logical flowchart illustrating the steps in one conversion cycle of a successive-approximation ADC.

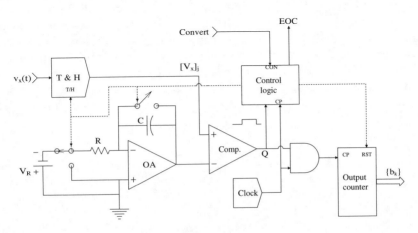

FIGURE 10.14
Block diagram of a single-slope integrating ADC.

for the next convert (CON) command. The leading edge of the CON command causes the counter to be reset; $v_x(t)$ to be held; the integrator to begin integrating V_R; and the counter to begin counting. Each completed conversion count, M, is proportional to that $[V_x]$. From the SSIDAC architecture, the jth conversion:

$$\frac{1}{RC}\int_0^{M_jT} V_R dt = [V_x]_j \tag{10.36}$$

$$\downarrow$$

$$M_j = \frac{[V_x]_j \, RC}{V_R T} \tag{10.37}$$

Suppose a 10-bit converter is desired and V_x ranges from 0 to 10 V. Let $V_R = 1.00$ V and $T = 10^{-6}$ sec. Then, from the preceding equation, it can be determined that $RC = 1.023 \times 10^{-4}$ sec, so if $C = 10^{-8}$ F, then $R = 1.023 \times 10^4\ \Omega$. With these parameters, the SSIADC will output $M_j = 2^{10} - 1$ when $[V_x]_j = 10.0$ V. Note that SSIADC conversion time is variable; the larger $[V_x]_j$ is, the longer it takes. When $[V_x]_j = 10$ V, conversion takes 1.023 MS. Thus, integrating ADCs (IADCs) are relatively slow, suitable for ECG and DC applications. Also, accuracy of the SSIADC depends on the stability of the RC product and clock period over time and temperature changes. To overcome these problems, the clever design of the dual-slope integrating ADC was developed.

Figure 10.15 illustrates a unipolar dual-slope integrating ADC. Note it does not require a DAC. On receiving the convert command, this ADC first resets its integrator output to $V_2 = 0$ and clears its counter to zero. S_1 connects the integrator to $V_x > 0$. V_x is integrated for 2^N clock cycles or $2^N T_c$ sec, causing V_2 to go negative. At the end of this integration time, the counter is again cleared and S_1 switches to $-V_R$, which is integrated, causing V_2 to ramp positively toward zero. During this interval, the counter counts up from zero because Q is high. When V_2 reaches zero, the comparator output Q goes from HI to LO, stopping the counter and signaling the end of the conversion cycle. Mathematically, the integrator output when the counter reaches $T_1 = 2^N T_c$ is:

$$V_2(2^N T_c) = -\frac{1}{RC}\left\{\int_0^{T_1} v_x(t)/(T_1)dt\right\}T_1 = \frac{-2^N T_c}{RC}\left\{\overline{V_x(T_1)}\right\} \tag{10.38}$$

In the second part of the conversion cycle, the integrator integrates until V_2 reaches zero. This takes M clock cycles. Mathematically:

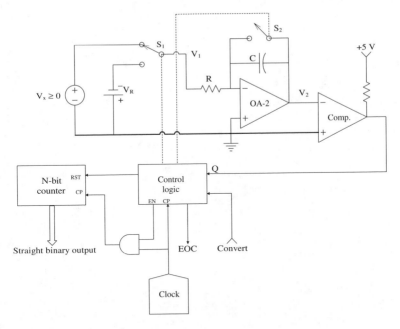

FIGURE 10.15
Block diagram of a unipolar-input dual-slope integrating ADC.

$$V_2 = 0 = \frac{-2^N T_c}{RC} \left\{ \overline{V_x(T_1)} \right\} + \frac{M T_c V_R}{RC} \tag{10.39}$$

$$\downarrow$$

$$M = \frac{\left\{ \overline{V_x(T_1)} \right\} 2^N}{V_R} \tag{10.40}$$

Therefore, the countdown time (and thus M) is proportional to the average of the input signal over $T_1 = 2^N T_c$ sec. Note that this ADC is independent of RC and T_c; these parameters are determined from practical considerations. Often T_1 is made $1/60$ sec to make the ADC reject 60-Hz hum on $v_x(t)$ (Northrop, 1990). Figure 10.16 illustrates the block diagram of a dual-slope integrating ADC (DSIADC).

This ADC gives an offset binary output code for bipolar DC input signals. When the convert command is given, the input is held, the counter is cleared (reset to zero), and V_2 is set to zero with S_2. Next, S_2 is opened and S_1 is set to integrate the output of OA-1, V_2, for a time equal to 2^N clock cycles ($T_1 = 2^N T_c$). V_2 goes positive, so $Q = $ LO, disabling the output counter. When $T_1 = 2^N T_c$, the counter is enabled and counts clock pulses, and S_1 is set to integrate $+V_R$. V_2 now ramps down to zero, which is sensed by the comparator output Q going HI. The number of clock cycles required for V_2 to go to 0 is M. The peak V_2 is found by:

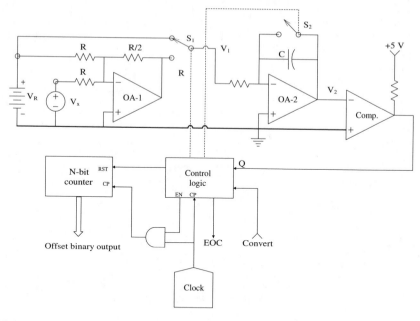

FIGURE 10.16
Block diagram of a bipolar-input dual-slope integrating ADC. The output is in offset binary code.

$$V_2\left(2^N T_c\right) = \frac{1}{2RC} \int_0^{2^N T_c} \left(V_R + [V_x]\right) dt = \frac{V_R 2^N T_c}{2RC} + \frac{[V_x] 2^N T_c}{2RC} \qquad (10.41)$$

The number of clock cycles required to integrate $V_2(2^N T_c)$ to zero is M:

$$\frac{V_R 2^N T_c}{2RC} + \frac{[V_x] 2^N T_c}{2RC} - \frac{V_R M T_c}{RC} = 0 \qquad (10.42)$$

Solving for M:

$$M = 2^{N-1}\left(1 + [V_x]/V_R\right) \qquad (10.43)$$

Note that when $[V_x] = -V_R$, $M = 0$, when $[V_x] = 0$, $M = 2^{N-1}$ (1 MSB), and when $[V_x] = +V_R$, $M = 2^N$, giving a true offset binary output code. Note that this dual-slope integrating ADC also has accuracy independent of RC and T_c.

10.5.5   Flash Converters

The fastest ADCs are flash converters (FADCs) that enable signal sampling in the ns range and thus are widely used in medical ultrasound systems,

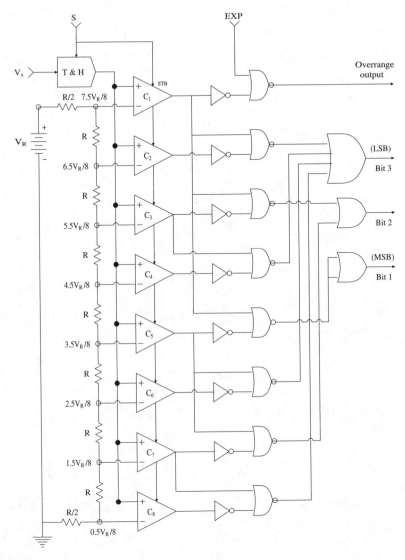

FIGURE 10.17
A 3-bit flash ADC.

sonar and radar data conversion, and certain communications applications. Data conversion rates into the hundreds of MSa/sec are typical. Figure 10.17 illustrates an $N = 3$-bit flash ADC with straight binary output. $2^N - 1 = 7$ voltage comparators are used for conversion; comparator C_1 is used to signal over-range. Thus, an 8-bit FADC uses 255 analog comparators, plus one for over-range. Figure 10.18 illustrates the transfer characteristic of the 3-bit FADC. The Analog Devices AD770 8-bit FADC uses three blocks of 64 comparators and one block of 65 comparators and two levels of bit decoding to

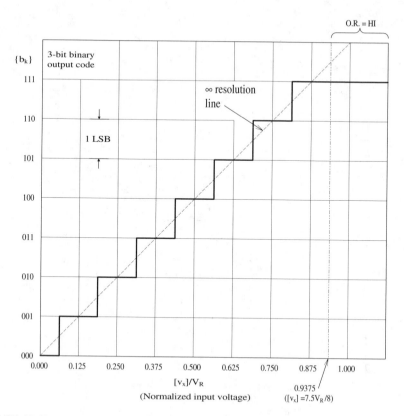

FIGURE 10.18
Transfer characteristic of an ideal 3-bit flash ADC.

obtain an 8-bit ECL-compatible, binary output with a guaranteed 200 MSa/sec rate.

One of the problems in realizing an 8-bit FADC is keeping the dc offset voltages of the 256 comparators small, with low, equal tempcos, and also keeping the resistors matched in the 2^N-resistor voltage divider. To realize flash conversions with resolutions greater than 8 bits, a two-step architecture can be used, as shown in Figure 10.19. For example, a 12-bit FADC can be made by letting $K = M = 6$ bits; thus, each subconverter needs only $2^6 = 64$ comparators. Assuming unipolar operation, $0 \leq v_x \leq V_{FS}$. The output of the K-MSB DAC following a conversion of $[v_x(nT)]$ is:

$$V_1 = V_{FS} \sum_{i=1}^{K} b_i/2^i \qquad (10.44)$$

The input to the M-lesser bits T and H and FADC is:

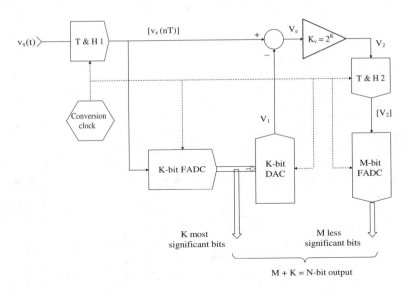

FIGURE 10.19

Architecture of a two-step flash ADC. This design is more efficient when $N \geq 8$ is desired.

$$V_2 = 2^K \left(\left[v_x(nT) \right] - V_{FS} \sum_{i=1}^{K} b_i / 2^i \right) \qquad (10.45)$$

The voltage difference in parentheses is V_e. Thus, the second FADC generates a binary code on the quantized remnant, V_e, to give a net $N = (K + M)$-bit output. Because the K- and M-bit FADCs use $(2^K - 1)$ and $(2^M - 1)$ comparators respectively, the system is generally less expensive and easier to build than a single N-bit FADC. The total coded output of the system is:

$$\left[v_x(nT) \right] = V_{FS} \left(\sum_{i=1}^{K} b_i / 2^i + \sum_{j=1}^{M} b_j / 2^j \right) = V_{FS} \sum_{k=1}^{N} b_k / 2^k \qquad (10.46)$$

When flash converters that sample at over 100 MSa/sec are used, special attention must be paid to how the digital data are handled. High-speed logic (e.g., ECL) must be used and data must be stored temporarily in shift registers and high-speed RAM before permanent recording can take place on a magnetic hard disk or optical disk. FADCs also are greedy for die size and operating power. For every bit increase in FADC resolution, the size of the ADC core circuitry (comparators, resistors, decoding logic) essentially doubles, as does the chip's power dissipation (Maxim, 2001). Conversion time, however, is independent of the bit resolution, N, and is fast; the state of the art for 2- and 4-bit FADCs is a sample rate of about 1 GSa/sec.

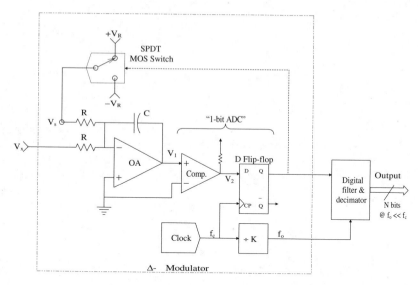

FIGURE 10.20

Block diagram of a first-order, delta–sigma ADC. The Δ–Σ modulator is in the dotted box.

10.5.6   Delta–Sigma ADCs

Delta–sigma ADCs are also called oversampled or noise-shaping converters. Oversampling ADCs are based on the principle of being able to trade off accuracy in time for accuracy in amplitude. Figure 10.20 illustrates the circuit of a first -order Δ–Σ ADC. The circuit in the box is a first-order Δ–Σ modulator. The digital filter and decimator produces the N-bit, digital output.

First, the operation of the Δ–Σ modulator in the time domain will be analyzed. Set $V_x \to 0$ and let the MOS switch apply $-V_R$ to the integrator so that its output, V_1, goes positive. The comparator output, V_2, applied to the D input of the D flip-flop (DFF) will be HI. At the rising edge of the next clock pulse, HI is seen at the Q output of the DFF. This HI causes the MOS switch to switch the integrator input to $+V_R$, so the integrator output V_1 begins to ramp down. When V_1 goes negative, the comparator output V_2 goes LO. Again when the clock pulse goes HI, the LO at D is sent to the DFF Q output. This LO again sets the MOS switch to $-V_R$, causing V_2 to ramp positively until it goes positive, setting V_2 HI, etc.

Figure 10.21 shows the Δ–Σ modulator's waveforms for $V_x = 0$. Q is the DFF output, which is the comparator output, V_2, latched in when the CP goes high. The peak-to-peak height of the steady-state triangle wave oscillation seen at V_1 can easily be shown to be equal to:

$$2V_{1m} = \frac{V_R T_c}{RC} \qquad (10.47)$$

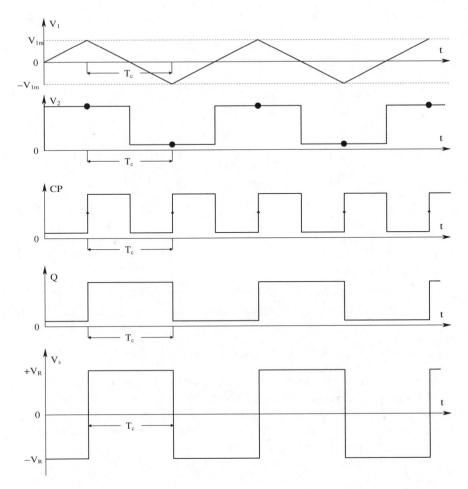

FIGURE 10.21
Waveforms in a first-order Δ–Σ modulator when $V_x = 0$.

where T_c is the DSDAC's clock period and the other parameters are given in the figure. The average value of $V_s = 0$.

Now set $V_x = +V_R/4$ and examine the Δ–Σ ADC's waveforms (refer to Figure 10.22). Let the system start with $V_1 = 0$ at $t = 0$ and begin to integrate V_x and $V_s = +V_R$. Initially, the integrator output V_1 ramps negative as $v_1(t) = -[5V_R/(4RC)]\,t$. At the first positive-going clock wave, the LO comparator output, V_2, is latched to the DFF's Q output, setting it low. When Q goes low, the MOS switch makes $V_s = -V_R$. Now the integrator output ramps upward with slope $+3V_R/(4RC)$. When V_1 goes positive, the second positive clock transition latches the HI V_2 to Q, setting V_s to $+V_R$. Now the integrator output, V_1, ramps down again with slope $-5V_R/(4RC)$.

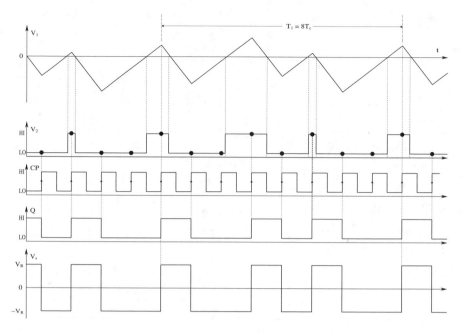

FIGURE 10.22
Waveforms in a first-order Δ-Σ modulator when $V_x = +V_R/4$.

When $V_1 < 0$, V_2 goes LO. The third positive clock transition latches this LO to the Q output of the DFF. As before, this sets V_s to $-V_R$, the integrator output again ramps positive, and the cycle repeats, etc. Note that there is a steady-state (SS) oscillation in V_1, V_2, Q, and V_s with a period of eight clock periods. The SS duty cycle of Q is 37.5%, and $\overline{V}_s = -\frac{1}{4}$.

It is also of interest to examine the Δ-Σ ADC's waveforms when $V_x = +V_R/2$. Now let the system start with $V_1 = 0$ at t = 0 and begin to integrate V_x with $V_s = +V_R$. Assuming V_x is constant, V_1 ramps negative as $v_1(t) = -3V_R\,t/(2RC)$, causing the comparator output, V_2, to be LO. At the first positive-going clock pulse, the DFF latches the low D input to Q, causing the MOS switch to make $V_s = -V_R$. Now the net input to the integrator is $-V_R/2$ and the integrator output begins to go positive with slope $+V_R/(2RC)$, as shown in Figure 10.23. When V_1 first goes positive, V_2 goes HI. At the third clock HI transition, the DFF output goes HI, setting the MOS switch to $-V_R$. Now the net input to the integrator is $+3V_R/2$, V_1 begins to ramp down again with slope $-3V_R/(2RC)$, and the ADC process repeats itself indefinitely until V_x changes. From the waveforms in this figure where $V_x = V_R/2$, it can be seen that the duty cycle of Q is 25% and $\overline{V}_s = -\frac{1}{2}$. From the three sets of V_s waveforms, it can be seen that, in general, $V_x = -V_R\,\overline{V}_s$.

Now consider the operation of first-order Δ-Σ ADC. If the number of ones in the output data stream (i.e., the DFF's Q output) is counted over a sufficient number of samples (clock cycles), the counter's digital output

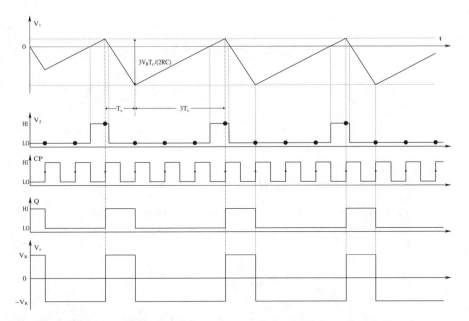

FIGURE 10.23
Waveforms in a first-order Δ–Σ modulator when $V_x = +V_R/2$.

will represent the digital value of the analog input, V_x. Obviously, this method of averaging will only work for DC or low-frequency V_x. In addition, at least 2^N clock cycles must be counted in order to obtain N-bit effective resolution. In the Δ–Σ ADC, the modulator's DFF Q output is the input to the block labeled "digital filter and decimator." The digital low-pass filter precedes the decimator and serves two functions: (1) it acts as an anti-aliasing filter for the final sampling rate, f_o, and (2) it filters out the higher frequency noise produced by the Δ–Σ modulator.

According to Analog Devices' AN-283 (Sigma–Delta ADCs and DACs):

> The final data rate reduction is performed by digitally resampling the filtered output using a process called decimation. The decimation of a discrete-time signal is shown in Figure ..., where the sampling rate of the input signal $x(n)$ is at a rate which is to be reduced by a factor of 4. The signal is resampled at the lower rate (the decimation rate), $s(n)$ [f_o]. Decimation can also be viewed as the method by which the redundant signal information introduced by the oversampling process is removed.

> In sigma–delta ADCs it is quite common to combine the decimation function with the digital filtering function. This results in an increase in computational efficiency if done correctly.

Figure 10.24 illustrates a heuristic frequency-domain block diagram approximation for a first-order Δ–Σ ADC. To appreciate what happens in the system in the frequency domain, find the transfer function for the analog

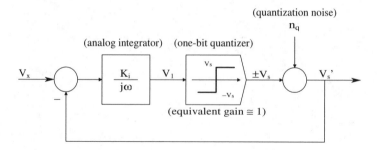

FIGURE 10.24
A heuristic frequency domain block diagram of a first-order Δ–Σ modulator.

input, V_x, and the internal quantization noise, n_q (see the following section). Assuming a linear system:

$$V_s' = \frac{V_x K_i}{j\omega + K_i} + \frac{j\omega n_q}{j\omega + K_i} \tag{10.48}$$

Thus the 1-bit quantization noise in the output is boosted at high frequencies so $V_s' \cong j\omega \, n_q / K_i$. The signal component in V_s' rolls off at –6 dB/octave above $\omega = K_i$ r/s. At low frequencies, the noise in V_s' is negligible and $V_s' \cong V_x$. Because the Δ–Σ modulator is really a sampled system at frequency f_c, the noise in V_s and Q has the root power density spectrum shown in Figure 10.25. Note that the broadband quantization noise is concentrated at the upper end of the root spectrum. The range from $0 \le f \le f_b$ is relatively free of noise. Operation in this range is achieved by first having the FIR LPF operate on the data stream from Q at clock rate, f_c, and then decimation, so $f_b = f_o/2$, the Nyquist frequency of the decimation frequency. Finally, the counter counts the decimated data for $2^N f_o$ clock periods.

10.6 Quantization Noise

This section describes an important source of noise in signals periodically sampled and converted to numerical form by an ADC. The numerical samples can then be digitally filtered or processed, and then returned to analog form, $v_y(t)$, by a digital-to-analog converter. Such signals include modern digital audio, video, and images. The noise created by converting from analog to digital form is called quantization noise (QN) and it is associated with the fact thatwhen a noise-free analog signal, $v_x(t)$, (with almost infinite resolution) is sampled and digitized, each $v_x^*(nT)$ is described by a binary number of finite length, introducing an uncertainty between the original $v_x(nT)$ and $v_x^*(nT)$. This uncertainty gives rise to the quantization noise, which

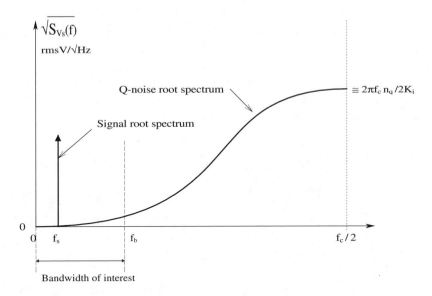

FIGURE 10.25
A typical root power density spectrum of signal and quantization noise in a first-order Δ–Σ modulator.

can be considered to be added to $v_y(t)$ or to $v_x(t)$. (A paper by Kollár (1986) has a comprehensive review of quantization noise. Also, Chapter 14 in the text by Phillips and Nagle (1994) has a rigorous mathematical treatment of QN.)

When a Nyquist band-limited analog signal is sampled and then converted by an N bit ADC to digital form, a statistical uncertainty in the digital signal amplitude exists that can be considered to be equivalent to a broadband quantization noise added to the analog signal input before sampling. In the quantization error-generating model of Figure 10.26, a noise-free Nyquist-limited analog signal, $v_x(t)$, is sampled and digitized by an N-bit ADC of the round-off type. The ADC's numerical output, $v_x^*(nT)$, is the input to an N-bit DAC. The quantization error, $e(n)$, is defined *at sampling instants* as the difference between the sampled analog input signal, $v_x(nT)$, and the analog DAC output, $v_y(nT)$. (From now on, the shorter notation, $x(n)$, $y(n)$, etc. will be used.) The ADC/DAC channel has unity gain. Thus the quantization error is simply:

$$e(n) = x(n) - y(n). \tag{10.49}$$

Figure 10.27 illustrates a bipolar rounding quantizer function relating analog sampler output, $x(n)$, to the binary DAC output, $x^*(n)$. In this example, $N = 3$. (This uniform rounding quantizer has 2^N levels and $(2^N - 1)$ steps.) When $y(n)$ is compared to the direct path, the error, $e(n)$, can range over

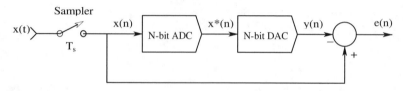

FIGURE 10.26
A quantization noise error-generating model for an ideal *N*-bit ADC driving an N-bit ideal DAC.

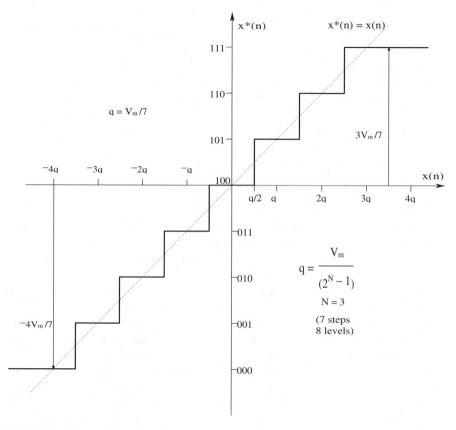

FIGURE 10.27
A 3-bit rounding quantizer I/O function.

$\pm q/2$ in the center of the range, where q is the voltage step size of the ADC/DAC. It is easy to see that for full dynamic range, q should be:

$$q = \frac{V_{xMAX}}{\left(2^N - 1\right)} \text{ volts} \tag{10.50}$$

where V_{xMAX} is the maximum (peak-to-peak) value of the input, $v_x(t)$, to the ADC/DAC system.

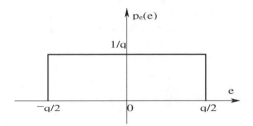

FIGURE 10.28
The rectangular probability density function generally assumed for quantization noise.

For example, if a 10-bit ADC is used to convert a signal ranging from −5 to +5 V, then by Equation 10.50, q = 9.775 mV. If $x(t)$ has zero mean and its probability density function (PDF) has a standard deviation $\sigma_x >$ q, then it can be shown that the PDF of $e(n)$ is well modeled by a uniform (rectangular) density, $f_e(e)$, over $e = \pm q/2$. This rectangular PDF is shown in Figure 10.28; it has a peak height of $1/q$. The mean-squared error voltage is found from the expectation:

$$E\{e^2\} = \overline{e^2} = \int_{-\infty}^{\infty} e^2 f_e(e)\,de = \int_{-q/2}^{q/2} e^2 f_e(e)\,de = \frac{(1/q)e^3}{3}\bigg|_{-q/2}^{q/2} = \frac{q^2}{12} = \sigma_q^2 \; \text{msV} \quad (10.51)$$

Thus, it is possible to treat quantization error noise as a zero-mean, broad-band noise with a standard deviation of $\sigma_q = q/\sqrt{12}$ V, added to the ADC/DAC input signal, $x(t)$. The QN spectral bandwidth is assumed to be flat over $\pm f_s/2$, where f_s is the sampling frequency, i.e., the Nyquist range.

In order to minimize the effects of quantization noise for an N-bit ADC, it is important that the analog input signal, $v_x(t)$, use nearly the full dynamic range of the ADC. In the case of a zero-mean, time-varying signal that is Nyquist band limited, gains and sensitivities should be chosen so that the peak expected $x(t)$ does not exceed the maximum voltage limits of the ADC.

If $x(t)$ is an SRV and has a Gaussian PDF with zero mean, the dynamic range of the ADC should be about ± 3 standard deviations of the signal. Under this particular condition, it is possible to derive an expression for the mean-squared signal-to-noise ratio of the ADC and its quantization noise. Let the signal have an RMS value σ_x volts. From Equation 10.50, the quantization step size can be written:

$$q \approx \frac{6\,\sigma_x}{(2^N - 1)} \; \text{volts,} \quad (10.52)$$

or

$$\sigma_x = q(2^N - 1)\big/6 \quad (10.53)$$

From which it can be seen that $\sigma_x > q$ for $N \geq 3$. Relation 10.52 for q can be substituted into Equation 10.51 for the variance of the quantization noise. Thus, the mean-squared output noise is:

$$N_o = \frac{q^2}{12} = \frac{36\,\sigma_x^2}{12\left(2^N - 1\right)} = \frac{3\,\sigma_x^2}{\left(2^N - 1\right)} = \sigma_q^2 \text{ MSV} \qquad (10.54)$$

Thus, the mean-squared signal-to-noise ratio of the N-bit rounding quantizer is:

$$\text{SNR}_q = \left(2^N - 1\right)/3 \ \text{MSV/MSV} \qquad (10.55)$$

Note that the quantizer SNR is independent of σ_x as long as σ_x is held constant under the dynamic range constraint described previously. In dB, $\text{SNR}q = 10 \log[(2^N - 1)/3]$. Table 10.1 summarizes the SNR_q of the quantizer for different bit values.

Because of their low quantization noise, 16- to 24-bit ADCs are routinely used in modern digital audio systems. Other classes of input signals to uniform quantizers, such as sine waves, triangle waves, and narrow-band Gaussian noise, are discussed by Kollár (1986).

Figure 10.29 illustrates a model whereby the equivalent QN is added to the ideal sampled signal at the input to some digital filter, $H(z)$. Note that the quantization error sequence, $e(n)$, is assumed to be from a wide-sense stationary white-noise process, where each sample, $e(n)$, is uniformly distributed over the quantization error. The error sequence is also assumed to be uncorrelated with the corresponding input sequence, $x(n)$. Furthermore, the input sequence is assumed to be a sample sequence of a stationary random process, $\{x\}$. Note that $e(n)$ is treated as white sampled noise (as opposed to sampled white noise). The auto-power density spectrum of $\mathbf{e}(n)$ is assumed to be flat (constant) over the Nyquist range: $-\pi/T \leq \omega \leq \pi/T$ r/s. (T is the sampling period.) $\mathbf{e}(n)$ propagates through the digital filter; in the time domain this can be written as a real discrete convolution:

TABLE 10.1

SNR Values for an N-Bit ADC Treated as a Quantizer

N	dB SNRq
6	31.2
8	43.4
10	55.4
12	67.5
14	79.5
16	91.6

Note: Total input range is assumed to be $6\,\sigma_x$ V. Note that about 6 dB of SNR improvement occurs for every bit added to the ADC word length.

$$y(n) = \sum_{m=-\infty}^{\infty} e(m)h(n - m) \qquad (10.56)$$

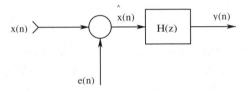

FIGURE 10.29

Block diagram of a model in which quantization noise is added to a noise-free sampled signal at the input to a digital filter.

σ_q^2 is the variance of the white quantization noise and the variance of the filter's output noise can be shown to be expressed as (Northrop, 2003):

$$\sigma_y^2 = \sigma_q^2 \sum_{k=0}^{\infty} h^2(k) \qquad (10.57)$$

10.7 Chapter Summary

Digital interfaces generate sampled data when they periodically convert an analog signal to numerical form or numerical data to an analog voltage or current. Sampled data are subject to the sampling theorem, which describes the conditions under which unwanted aliasing can take place. This chapter described sampling as impulse modulation and showed how sampled data can be described in the frequency domain by a repeated spectrum Poisson sum. In the frequency domain, aliasing was shown to exist when the edges of the repeated spectra in the Poisson sum over-lapped. This overlapping occurred when the power density spectrum of the sampled analog signal contained significant power above one half the sampling frequency, also known as the Nyquist frequency.

Digital-to-analog converters (DACs) were next covered and their circuit architecture and factors affecting the speed of conversion were described. Hold circuits were also described; the transfer function of the zero-order hold and a simple extrapolator hold were derived.

Many types of analog-to-digital converters (ADCs) were described, including the tracking or servo ADC; the successive approximation ADC; integrating ADCs; and flash ADCs. Flash ADCs were seen to be the fastest because they convert in parallel.

Finally, quantization noise was described and an expression for ADC SNR due to quantiza;-tion noise was derived as a function of the number of binary bits in the converted signal. The more bits there are, the higher the ADC's SNR is.

Home Problems

10.1 A 16-bit ADC is used to convert an audio signal ranging over ± 1 V.

   a. Find the size of the quantization step, q, required.

   b. Find the RMS quantization noise associated with full-scale operation of this ADC.

   c. Let $v_{in}(t) = 1 \sin(\omega_o t)$. Find the RMS SNR at the ADC output in decibels.

10.2 Consider the 4-bit resistive ladder DAC shown in Figure P10.2.

   a. Use superposition to find an expression for $V_o = f(I_o, I_1, I_2, I_3)$. Let $R = 1$ kΩ and $I_o = 1$ mA dc.

   b. What values should I_1, I_2, and I_3 have to make a binary DAC? What is the max. V_o?

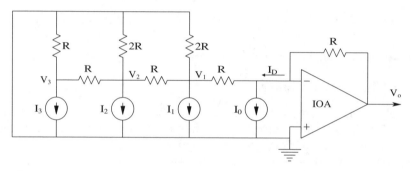

FIGURE P10.2

10.3 Refer to the text Figure 10.5 for the switched weighted capacitor DAC; in this problem you will examine the dynamics of this system. A simplified circuit is shown in Figure P10.3. In this circuit, $k = 0, 1, 2, ..., N - 1$. The op amp is characterized by $R_{in} = \infty$; $I_B = V_{os} = R_{out} = 0$; and $V_o = (-K_{vo} \, \omega_b)/(s + \omega_b)$.

   a. Find an algebraic expression for $V_o/V_R(s)$.

   b. Assume $V_R(s) = V_{Ro}/s$ (step input). Give an expression for $V_o(s)$. Plot and dimension a general $v_o(t)$.

   c. Let $k = 0, N = 8$; sketch and dimension $v_o(t)$.

   d. Let $k = N - 1 = 7$; sketch and dimension $v_o(t)$.

   e. Find a general expression for the maximum slope of $v_o(t)$ in terms of k and other system parameters.

   f. Let $V_{Ro} = 1$ V and the op amp's GBWP $= K_{vo} \, \omega_b = 3 \times 10^8$. Find $\overset{\circ}{V}_{omax}$ for $k = 0$ and $k = 7$. What must the op amp's slew rate be to avoid slew-rate limiting of $V_o(t)$?

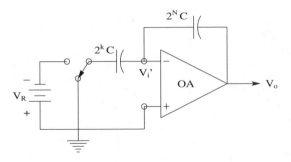

FIGURE P10.3

10.4 Figure P10.4 illustrates an $N = 8$-bit MOSFET current-scaling DAC. The feedback action of the left-hand op amp forces the Q_1 drain current to be $I_D = V_R/(2^N R)$. The left-hand op amp also puts all the connected FET gates at virtual ground (0). The right-hand op amp forces the FET drains connected to it to be at virtual ground (0). Because all of the MOSFETs are matched and they all have the same drain, gate, and source voltage, they all have the same drain current, I_D. Write an expression for $V_o = f(\{b_k\}, V_R)$.

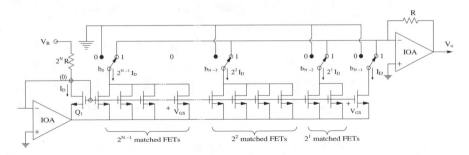

FIGURE P10.4

10.5 Figure P10.5 illustrates an N-bit binary-weighted charge amplifier DAC. Note that the ideal op amp's summing junction is at virtual ground, so the net charge flowing into the kth input capacitor when $b_k = 1$ must also equal the charge accumulated in $C_F = 2C/K$. That is, $Q_k = V_R C/2^k = Q_F = V_o 2C/K$. Write an expression for $V_o = f(\{b_k\}, V_R, K)$; use superposition.

10.6 An 8-bit successive approximation ADC has a reference voltage, V_R, set to 10.0 V at 25°C. Find the maximum allowable temperature coefficient of V_R in $\mu V/°C$ that will allow an error of no more than plus or minus one half LSB over an operating temperature range of 0 to 50°C.

10.7 A 100-mV peak-to-peak sinusoidal signal is the input to a 12-bit ADC that has a bipolar offset binary output and a full-scale input range of ±2.5 V.

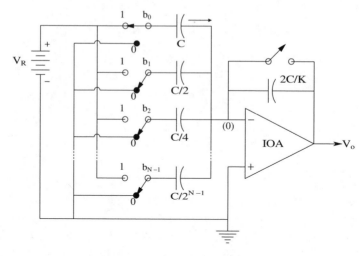

FIGURE P10.5

    a. Find the output RMS SNR in decibels when the input is a 2.5-V peak sinewave.

    b. Find the output RMS SNR in decibels when the input is a 50-mV peak sinewave.

10.8   A unipolar 3-bit successive-approximation ADC has $V_R = 8.0$ V and a ½ LSB offset as shown in text Figure 10.27. $V_{in} = 2.832$ V. Find the LSB voltage as well as the intermediate and final DAC output voltages during conversion.

10.9   Explain the differences between Nyquist-rate data converters and oversampling data converters.

10.10 Find the maximum magnitude of quantization error for a 10-bit ADC with $V_R = 10$ V and one half LSB absolute accuracy.

11

Modulation and Demodulation of Biomedical Signals

11.1 Introduction

In general, modulation is a process by which a dc or low-frequency signal of interest is combined nonlinearly with a high-frequency carrier wave to form a modulated carrier suitable for transmission to a receiver/demodulator where the signal is recovered. Modulators and demodulators form essential components of most communication and data transmission systems. Some modulation schemes involve multiplication of the carrier with a function of the modulating signal.

In biomedical engineering, recorded physiological signals are modulated because modulation permits robust transmission by wire or coaxial cable, fiber optic cable, or radio (telemetry by electromagnetic waves) from the recording site to the site where the signal will be demodulated, processed, and stored. As an example, in biotelemetry, physiological signals such as the ECG and blood pressure modulate a carrier sent as an FM radio signal from an ambulance to a remote receiver (in a hospital ER) where the signals are demodulated, interpreted, filtered, digitized, and stored. Five major forms of modulation involve altering a high-frequency sinusoidal carrier wave: (1) amplitude modulation (AM); (2) single-sideband AM (SSBAM); (3) frequency modulation (FM); (4) phase modulation (PhM); and (5) double-sideband, suppressed-carrier modulation (DSBSCM).

Modulation can also be done using a square wave (or TTL) carrier and can involve FM, NBFM, and PhM. Delta modulation, pulse-position modulation (PPM), and pulse-width modulation (PWM) at constant frequency are done with digital carrier. AM, FM, and DSBSCM are expressed mathematically below for a sinusoidal carrier. $v_m(t)$ is the actual physiological signal. The maximum frequency of $v_m(t)$ must be $\ll \omega_c$, the carrier frequency. The normalized modulating signal, $m(t)$, is defined by the following equation:

$$m(t) = \frac{v_m(t)}{v_{m\max}},\ 0 \le |m(t)| \le 1 \qquad \text{Normalized modulating signal} \quad (11.1\text{A})$$

$$y_m(t) = A[1 + m(t)]\cos(\omega_c t) \qquad \text{AM} \qquad (11.1\text{B})$$

$$y_m(t) = A\,m(t)\cos(\omega_c t) \qquad \text{DSBSCM} \qquad (11.1\text{C})$$

$$y_m(t) = A\,\cos\left[\omega_c t + K_f \int^t m(t)\,dt\right] \qquad \text{FM} \qquad (11.1\text{D})$$

$$y_m(t) = A\,\cos\left[\omega_c t + K_p m(t)\right] \qquad \text{PhM} \qquad (11.1\text{E})$$

11.2   Modulation of a Sinusoidal Carrier Viewed in the Frequency Domain

It is interesting to examine the frequency spectrums of the modulated signals. For illustrative purposes, let the modulating signal be a pure cosine wave, $v_m(t) = m_o \cos(\omega_m t)$, $0 < m_o \le 1$. Thus, by using Equation 11.1B and a trig. identity, the amplitude modulated (AM) signal can be rewritten:

$$y_m(t) = A\,\cos(\omega_c t) + (A\,m_o/2)\big[\cos((\omega_c + \omega_m)t) + \cos((\omega_c - \omega_m)t)\big] \quad (11.2)$$

Thus, the AM signal has a carrier component and two sidebands, each spaced by the amount of the modulating frequency above and below the carrier frequency. In SSBAM, a sharp cut-off filter is used to eliminate the upper or the lower sideband; the information in both sidebands is redundant, so removing one means less bandwidth is required to transmit the SSBAM signal. SSBAM signals are more noise resistant than conventional AM because they require less bandwidth to transmit the same m(t).

FM and PhM are subsets of angle modulation. FM can be further classified as broadband (BBFM) or narrowband FM (NBFM). In BBFM, $K_f \equiv 2\pi f_d$, where f_d is called the frequency deviation constant. In NBFM, $f_d/f_{mmax} \ll 1$ f_{mmax} is the highest expected frequency in $v_m(t)$, which is bandwidth-limited. Unlike AM, the frequency spectrum of an FM carrier is tedious to derive. Using $m(t) = m_o \cos(\omega_m t)$, the FM carrier can be written as:

$$y_m(t) = A\,\cos\left[\overset{\alpha}{\omega_c t} + \left(K_f/\omega_m\right)\overset{\beta}{m_o}\sin(\omega_m t)\right] \qquad (11.3)$$

Using the trigonometric identity $\cos(\alpha + \beta) = \cos(\alpha)\cos(\beta) - \sin(\alpha)\sin(\beta)$, Equation 11.3 can be written as:

$$y_m(t) = A\cos(\omega_c t)\cos\left[\left(K_f/\omega_m\right)m_0\sin(\omega_m t)\right]$$
$$- A\sin(\omega_c t)\sin\left[\left(K_f/\omega_m\right)m_0\sin(\omega_m t)\right] \tag{11.4}$$

Now the $\cos[(K_f/\omega_m)m_0\sin(\omega_m t)]$ and $\sin[(K_f/\omega_m)m_0\sin(\omega_m t)]$ terms can be expressed as two Fourier series whose coefficients are ordinary Bessel functions of the first kind and argument β (Clarke and Hess, 1971); note that $\beta \equiv m_0 2\pi f_d/\omega_m$:

$$\cos\left[\beta\sin(\omega_m t)\right] = J_0(\beta) + 2\sum_{n=1}^{\infty} J_{2n}(\beta)\cos(2n\omega_m t) \tag{11.5A}$$

$$\sin\left[\beta\sin(\omega_m t)\right] = 2\sum_{n=0}^{\infty} J_{2n+1}(\beta)\sin(2(n+1)\omega_m t) \tag{11.5B}$$

The two Bessel sum relations for $\cos[\beta\sin(\omega_m t)]$ and $\sin[\beta\sin(\omega_m t)]$ can be recombined with Equation 11.4 using the trigonometric identities $\cos(x)$ $\cos(y) = \frac{1}{2}[\cos(x+y) + \cos(x-y)]$ and $\sin(x)\sin(y) = \frac{1}{2}[\cos(x-y) - \cos(x+y)]$, and one can finally write for the FM carrier spectrum, letting $m_0 = 1$:

$$y_m(t) = A\Big\{J_0(\beta)\cos(\omega_c t) + J_1(\beta)\left[\cos((\omega_c + \omega_m)t) - \cos((\omega_c - \omega_m)t)\right]$$
$$+ J_2(\beta)\left[\cos((\omega_c + 2\omega_m)t) + \cos((\omega_c - 2\omega_m)t)\right]$$
$$+ J_3(\beta)\left[\cos((\omega_c + 3\omega_m)t) + \cos((\omega_c - 3\omega_m)t)\right] \tag{11.6}$$
$$+ J_4(\beta)\left[\cos((\omega_c + 4\omega_m)t) + \cos((\omega_c - 4\omega_m)t)\right]$$
$$+ J_5(\beta)\left[\cos((\omega_c + 5\omega_m)t) + \cos((\omega_c - 5\omega_m)t)\right] + ...\Big\}$$

At first inspection, this result appears quite messy. However, it is evident that the numerical values of the Bessel terms tend to zero as n becomes large. For example, let $\beta = 2\pi f_d/\omega_m = 1$; then $J_0(1) = 0.7852$; $J_1(1) = 0.4401$; $J_2(1) = 0.1149$; $J_3(1) = 0.01956$; $J_4(1) = 0.002477$; $J_5(1) = 0.0002498$; $J_6(1) = 0.00002094$; etc. Bessel constants $J_n(1)$ for $n \geq 4$ contribute less than 1% each to the $y_m(t)$ spectrum, so they can be neglected. Thus, the practical bandwidth of the FM carrier, $y_m(t)$, for $\beta = 1$ is $\pm 3\omega_m$ around the carrier frequency, ω_c. In general, as β increases, so does the effective bandwidth of the FM $y_m(t)$. For example, when $\beta = 5$, the bandwidth becomes $\pm 8\omega_m$ around ω_c and when $\beta = 10$, the bandwidth required is $\pm 14\omega_m$ around ω_c (Clarke and Hess, 1971).

In the case of NBFM, $\beta \ll 1$. Thus, the modulated carrier can be written:

$$y_m(t) = A \cos\left[\overset{\alpha}{\omega_c t} + \overset{\beta}{\left(K_f/\omega_m\right)\sin\left(\omega_m t\right)}\right] \qquad (11.7A)$$

$$\downarrow$$

$$y_m(t) = A\left\{\cos\left(\omega_c t\right)\cos\left[\beta\sin\left(\omega_m t\right)\right] - \sin\left(\omega_c t\right)\sin\left[\beta\sin\left(\omega_m t\right)\right]\right\}$$

$$\cong A\left\{\cos\left(\omega_c t\right)(1) - \sin\left(\omega_c t\right)\left[\beta\sin\left(\omega_m t\right)\right]\right\} \qquad (11.7B)$$

$$= A\left\{\cos\left(\omega_c t\right) - \left(\beta/2\right)\left[\cos\left(\left(\omega_c - \omega_m\right)t\right) - \cos\left(\left(\omega_c + \omega_m\right)t\right)\right]\right\}$$

With the exception of signs of the sideband terms, the NBFM spectrum is very similar to the spectrum of an AM carrier (Zeimer and Tranter, 1990); sum and difference frequency sidebands are produced around a central carrier.

The spectrum of a double-sideband suppressed carrier (DSBSCM) signal is given by:

$$y_m(t) = A\,m_o\cos\left(\omega_m t\right)\cos\left(\omega_c t\right)$$

$$= \left(A\,m_o/2\right)\left[\cos\left(\left(\omega_c + \omega_m\right)t\right) + \cos\left(\left(\omega_c - \omega_m\right)t\right)\right] \qquad (11.8)$$

i.e., ideally, the information is contained in the two sidebands; there is no carrier.

DSBSCM is widely used in instrumentation and measurement systems. For example, it is the natural result when a light beam is chopped in a photonic instrument such as a spectrophotometer; it also results when a Wheatstone bridge is given ac (carrier) excitation and nulled, then one or more arm resistances are slowly varied in time around its null value (see Figure 11.1(A)). DSBSCM is also present at the output of an LVDT (linear variable differential transformer) length sensor as the core is moved in and out (Northrop, 1997). Figure 11.1(B) illustrates a simple system used to demodulate DSBSCM signals.

11.3 Implementation of AM

11.3.1 Introduction

Equation 11.1B indicates that multiplication is inherent in the AM process. In practice, an actual analog multiplier can be used or effective multiplication

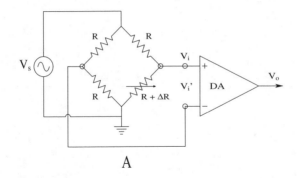

A

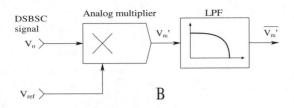

B

FIGURE 11.1
(A) A one-active arm Wheatstone bridge. When ac excitation is used, the output is a double-sideband, suppressed-carrier modulated carrier. (B) The use of an analog multiplier and low-pass filter to demodulate a DSBSC signal.

can be realized by passing $v_c(t)$ and $[1 + m(t)]$ through a square-law nonlinearity, such as a field-effect transistor. Note that, in Equation 11.1B, $|m(t)| \leq 1$, so $[1 + m(t)] \geq 0$. If $[1 + m(t)]$ were to go <0, a 180° phase-shift would take place in the AM output, which is an undesirable condition called *overmodulation*. This condition also occurs when the modulator output stage is driven so hard that the output transistor stage is cut off, giving zero output for several carrier cycles. Hard cut-off also distorts the AM carrier and produces unwanted harmonics in the demodulated signal. Many types of circuits have been devised to do AM. Although all of them cannot be examined here, several are described in the next section.

11.3.2 Some Amplitude Modulation Circuits

Figure 11.2 illustrates the use of a JFET as a square-law modulator. The gate–source voltage is the sum of a dc bias voltage, which places the quiescent operating point of the JFET at the center of its saturated channel region, plus the carrier signal and the modulating signal. In this and the following examples, $\omega_m \ll \omega_c$ is asserted.

$$v_{GS} = -\left|V_p/2\right| + V_c \cos(\omega_c t) + V_m \cos(\omega_m t) \qquad (11.9)$$

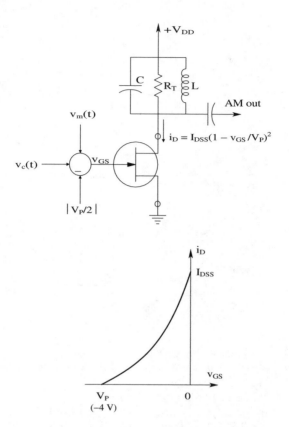

FIGURE 11.2
Top: schematic of a tuned-output JFET square-law amplitude modulator. Bottom: square-law drain current vs. gate-source voltage curve for a JFET operated under saturated drain conditions $[v_{DS} > |v_{GS} + V_P|]$.

The JFET's drain current is then:

$$i_D = I_{DSS}\left(1 - \frac{-|V_P/2| + V_c \cos(\omega_c t) + V_m \cos(\omega_m t)}{V_P}\right)^2 \tag{11.10A}$$

$$= I_{DSS}\left(1 + \frac{-|V_P/2| + V_c \cos(\omega_c t) + V_m \cos(\omega_m t)}{|V_P|}\right)^2 \tag{11.10B}$$

$$= I_{DSS}\left(\frac{|V_P/2| + V_c \cos(\omega_c t) + V_m \cos(\omega_m t)}{|V_P|}\right)^2 \tag{11.10C}$$

$$= \left(I_{DSS}/V_P^2\right)\left(V_P^2/4 + V_c^2\cos^2(\omega_c t) + V_m^2\cos^2(\omega_m t)+ \right. \tag{11.10D}$$

$$\left. V_P\left[V_c\cos(\omega_c t) + V_m\cos(\omega_m t)\right] + 2V_cV_m\left[\cos(\omega_c t)\cos(\omega_m t)\right] \right.$$

$$i_D = \left(I_{DSS}/V_P^2\right)\left\{\left(V_P^2/4 + V_c^2\,\tfrac{1}{2}\left[1 + \cos^2(2\omega_c t)\right] + V_m^2\,\tfrac{1}{2}\left[\cos^2(2\omega_m t)\right]+ \right.\right. \tag{11.10E}$$

$$\left.\left. V_P\left[V_c\cos(\omega_c t) + V_m\cos(\omega_m t)\right] + V_cV_m\left[\cos((\omega_c t)t) + \cos((\omega_m ta)t)\right]\right]\right\}$$

Equation 11.10E shows that the drain current has dc terms, terms at ω_m and $2\omega_m$, terms at ω_c and $2\omega_c$, and the sideband terms at $\omega_c + \omega_m$ and $\omega_c - \omega_m$. The dc terms are eliminated by the output coupling capacitor. The RLC "tank" circuit is resonant around ω_c and so selects the ω_c and sideband terms. The AM output voltage is approximately:

$$\tag{11.11}$$

$$v_o \cong -R_T\left(I_{DSS}/V_P^2\right)\left\{V_PV_c\cos(\omega_c t) + V_cV_m\left[\cos((\omega_c + \omega_m)t) + \cos((\omega_c - \omega_m)t)\right]\right\}$$

i.e., the resonant circuit attenuates all frequencies not immediately around ω_c.

Figure 11.3 illustrates the architecture of a class C MOSFET RF power amplifier with a high Q output resonant circuit. The modulating signal, $v_m(t)$, is added to a dc gate bias and the RF carrier source. The radio-frequency chokes (RFC) are inductors with very high reactance around ω_c; they pass currents from dc to ω_{mmax}. The principle of sideband generation is very similar to the preceding JFET example. JFETs and MOSFETs have square-law i_D vs. v_{GS} curves.

The BJT circuit of Figure 11.4 illustrates another amplitude modulator architecture. Q3 and Q4 modulate the collector currents in Q1 and Q1 by changing the g_m of these transistors; for example, $g_{m1} = I_{CQ1}/V_T$. The operating points of Q1 and Q2 are identical and are affected by $I_{C4} = I_{E1} + I_{E2}$, which is in turn a function of the modulating signal, $v_m(t)$. Clarke and Hesse (1971) give a detailed analysis of this transconductance modulator.

Still another approach to AM generation is illustrated in the block diagram of Figure 11.5. This system is basically a quarter square multiplier, except the nonlinearities contain a linear (a_1) term as well as the square-law (a_2) term. The signals are:

$$w(t) = V_c\cos(\omega_c t) + \left[1 + m(t)\right], \; |m_{max}| \le 1. \tag{11.12A}$$

$$z(t) = V_c\cos(\omega_c t) - \left[1 + m(t)\right], \tag{11.12B}$$

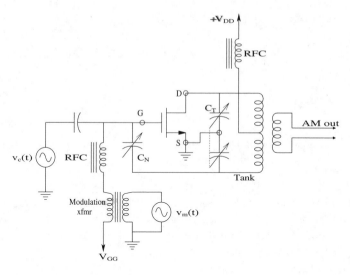

FIGURE 11.3
A class C MOSFET tuned RF power amplifier in which the low-frequency modulating signal is added to the carrier voltage at the gate. Miller input capacitance at the gate is cancelled by positive feedback through the small neutralizing capacitor, C_N.

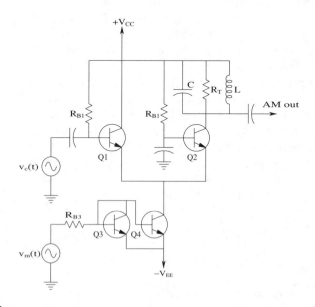

FIGURE 11.4
A transconductance-type amplitude modulator using *npn* BJTs. The circuit effectively multiplies the carrier by the modulating signal, producing an AM output.

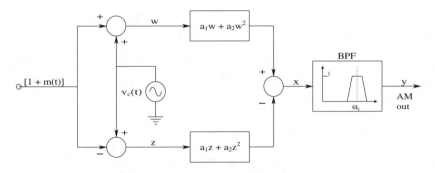

FIGURE 11.5
Block diagram of a quarter-square multiplier used for amplitude modulation.

$$u(t) = a_1 V_c \cos(\omega_c t) + a_1[1 + m(t)] +$$
$$a_2\left\{V_c^2 \cos^2(\omega_c t) + 2V_c[1 + m(t)]\cos(\omega_c t) + [1 + 2m(t) + m^2(t)]\right\}$$

(11.12C)

$$v(t) = a_1 V_c \cos(\omega_c t) - a_1[1 + m(t)] +$$
$$a_2\left\{V_c^2 \cos^2(\omega_c t) - 2V_c[1 + m(t)]\cos(\omega_c t) + [1 + 2m(t) + m^2(t)]\right\}$$

(11.12D)

$$x = u - v$$

(11.12E)

$$x(t) = 2a_1 + 2a_1 m_c \cos(\omega m t) + (4a_2 V_c)\cos(\omega_c t) +$$
$$(4a_2 V_c)\tfrac{1}{2}\left\{\cos[(\omega_c + \omega_m)t] + \cos[(\omega_c - \omega_m)t]\right\}$$

(11.12F)

The band-pass filter around $(\omega_c - \omega_m)$ to $(\omega_c + \omega_m)$ selects the AM output and blocks dc and ω_m. Many other AM circuits exist; some are practical for high-power RF output while others assume the AM output will be amplified by a linear RF amplifier.

Double-sideband suppressed carrier modulation (DSBSCM) is another form of AM in which little or no carrier frequency power occurs in the output spectrum. Ideally, DSBSCM follows Equation 11.1C, i.e., DSBSCM results as the product of a low-frequency modulating signal multiplying a high-frequency carrier voltage.

Many processes are inherent generators of DSBSCM. For example, see Figure 11.1(A) for a Wheatstone bridge initially nulled, whose output depends on $\Delta R/R$. The bridge is given ac excitation so that its sensitivity will be enhanced. Developing an expression for V_o using voltage-divider relations,

$$V_i = V_s \frac{R + \Delta R}{2R + \Delta R}$$

(11.13)

$$V_i' = V_s \frac{R}{2R} \tag{11.14}$$

The output is found by subtracting V_i' from V_i and multiplying the difference by the DA's gain, K_D.

$$V_o = K_D V_s \left[\frac{\Delta R}{4R + 2\Delta R} \right] \cong K_D V_s [\Delta R/4R] = (K_D V_s/4R)[\Delta R(t)\cos(\omega_c t)] \tag{11.15}$$

The quantity in the brackets is the DSBSCM product. $\Delta R(t)$ varies at ω_m.

DSBSCM occurs for light-beam chopping in photonic systems, as well as for the output of the linear variable differential transformer (LVDT) linear position sensor. A schematic of an LVDT is shown in Figure 11.6. Seen on end, an LVDT is a cylinder with a tube in the center running the length of the cylinder. In the center of the tube slides a cylindrical, high-permeability magnetic core that couples magnetic flux from the excitation core to the two secondary coils, which are wound in opposite directions with the same number of turns. When the core is centered ($x = 0$), equal flux intercepts the winding of both secondary coils and the output EMF is zero. If the core position is up ($x = +x_m$), most of the flux is coupled to the upper secondary coil and $|V_o|$ is maximum, having the same phase as V_c. If $x = -x_m$, $|V_o|$ is maximum and the phase is 180° from V_o with $x = +x_m$. In general, the linear part of the output can be written as:

$$V_o = N\left(\mathring{\varphi}_u - \mathring{\varphi}_1 \right) = K x(t) V_c \cos(\omega_c t) \tag{11.16}$$

where $\mathring{\varphi}_u$ is the time rate of change of the ac flux intercepting the N turns of the upper secondary coil and K is the slope of the linear V_o vs. x curve.

Refer to Figure 11.5. If $[1 + m(t)]$ is replaced by $v_m(t)$, it is easy to see that the output $x(t)$ is given by:

$$x(t) = u(t) - v(t) = 2a_1 v_m(t) + 4a_2 v_c(t) v_m(t) \tag{11.17}$$

$$= 2a_1 V_m \cos(\omega_m t) + 2a_2 V_c V_m \left[\cos\left((\omega_c + \omega_m)t\right) + \cos\left((\omega_c - \omega_m)t\right) \right]$$

The BPF centered on ω_c removes the $2a_1 V_m \cos(\omega_m t)$ term, leaving the DSBSCM output; thus,

$$y(t) = 2a_2 V_c V_m \left[\cos\left((\omega_c + \omega_m)t\right) + \cos\left((\omega_c - \omega_m)t\right) \right] \tag{11.18}$$

DSBSCM is widely encountered in all phases of instrumentation and measurement systems; it is the direct result of multiplying the carrier times the modulating signal.

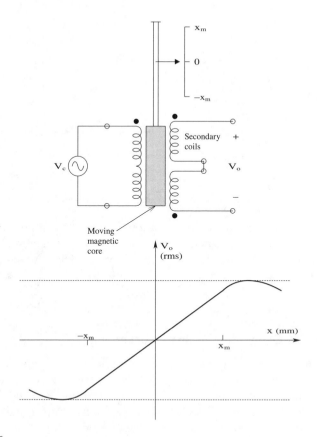

FIGURE 11.6
Top: cross-sectional schematic of an LVDT. The output is a DSBSC modulated carrier. Bottom: transfer curve of the RMS voltage output of the LVDT vs. core position. A 180° phase shift in the output is signified by $V_o(x) < 0$.

11.4 Generation of Phase and Frequency Modulation

11.4.1 Introduction

Phase and frequency modulation are subsets of angle modulation, which has the general form:

$$y_m(t) = A \cos[\omega_c t + \Phi(t)] \qquad (11.19)$$

The phase argument of the modulated carrier is $[\omega_c t + \Phi(t)]$ radians and the frequency of the modulated carrier is $[\omega_c + \overset{\circ}{\Phi}]$ r/s. When $\Phi(t) = K_f \int^t \dot{m}(t)\, dt$, FM is obtained; when $\Phi(t) = K_p\, m(t)$, PhM is the result. Many practical angle modulation and demodulation circuits have been developed since Edwin H.

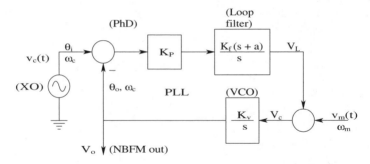

FIGURE 11.7
Block diagram of a phase-locked loop used to generate narrowband FM.

Armstrong invented frequency modulation in 1933. Like many innovations in technology, FM did not "catch on" at once; it did not become widely used commercially until after World War II (Stark et al., 1988). A useful practical source of PhM and FM circuits can be found in the ARRL's *Radio Amateur's Handbook*, 1953.

11.4.2 NBFM Generation by Phase-Locked Loop

Figure 11.7 illustrates at the systems level the processes of generating NBFM using a phase-locked loop (PLL) IC. A PLL is a type 1 negative feedback system that continually tries to match the phase of the periodic output of a voltage-controlled oscillator (VCO) to the phase of its input signal (Northrop, 1990). A basic PLL consists of a phase detector, loop filter, and VCO. The VCO output may be sinusoidal or digital. (PLLs are covered in detail in Chapter 12.) The frequency output of the VCO is given by $\omega_o = K_v V_c$. However, it is the VCO's phase that is compared with the carrier's input phase by a phase detector (PhD) with gain, $V_p = K_P (\theta_i - \theta_o)$. Note that phase is the integral of frequency $\theta_o = V_c (K_v/s)$. When a PLL is locked, the frequency and phase of the VCO equal the frequency and phase of the input signal.

Examine the transfer function between the VCO's output phase and the modulating signal, $v_m(t)$:

$$\frac{\theta_o}{V_m}(s) = \frac{K_v/s}{1 + K_P K_f K_v (s+a)/s^2} \tag{11.20}$$

To optimize the dynamics of the closed-loop PLL, it is prudent to make $K_P K_f K_v = 2a$ (Northrop, 1990). Thus, the output phase frequency response can be written:

$$\frac{\theta_o}{V_m}(j\omega) = \frac{j\omega K_v/2a^2}{(j\omega)^2/2a^2 + (j\omega)/a + 1} \tag{11.21}$$

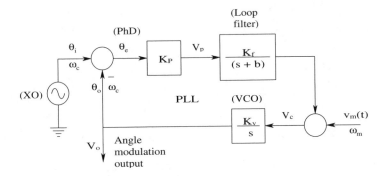

FIGURE 11.8
A PLL used for a frequency-dependent angle modulator.

Note that ω in this frequency response function is the radian frequency of the modulating signal. Now for $\omega_m > 2a\sqrt{2}$, the VCO's output phase is approximately:

$$\frac{\boldsymbol{\theta}_o}{V_m}(j\omega_m) \cong \frac{K_v}{j\omega_m} \tag{11.22}$$

Equation 11.22 implies that the phase of the constant-amplitude VCO output is proportional to the integral of $v_m(t)$, which is the condition present in FM. The VCO frequency when $v_m(t) = 0$ is simply that of the carrier input oscillator (XO), ω_c. The PLL is a compact, useful way of generating NBFM for a variety of communications applications. The NBFM output of the PLL can be conditioned by a linear RF amplifier to boost its power level or can be amplified by a frequency multiplier to convert it to wideband FM (Stark et al., 1988). Note that if the modulation input signal to the PLL is the derivative of $v_m(t)$, PhM results for $\omega_m > 2a\sqrt{2}$ r/s.

Figure 11.8 illustrates another PLL angle modulator system. Inspection of the figure gives the transfer function for the phase, θ_o, of the VCO output as a function of V_m.

$$\frac{\boldsymbol{\theta}_o}{V_m}(s) = \frac{K_v/s}{1 + K_p K_f K_v / [s(s+b)]} = \frac{K_v(s+b)}{s^2 + sb + K_p K_f K_v} \tag{11.23}$$

Now, for the closed loop system to have a damping factor of $\xi = 0.707$, the gain product, $K_p K_f K_v$, must equal $b^2/2$. Thus, the frequency response function of the PLL angle modulator can be written:

$$\frac{\boldsymbol{\theta}_o}{V_m}(j\omega) = \frac{(2K_v/b)(j\omega/b + 1)}{(j\omega)^2/(b^2/2) + j\omega 2/b + 1} \tag{11.24}$$

In the modulating signal frequency range from $0 \leq \omega_m \leq b/2$ r/s, $\theta_o/V_m \cong 2K_v/b$. That is, θ_o is proportional to V_m and phase modulation occurs. In the frequency range $2b/\sqrt{2} \leq \omega_m \leq \infty$, the VCO output phase is given by:

$$\frac{\theta_o}{V_m} = K_v/(j\omega_m) \tag{11.25}$$

Because the phase is proportional to the integral of $v_m(t)$, FM again takes place in this frequency range.

Although the PLL method of generating PhM and FM can produce a modulated sinusoidal carrier, it is often desirable to generate an angle-modulated TTL wave or pulse train.

11.4.3 Integral Pulse Frequency Modulation as a Means of Frequency Modulation

A systems model for a two-sided integral pulse frequency modulation (IPFM) system is shown in Figure 11.9. A positive modulating signal, v_m, is integrated; the integrator output, v, is sent to two threshold nonlinearities. When v reaches the positive threshold, φ_+, the nonlinearity's output, w^+, jumps to +1. This step is differentiated to make a positive unit impulse at time t_k, $\delta(t - t_k)$. This impulse is fed back, given a weight of φ/K_i, and subtracted from the input to form $e(t_k) = v_m(t_k) - (\varphi/K_i)\delta(t - t_k)$. When integrated, this $e(t_k)$ resets the integrator output to zero and the process repeats. If $v_m < 0$, v approaches the negative threshold φ^-. When φ^- is reached, the output from the two-sided IPFM system is a negative unit impulse that is also fed back to reset the integrator. The net output from the two-sided IPFM system can be written as a superposition of the positive and negative impulse outputs:

$$y(t) = \sum_{k=1}^{\infty} \delta(t - t_k) - \sum_{j=1}^{\infty} \delta(t - t_j) \tag{11.26}$$

where $\{t_k\}$ are the times that positive pulses are emitted and $\{t_j\}$ are the times that negative pulses occur.

A simpler way of dealing with negative $v_m(t)$ is to add a dc bias V_B to $v_m(t)$ so that $[V_B + v_m(t)]$ is always >0. Now the negative pulse generation and integrator reset channel can be eliminated. Many low-frequency physiological signals such as body temperature and blood pressure are always positive, so the negative pulse channel on the IPFM system can be deleted and V_B set to 0 in a one-sided system.

Note that a one-sided IPFM system behaves like a classical pulse FM system given a positive modulating signal input and zero carrier frequency. If the modulating signal is small, the output pulse rate will be low and the

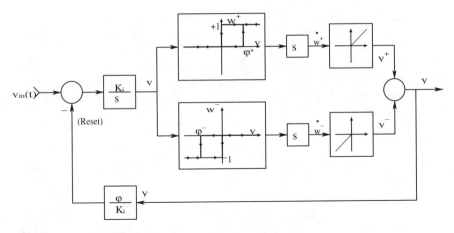

FIGURE 11.9
Block diagram of a two-sided, integral pulse frequency modulation (IPFM) system.

IPFM system will be poor at following high-frequency components of $v_m(t)$. By establishing a carrier frequency with input bias voltage, V_B, a classic pulse FM system with a carrier frequency, r_c pps, results. A carrier FM system is better able to follow high-frequency changes in small v_m. One-sided IPFM can be described mathematically by a set of integral equations:

$$v = \int K_i\, e(t)\, dt \qquad (11.27)$$

$$\varphi = \int_{t_{k-1}}^{t_k} K_i\, e(t)\, dt, \quad k = 2, 3, \ldots, \infty \qquad (11.28)$$

where K_i is the integrator gain; $e(t)$ is its input; and $e(t) = [v_m(t) + V_B]$ for $t_{k-1} < t < t_k$. t_k is the time the kth output pulse occurs. $v(t_{k-1}) = 0$, due to the feedback pulse resetting the integrator. Thus, Equation 11.28 can be rewritten as:

$$r_k = \frac{1}{t_k - t_{k-1}} = (K_i/\varphi)\frac{1}{t_k - t_{k-1}} \int_{t_{k-1}}^{t_k} e(t)\, dt, \quad k = 2, 3, \ldots \qquad (11.29)$$

Here r_k is the kth element of instantaneous frequency, defined as the reciprocal of the interval between the kth and $(k-1)^{th}$ output pulses, $\tau_k = (t_k - t_{k-1})$. Thus, the kth element of instantaneous (pulse) frequency is given by:

$$r_k \equiv 1/\tau_k = (K_i/\varphi)\overline{\{e\}}_{\tau^k} \qquad (11.30)$$

If v_m is zero and the input to the IPFM system is a constant $V_B \geq 0$, $r_c = (K_i/\varphi) V_B$ pps. That is, the IPFM output carrier center frequency, r_c, is proportional to the bias, V_B.

As an example of finding the pulse emission times for a one-sided IPFM system, consider the input, $v_m(t) = (4 e^{-7t}) U(t)$, the threshold $\varphi = 0.025$ V, $K_i = 1$, and $V_B = 0$. The first pulse is emitted at t_1, which is found from the definite integral:

$$\varphi = \int_0^{t_1} v_m(t)\,dt \rightarrow 0.025 = \int_0^{t_1} \frac{4(e^{-7t})(-7)\,dt}{(-7)} \rightarrow \frac{0.025(-7)}{4} = \left(e^{-7t_1} - 1\right) \rightarrow \quad (11.31)$$

$$e^{-7t_1} = 1 - \frac{7 \times 0.025}{4} = 0.95625 \xrightarrow{\ln(*)} -7t_1 = -4.47359 \times 10^{-2} \quad (11.32)$$

The time the first pulse is emitted, t_1, is found to be at 6.391×10^{-3} sec. The general pulse emission time, t_k, is found by recursion. For example, once t_1 is known, t_2 is found by solving:

$$\varphi = \int_{t_1}^{t_2} v_m(t)\,dt \quad (11.33)$$

In this simple case $t_2 = 13.081$ E–3 sec. Induction is used to find a general formula for t_k:

$$t_k = (-1/7)\ln\left[1 - \frac{k \times 7 \times 0.025}{4}\right] \quad (11.34)$$

From Equation 11.34, it can be seen that t_k is only defined for a positive $ln[*]$ argument, i.e., for

$$k \leq \frac{4}{7 \times 0.025} = 22.875 \quad (11.35)$$

Thus, $k_{max} = 22$; only 22 pulses are emitted.

Demodulation of IPFM positive pulse trains can be done by passing the pulses through a low-pass filter or by actually calculating the pulse train's instantaneous frequency by taking the reciprocal of the time interval between any two pulses and holding that value until the next pulse [(k + 1)th] occurs in the sequence, then repeating the operation. Stated mathematically, instantaneous pulse frequency demodulation (IPFD) can be written:

$$\hat{v}_m(t) = \sum_{k=2}^{\infty} \tau_k \left\{ U(t - t_k) = U(t - t_{k+1}) \right\}$$ (11.36)

where

$$\tau_k \equiv 1/\tau_k = \frac{1}{t_k - t_{k-1}}, \quad k = 2, 3, \ldots$$ (11.37)

Note that two pulses ($k = 2$) are required to define the first pulse interval.

$\hat{v}_m(t)$ is a series of steps and the height of each is the (previous) r_k. Note that the IPFD is not limited to the demodulation of IPFM; it has been experimentally applied as a descriptor to actual neural spike signals (Northrop, 2001).

11.5 Demodulation of Modulated Sinusoidal Carriers

11.5.1 Introduction

Of equal importance in the discussion of modulation is the process of demodulation or detection, in which the modulating signal, $v_m(t)$, is recovered from the modulated carrier, $y_m(t)$. Generally, several circuit architectures can be used to modulate a given type of modulated signal and several ways can be used to demodulate it. In the case of AM (or single-sideband AM), the signal recovery process is called *detection*.

11.5.2 Detection of AM

There are several practical means of AM detection (Clarke and Hess, 1971, Chapter 10). One simple form is to rectify and low-pass filter $y_m(t)$. Because rectification is difficult at high radio frequencies, heterodyning or mixing the incoming high-frequency AM signal with a local oscillator (in the receiver) whose frequency is separated by a fixed interval, Δf, from that of the incoming signal produces mixing frequencies of $(f_c - f_{lo}) = \Delta f$. Δf is called the intermediate frequency of the receiver and is typically 50 to 455 kHz, or 10.7 MHz in commercial FM receivers. High-frequency selectivity IF transformers are used that have tuned primary and secondary windings. Very high IF frequency selectivity can be obtained with piezoelectric crystal filters or surface acoustic wave (SAW) tuned IF filters.

Another form of AM detection passes $y_m(t)$ through a square-law nonlinearity followed by a low-pass filter; however, the square-law detector suffers

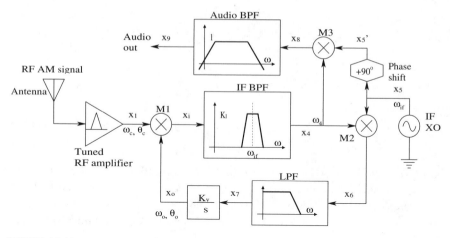

FIGURE 11.10
Block diagram of a PLL system used to demodulate AM audio signals. Note that three mixers (multipliers) are used; M_1 is the quadrature phase detector of the PLL.

from the disadvantage that it generates a second harmonic component of the recovered modulating signal. A third way to demodulate an AM carrier of the form given by Equation 11.1B is to mix (multiply) it by a sinusoidal signal of the same frequency and phase as the carrier component of the $y_m(t)$. A phase-locked loop system architecture can be used for this purpose; see Figure 11.10 (Northrop, 1990). This PLL system uses three multiplicative mixers. The AM input after RF amplification is:

$$x_1 = A\big[1 + m(t)\big]\sin\big(\omega_c t + \theta_c\big) \tag{11.38}$$

Mixer $M1$ effectively multiplies $x_1 \times x_o$. x_o is the output of the PLL's VCO. Thus,

$$x_i = A\big[1 + m(t)\big]\sin\big(\omega_c t + \theta_c\big) \times X_o \cos\big(\omega_o t + \theta_o\big) \tag{11.39}$$

$$= \big[A X_o \big[1 + m(t)\big]/2\big]\big\{\sin\big[(\omega_c + \omega_o)t + \theta_c + \theta_o\big] + \sin\big[(\omega_c - \omega_o)t + \theta_c - \theta_o\big]\big\}$$

The IF band-pass filter selects the second term, which has frequency close to ω_{if} when the PLL is near lock. This means that x_4 is:

$$x_4 = \big[K_i A X_o \big[1 + m(t)\big]/2\big]\sin\big[(\omega_c - \omega_o)t + \theta_c - \theta_o\big] \tag{11.40}$$

Also, the output of the crystal-controlled oscillator (XO) is:

$$x_5 = X_5 \cos(\omega_{if} t) \tag{11.41}$$

Mathematically, the product, $x_6 = x_4 \times x_5$ is formed:

$$x_6 = \left[K_i A X_o \left[1 + m(t)\right]/2\right] \sin\left[\left(\omega_c - \omega_o\right)t + \theta_c - \theta_o\right] \times X_5 \cos\left(\omega_{if} t\right) \quad (11.42\text{A})$$

$$x_6 = X_5 \left[K_i A X_o \left[1 + m(t)\right]/4\right] \sin\left[\left(\omega_c - \omega_o + w_{if}\right) + \theta_c - \theta_o\right]$$
$$+ \sin\left[\left(\omega_c - \omega_o - \omega_{if}\right) + \theta_c - \theta_o\right] \quad (11.42\text{B})$$

At lock, $(\omega_c - \omega_o) = \omega_{if}$ r/s and $(\theta_c - \theta_o) \rightarrow 0$. The low-pass filter acts on x_6; its output is the zero-frequency component of x_6. Thus:

$$X_7 = X_5 \left[K_i A X_o \left[1 + m(t)\right]/4\right] \sin\left[\left(\omega_c - \omega_o - \omega_{if}\right) + \theta_c - \theta_o\right] \quad (11.43)$$

Note that $x_7 \rightarrow 0$ at lock. Now, $x_5' = X_5 \sin(\omega_{if} t)$, so x_8 can be written:

$$x_8 = x_4 \times x_5' = \left[K_i A X_o \left[1 + m(t)/2\right]\right] \sin\left[\left(\omega_c - \omega_o\right)t + \theta_c - \theta_o\right] \times$$
$$X_5 \sin\left(\omega_{if} t\right) \quad (11.44\text{A})$$

$$x_8 = \left[X_5 K_i A X_o \left[1 + m(t)/4\right]\right]$$
$$\left\{\cos\left[\left(\theta_c - \theta_o - \omega_{if}\right)t + \theta_c - \theta_o\right] - \cos\left[\left(\theta_c - \theta_o + \omega_{if}\right)t + \theta_c - \theta_o\right]\right\} \quad (11.44\text{B})$$

Again, at lock:

$$x_8 = \left[X_5 K_i A X_o \left[1 + m(t)/4\right]\right]\left\{\cos(0) - \cos\left[\left(2\omega_{if}\right)t + \theta c - \theta_o\right]\right\} \quad (11.44\text{C})$$

The band-pass filter cuts the dc term in x_8 and also the $2\omega_{if}$ term; therefore, the output of the BPF is proportional to the modulating signal:

$$x_9 = X_5 K_i A X_o m(t)/4 \quad (11.45)$$

Thus, the normalized modulating signal, $[m_o \cos(\omega_m t)]$, is recovered, times a scaling constant.

A fourth kind of AM demodulation can be accomplished by finding the magnitude of the modulated signal's analytical signal (Northrop, 2003).

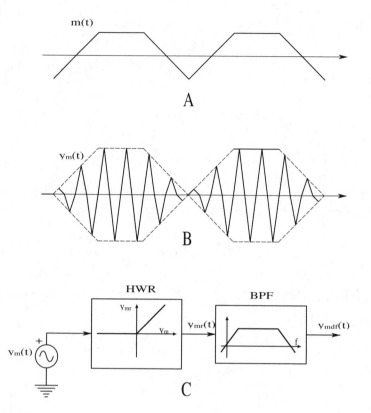

FIGURE 11.11
AM detection by simple half-wave rectification. (A) The modulating signal. (B) The AM carrier (drawn as a triangle wave instead of a sinusoid). (C) An ideal half-wave rectifier followed by an audio band-pass filter.

Examine the widely used rectifier + low-pass filter (average envelope) AM detector. Figure 11.11(A) illustrates a low-frequency modulating signal, $m(t)$. Figure 11.11(B) shows the amplitude-modulated carrier (the sinusoidal carrier is drawn with straight lines for simplicity). Figure 11.11(C) illustrates the block diagram of a simple half-wave rectifier circuit followed by a band-pass filter to exclude dc and terms of carrier frequency and higher. The half-wave rectification process can be thought of as multiplying the AM $y_m(t)$ by a 0,1 switching function, $Sq(t)$, in phase with the carrier. Mathematically, this can be stated as:

$$y_{mr}(t) = A\left[1 + m\cos(\omega_m t)\right]\cos(\omega_c t)Sq(t)$$

$$= A\cos(\omega_c t)Sq(t) + A m_o \cos(\omega_m t)\cos(\omega_c t)Sq(t)$$

(11.46)

$Sq(t)$ can be written as a Fourier series (Northrop, 2003):

$$Sq(t) = \tfrac{1}{2} + (2/\pi)\sum_{n=1}^{\infty}(-1)^{n+1}\frac{\cos\left[(2n-1)\omega_c t\right]}{(2n-1)} \tag{11.47A}$$

$$\downarrow$$

$$Sq(t) = \tfrac{1}{2} + (2/\pi)\left\{\cos(\omega_c t) - (1/3)\cos(3\omega_c t) + (1/5)\cos(5\omega_c t) - ...\right\} \tag{11.47B}$$

Now multiply the Fourier series by the terms of Equation 11.46:

$$y_d(t) = \tfrac{1}{2}A\cos(\omega_c t) + (2/\pi A\left\{\cos^2(\omega_c t) - (1/3)\cos(\omega_c t)\cos(3\omega_c t) + \right.$$

$$\left. + (1/5)\cos(\omega_c t)\cos(5\omega_c t) - ...\right\} + \tfrac{1}{2}A m_o \cos(\omega_m t)\cos(\omega_c t)$$

$$+ (2A m_o/\pi)\cos(\omega_m t)\cos^2(\omega_c t) - (2A m_o/3\pi)\cos(\omega_m t)\cos(\omega_c t)\cos(3\omega_c t)$$

$$+ (2A m_o/5\pi)\cos(\omega_m t)\cos(\omega_c t)\cos(5\omega_c t)$$

$$- (2A m_o/7\pi)\cos(\omega_m t)\cos(\omega_c t)\cos(7\omega_c t) + ... \tag{11.48}$$

and examine what happens when the terms of Equation 11.48 are passed through a band-pass filter that attenuates to zero dc and all terms at above $(\omega_c - \omega_m)$. Trigonometric expansions of the form $\cos(x)\cos(y) = (1/2)[\cos(x + y) + \cos(x - y)]$ are used. Let the BPF's output be $y_{mdf}(t)$:

$$y_{mdf}(t) = (A/\pi) + (A/\pi)\left[m_o \cos(\omega_m t)\right] \tag{11.49}$$

The BPF output contains a dc term plus a term proportional to the desired $m_o \cos(\omega_m t)$. Because AM radio is usually used to transmit audio signals that do not extend to zero frequency, the band-pass filter blocks the dc but passes modulating signal frequencies. Thus, $y_{mdf}(t) \propto m_o \cos(\omega_m t)$. Several other AM detection schemes exist, including peak envelope detection and synchronous detection, described later in the detection of DSBSCM signals; the interested reader can find a good description of these modes of AM detection in Clarke and Hess (1971).

11.5.3   Detection of FM Signals

When modulating and transmitting signals with a dc component, FM is the desired modulation scheme because a dc signal, V_m, produces a fixed frequency deviation from the carrier at ω_c given by:

$$\Delta\omega = K_f V_m \tag{11.50}$$

As in the case of AM, FM demodulation can accomplished by several means. The first step in any FM demodulation scheme is to limit the received signal. Mathematically, limiting can be represented as passing the sinusoidal FM $y_m(t)$ through a signum function (symmetrical clipper); the clipper output is a square wave of peak height, $y_{mcl}(t) = B\ sgn[y_m(t)]$. (The $sgn(y_m)$ function is 1 for $y_m \geq 0$, and -1 for $y_m < 0$.) Clipping removes most unwanted amplitude modulation, including noise on the received $y_m(t)$; this is one reason why FM radio is free of noise compared to AM. The frequency argument of $y_{mcl}(t)$ is the same as for the FM sinusoidal carrier, i.e., $\omega_{FM} = \omega_c + K_f v_m(t)$.

Once limited, several means of FM demodulation are now available, including the phase-shift discriminator; the Foster–Seely discriminator; the ratio detector; pulse averaging; and certain phase-locked loop circuits (Chirlian, 1981; Northrop, 1990). It is beyond the scope of this text to describe all of these FM demodulation circuits in detail, so the simple pulse averaging discriminator will first be examined.

In this FM demodulation means, the limited signal is fed into a one-shot multivibrator that triggers on the rising edge of each cycle of $y_{mcl}(t)$, producing a train of standard TTL pulses, each of fixed width $\delta = \pi/\omega_c$ sec. For simplicity, assume the peak height of each pulse is 5 V and low is 0 V. Now the average pulse voltage is $v_{av}(t)$:

$$v_{av}(t) = \frac{1}{T}\int_0^\delta 5\ dt = \frac{\omega_c + K_f v_m}{\pi}\int_0^{\pi/\omega_c} 5\ dt = (5/2)\left(1 + K_f v_m/\omega_c\right) \tag{11.51}$$

Thus, recovery of $v_m(t)$, even a dc v_m, requires the linear operation:

$$v_m(t) = \left[(2/5)v_{av}(t) - 1\right]\left(\omega_c/K_f\right) \tag{11.52}$$

In practice, the averaging is done by a low-pass filter with break frequency $\omega_{mmax} \ll \omega_f \ll \omega_c$.

In phase modulation, the modulated carrier is given by:

$$y_m(t) = A\ \cos\left[\omega_c t + K_p v_m(t)\right] \tag{11.53}$$

Because the frequency of the PhM carrier is the derivative of its phase,

$$\omega_{PhM} = \omega_c + K_p \dot{v}_m(t) \tag{11.54}$$

PhM carriers can be generated and demodulated using phase-locked loops (Northrop, 1989).

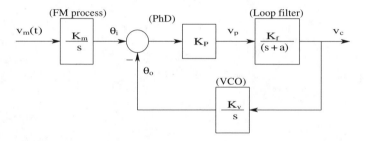

FIGURE 11.12
A PLL used to demodulate an NBFM carrier.

Figure 11.12 illustrates an example of a PLL used to recover the modulating signal, $v_m(t)$, in an NBFM carrier. Note that the PLL input is the phase of the NBFM signal, θ_i, which is proportional to the integral of $v_m(t)$. The PLL tries to track $\theta_i(t)$ and in doing so generates the VCO control signal, $v_c(t)$, that is of interest. The frequency in the transfer function of the PLL is the frequency of $v_m(t)$, not ω_c. The loop gain of the PLL is:

$$A_L(s) = -\frac{K_p K_f K_v}{s(s+b)} \tag{11.55}$$

To give the closed-loop PLL a damping of $\xi = 0.707$, it is easy to show, using root locus, that $K_p K_f K_v = b^2/2$ and the undamped natural frequency of the PLL is $\omega_n = b\sqrt{2}/2$ r/s. The frequency response function for the PLL demodulator can be shown to be:

$$\frac{\mathbf{V_c}}{\mathbf{V_m}}(j\omega) = \frac{(K_m/j\omega)K_p K_f/(j\omega+b)}{1 + K_p K_f K_v/[j\omega(j\omega+b)]} = \frac{K_m/K_v}{(j\omega)^2/(b^2/2) + j\omega(2/b) + 1} \tag{11.56}$$

Thus, at signal frequencies below the loop's $\omega_n = b\sqrt{2}/2$ r/s, the PLL demodulates the NBFM input; the output is proportional to $v_m(t)$. That is:

$$v_c(t) \cong (K_m/K_v)v_m(t) \tag{11.57}$$

Therefore, the loop filter output is proportional to $v_m(t)$ for v_m frequencies between zero and about $\omega_n/2$.

11.5.4 Demodulation of DSBSCM Signals

The demodulation of DSBSCM carriers is generally done by a phase-sensitive rectifier (PSR) (also known as a synchronous rectifier) followed by a low-pass filter. One version of this system is shown in Figure 11.13. In this op amp

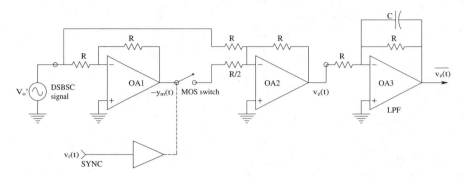

FIGURE 11.13
Schematic of a three-op amp synchronous (phase-sensitive) rectifier used to demodulate a
DSBSC-modulated carrier.

version of a PSR, an analog MOS switch is made to close for the positive
half-cycles of the reference signal that has the same frequency and phase as
the unmodulated carrier. Figure 11.14 illustrates a low-frequency modulating
signal, $v_m(t)$, from there, the DSBSCM signal, and, finally, $V_z(t)$, the unfiltered
output of the PSR. Note that "c" means the MOS switch is closed and "o"
means it is open. The simple op amp low-pass filter also inverts, so its output
$\overline{V_z}$ is proportional to $-v_m(t)$.

Another means of demodulating a DSBSC signal is by an analog multiplier
followed by an LPF. In the latter means, the multiplier output voltage, $V_o'(t)$,
is the product of a reference carrier and the DSBSCM signal:

$$V_o'(t) = (0.1)B\cos(\omega_c t) \times (Am_o/2)\left[\cos((\omega_c + \omega_m)t) + \cos((\omega_c - \omega_m)t)\right] \quad (11.58)$$

The 0.1 constant is inherent to all analog multipliers. By trigonometric
identity, noting that $\cos\theta$ is an even function, the multiplier output can be
written:

$$V_o'(t) = (0.1)(Am_o B/4)\left[\cos((2\omega_c + \omega_m)t) + \cos(\omega_m t)\right] \quad (11.59)$$

After unity-gain low-pass filtering,

$$\overline{V_o'}(t) = (0.1)(AB/4)m_o \cos(\omega_m t) \quad (11.60)$$

which is certainly proportional to $v_m(t)$.

Still another way to demodulate DSBSC signals is by a special PLL architecture called the Costas loop (Northrop, 1990), shown in Figure 11.15. Its
successful operation requires that the modulating signal, $vm(t)$, be nonzero

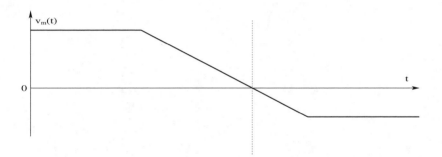

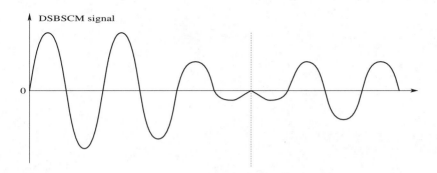

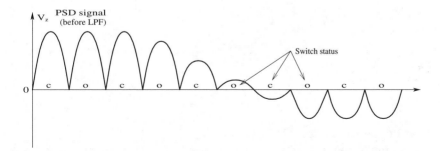

FIGURE 11.14
Waveforms relevant to the operation of the synchronous rectifier of Figure 11.13. Top: Modulating signal. Middle: DSBSC signal. Bottom: Detected signal before LPF.

only for short intervals so that the PLL does not lose lock. The input DSBSCM signal can be written:

$$x_1 = v_m(t) \, V_c \cos(\omega_c t + \theta_c) \tag{11.61}$$

The output of the PLL's VCO is:

$$x_6 = X_6 \cos(\omega_o t + \theta_o) \tag{11.62}$$

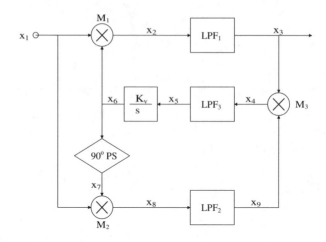

FIGURE 11.15
Block diagram of a simple Costas PLL.

and the output of mixer $M1$ is:

$$x_2 = x_1 \times x_6 = v_m(t) V_c X_6 \cos(\omega_c t + \theta_c) \cos(\omega_o t + \theta_o) \tag{11.63}$$

$$= [v_m(t) V_c X_6/2]\{\cos[(\omega_c + \omega_o)t + \theta_c + \theta_o] + \cos[(\omega_c - \omega_o)t + \theta_c - \theta_o]\}$$

At lock, $\omega_o \rightarrow \omega_c$ and $\theta_o \rightarrow \theta_c$, and LPF1 passes only the low-frequency components of x_2. Thus:

$$x_3 = v_m(t) \, V_c \, X_6/2 \tag{11.64}$$

which is the desired output.

Now examine how the other signals in the Costas loop contribute to its operation. By trigonometric identity, the output of the quadrature phase shifter is:

$$x_7 = -X_6 \sin(\omega_o t + \theta_o) \tag{11.65}$$

The output of the second mixer is thus:

$$x_8 = -X_6 v_m(t) V_c \sin(\omega_o t + \theta_o) \cos(\omega_c t + \theta_c) \tag{11.66A}$$

$$x_8 = [-X_6 v_m(t) V_c/2]\{\sin[(\omega_0 + \omega_c)t + \theta_o + \theta_c] + \sin[(\omega_o - \omega_c)t + \theta_o - \theta_c]\} \tag{11.66B}$$

Near lock, at the output of LPF2,

$$x_9 \cong \left[-X_6 v_m(t) V_c / 2\right]\left[(\omega_o - \omega_c)t + \theta_o - \theta_c\right] \tag{11.67}$$

so the output of mixer M3 is:

$$
\begin{aligned}
x_4 = x_9 \times x_3 &= \left[-X_6 v_m(t) V_c / 2\right]\left[v_m(t) V_c X_6 / 2\right]\left[(\omega_o - \omega_c)t + \theta_o - \theta_c\right] \\
&= -\left[v_m(t) V_c X_6 / 2\right]^2 \left[(\omega_o - \omega_c)t + (\theta_o - \theta_c)\right]
\end{aligned}
\tag{11.68}
$$

x_4 tends to zero when the loop locks, leaving the VCO with phase $\theta_o = \theta_c$ and $\omega_o = \omega_c$.

11.6 Modulation and Demodulation of Digital Carriers

11.6.1 Introduction

TTL NBFM carriers can be modulated using voltage-to-frequency converter or voltage-controlled oscillator (VCO) integrated circuits. The frequency output of such an IC is given by:

$$f_o = k_1 + K_v\, v_m(t)\ \text{Hz} \tag{11.69}$$

Obviously, $k_1 = f_c$, the unmodulated carrier frequency. Many VCO ICs will give simultaneous TTL, triangle, and sinusoidal wave outputs over a sub-hertz to +10-MHz range.

One way to produce a TTL wave whose duty cycle is modulated by $v_m(t)$ is to begin with a constant-frequency, zero-mean, symmetrical triangle wave, $v_T(t)$, as shown in Figure 11.16. $v_T(t)$ is one input to an analog comparator with TTL output; the other input is $v_m(t)$. As $v_m(t)$ approaches the peak voltage of the triangle wave, V_p, the duty cycle, η, of the TTL wave approaches unity; similarly, as $v_m(t) \to -V_p$, $\eta \to 0$. Mathematically, the duty cycle is defined as the positive pulse width, δ, divided by the triangle wave period, T. In other words, the comparator TTL output is HI for $v_m(t) > v_T(t)$.

From the foregoing, it is easy to derive the TTL wave's duty cycle:

$$\eta = \delta/T = \tfrac{1}{2}\left[1 + v_m(t)/V_p\right] \tag{11.70}$$

Here $v_m(t)$ is assumed to be changing slowly enough to be considered constant over $T/2$. Demodulation of a pulse width-modulated TTL carrier is

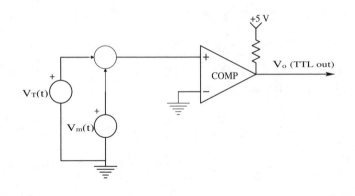

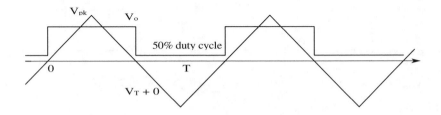

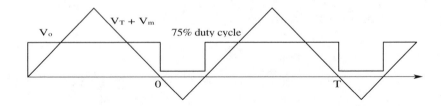

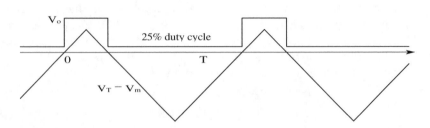

FIGURE 11.16
A simple pulse-width modulator and waveforms.

done by averaging the TTL pulse train and subtracting the dc component present when $v_m = 0$.

11.6.2 Delta Modulation

Now consider delta modulation (DM) and demodulation. A delta modulator is also known as a 1-bit differential pulse code modulator (DPCM). The output of a delta modulator is a clocked (periodic) train of TTL pulses with amplitudes that are HI or LO, depending on the state of the comparator output shown in Figure 11.17. The DM output basically tracks the derivative of the input signal. The comparator output is TTL HI if $e(t) = [v_m(t) - v_r'(t)] > 0$ and LO if $e < 0$. The D flip-flop's (DFF) complimentary output ($\overline{Q} = V_o$) is LO if the comparator output is HI at a positive transition of the TTL clock signal. The LO output of the DFF remains LO until the next positive transition of the clock signal; then, if the comparator output has gone LO, V_o goes high for one clock period (T_c), etc. $v_r'(t)$ is the output of the analog integrator offset by V_{bias}, which is one half the maximum v_r ramp height over one clock period. V_{bias} can be shown to be $1.1T_c/(RC)$ volts.

With this V_{bias}, when $v_m(t) = 0$, $v_r'(t)$ will oscillate around zero with a triangle wave with zero mean and peak height $1.1T_c/(RC)$ volts. Note that the $\overline{Q}$ output of the DFF must be used because the integrator gain is negative (i.e., $-1/RC$): a HI V_o will cause v_r' to go negative and a low V_o will make v_r' go positive. Note that $v_r'(t)$ is slew rate limited at $\pm(2.2 \text{ V}/RC)$ volts/second and, if the slope of $v_m(t)$ exceeds this value, a large error will accumulate in the demodulation operation of the DM signal. (Slew rate is simply the magnitude of the first derivative of a signal, i.e., its slope.) When a DM system is tracking $v_m = 0$, $v_r'(t)$ oscillates around zero and the DM output is a periodic square-wave 1-bit "noise."

In adaptive delta modulation (ADM), the magnitude of the error is used to adjust the effective gain of the integrator to increase the slew rate of $v_r'(t)$ to track rapidly changing $v_m(t)$ better. One version of an ADM system is shown in Figure 11.18. Note that, ideally, the comparator should perform the signum operation; therefore, the dc value (mean) of the TTL wave must be subtracted before it is filtered, absval'd, and used to modulate the size of the square wave input to the integrator. A conventional analog multiplier is used as a modulator.

If a large error occurs as a result of poor tracking due to low slew rate in $v_r'(t)$, the comparator output will remain HI (or LO) for several clock cycles. This condition produces a nonzero signal at v_f, which in turn increases the amplitude of the symmetrical pulse input to the integrator. When the ADM is tracking well, so that $v_r'(t)$ oscillates around a nearly constant v_m level, then $v_f \rightarrow 0$ and the peak amplitude of the error remains small. In summary, the ADM acts to minimize the mean squared error between $v_m(t)$ and $v_r'(t)$.

There are other variations on DM (e.g., sigma–delta modulation) and other types of nonlinear adaptive DM designs in addition to the one shown here.

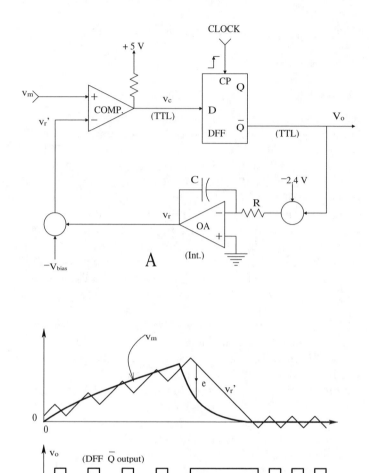

FIGURE 11.17
Block diagram and waveforms of a simple delta modulator.

Much of the interest in efficient, simple, low-noise modulation schemes has been driven by the need to transmit sound and pictures over the Internet. Medical signals such as ECG and EEG also benefit from this development because of the need to transmit them from the site of the patient to a diagnostician. Biotelemetry is an important technology in the wireless monitoring of internal physiological states, sports medicine, and emergency medicine, and in ecological studies.

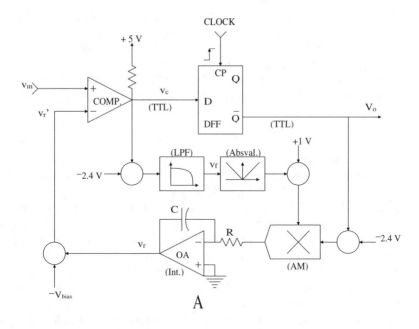

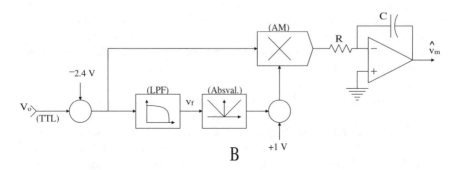

FIGURE 11.18
(A) Circuit for an adaptive delta modulator. (B) Demodulator for ADM. A long time-constant LPF is generally used instead of an ideal integrator for filtering v_m.

11.7 Chapter Summary

Broadly speaking, modulation is a process in which a low-frequency modulating signal acts on a high-frequency carrier wave in some way so that the high-frequency modulated carrier can be transmitted (e.g., as radio waves, ultrasound waves, light waves, etc.) to a suitable receiver; after this the process of demodulation occurs, recovering the modulating signal. In the frequency domain, the low-frequency power spectrum of the signal is translated upward in frequency to lie around the carrier frequency. A major purpose of modulation is to permit long-range transmission of the modulating signal by a relatively noise-free modality.

Why transmit modulated carriers? After all, traditional short-distance telephony transmits audio information directly on telephone lines. The answer lies in the signal spectrum. The low frequencies associated with many endogenous physiological signals cannot be transmitted by conventional voice telephony; modulation must be used. The carrier modality can be radio waves, ultrasound, or light on fiber optic cables. For example, when the modulating signal is an ECG, its power spectrum is too low for direct transmission by telephone lines. However, the ECG can narrow-band frequency-modulate (NBFM) an audio-frequency carrier that can be transmitted on phone lines and demodulated at the receiver. In a case in which an ambulance is en route carrying a patient, the ECG can directly NBFM an RF carrier, which is received and demodulated at the hospital's ER.

Subcarrier modulation can be used as well. Here several low-frequency physiological signals such as ECG, blood pressure, and respiration can NBFM an audio subcarrier, each with a different frequency. The modulated subcarriers are added together and used to modulate amplitude of frequency of an RF carrier, which is transmitted. Subcarrier FM can also be used with ultrasonic "tags" to monitor marine animals such as whales and dolphins. The tag is attached to the animal and reports such parameters as depth, water temperature, heart rate, etc. The subcarriers are separated following detection at the receiver by band-pass filters and then demodulated.

The section about AM examined the process in the frequency domain and gave examples of selected circuits used in AM and single-sideband AM. Double-sideband, suppressed-carrier AM was shown to be the simple result of multiplying the carrier by the modulating signal. Examples of DSBSCM were shown to include Wheatstone bridge outputs given ac carrier excitation and the output of an LVDT. Broadband and narrowband FM were examined theoretically; circuits and systems used to generate NBFM, such as the phase-locked loop (PLL), were described as well. Integral- and relaxation-pulse frequency modulation were introduced.

The section on demodulation illustrated circuits and systems used to demodulate AM, DSBSCM, FM, and NBFM signals. Again, the PLL was shown to be effective at demodulation. Modulation of digital (e.g., TTL, ECL) carriers includes FM and Σ–Δ (sigma–delta) modulation, pulse-width or duty-cycle modulation, and adaptive delta modulation. Means of demodulating digital modulated signals were described.

Home Problems

11.1   An analog pulse instantaneous pulse frequency demodulator (IPFD) must generate a hyperbolic (not exponential) capacitor discharge waveform in order to convert interpulse intervals to elements of instantaneous frequency

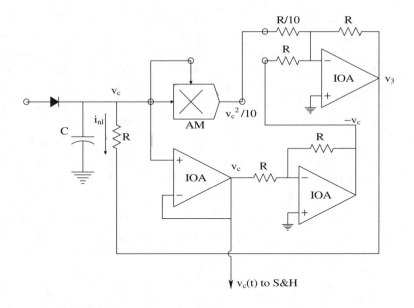

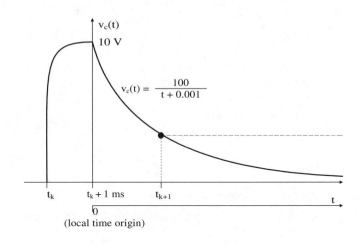

FIGURE P11.1

(IF). IF is defined as the reciprocal of the interval between two adjacent impulses in a sequence of pulses. When the $(k + 1)^{th}$ pulse in a sequence occurs, the kth hyperbolic waveform voltage is sampled and held, generating the kth element of IF, which is held until the $(k + 2)^{th}$ pulse occurs, etc. The capacitor discharge will be a portion of a hyperbola for $t \geq 1$ MS following the occurrence of each pulse. Mathematically, this can be stated:

$$v_c(t) = \frac{C/\beta}{t + \tau_o}$$

where V_{cmax} = 10 V; C = 1 μF; and $τ_o$ = $C/(βV_{cmax})$ = 0.001 sec. It can be shown that if the capacitor is allowed to discharge into a nonlinear conductance so that: $i_{nl}(t) = β\,v_c(t)^2$, the preceding hyperbolic $v_c(t)$ will occur (Northrop, 1997). Time t is measured from $(t_k + 0.001)$ sec (see the timing diagram below the schematic). This means that if $t_{k+1} = (t_k + 0.001)$, $v_c(0) =$ 10 V for an IF of 1000 pps. Note that prior to each discharge cycle, C is charged through the diode to +10 V.

In this problem, you are to analyze and design the active circuit of Figure P11.1 that causes $i_{nl}(t) = βv_c(t)^2$ and generates the hyperbolic $v_c(t)$ described. That is, find the numerical value of R required, given the preceding parameter values. Also find the numerical values for $β$ and the peak $i_{nl}(t)$.

11.2   Show that the PLL circuit of Figure P11.2 generates FM. Show that the phase output of the VCO is true wideband FM. (Hint: find the transfer function, $θ_o/X_m$.)

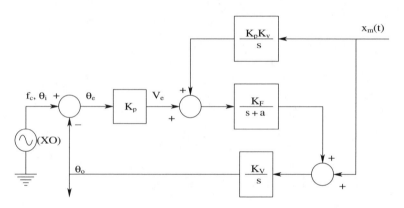

FIGURE P11.2

11.3   Make a Bode plot of $θ_o/X_m$ for the system of Figure P11.3. Show the frequency range(s) at which FM is generated and phase modulation is generated.

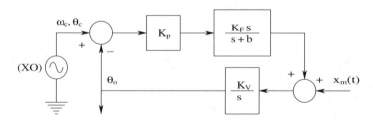

FIGURE P11.3

11.4   The system illustrated in Figure P11.4 is an FM demodulator. The K_m/s block represents the operation on the phase of the carrier by an ideal FM modulator.

Make a Bode plot of V_c/X_m and show the range of frequencies (of $x_m(t)$) where ideal FM demodulation occurs (i.e., where $V_c \propto x_m$).

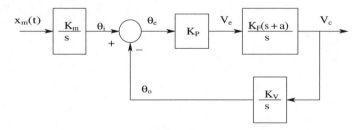

FIGURE P11.4

11.5 A quarter-square multiplier, shown in Figure P11.5, is used to demodulate a double-sideband, suppressed-carrier modulated cosine wave. The modulated wave is given by $v_m(t) = A \, x_m(t) \cos(\omega_c t)$. Write expressions for w, aw^2, y, ay^2, z and $\bar{z}$, and show $\bar{z} \propto x_m(t)$. Assume that the LPF totally attenuates frequencies at and above ω_c.

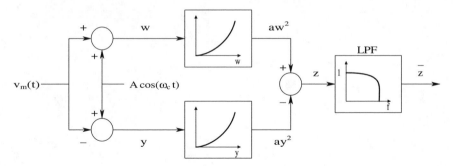

FIGURE P11.5

11.6 An analog multiplier (AM) followed by a low-pass filter (LPF) is used to demodulate a DSBSC signal, $v_m(t) = A \, x_m(t) \cos(\omega_c t)$, as shown in Figure P11.6. Give algebraic expressions for z and $\bar{z}$. Assume that the LPF totally attenuates frequencies at and above ω_c.

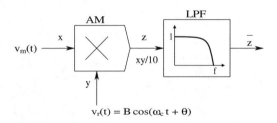

FIGURE P11.6

12

Examples of Special Analog Circuits and Systems in Biomedical Instrumentation

12.1 Introduction

Biomedical engineers may be expected to understand many specialized integrated circuits and be able to incorporate them effectively into biomedical measurement system designs. These integrated circuits include but are not limited to:

- Phase-sensitive rectifiers
- Phase detectors
- Voltage- and current-controlled oscillators
- Phase-locked loops
- True-RMS converters
- IC thermometers

Most designers and vendors of analog ICs, such as Analog Devices, Burr–Brown, Maxim, National, etc., make one or more of the preceding ICs. In describing them, this chapter will stress application as well as design.

12.2 The Phase-Sensitive Rectifier

12.2.1 Introduction

The phase-sensitive rectifier (PSR) is also known as the *phase-sensitive detector*, the *synchronous rectifier or detector*, or the *balanced demodulator*. Its primary role is to recover the modulating signal in a double-sideband, suppressed-carrier (amplitude) modulated carrier. The PSR is also at the heart of the lock-in amplifier, which is widely used in photonics and in certain applications in physics to recover a low-frequency modulating signal. A PSR will also demodulate ordinary AM. The four major embodiments of the PSR are the (1) analog multiplier/low-pass filter (LPF) PSR; (2) switched op amp PSR; (3) electromechanical chopper PSR; and (4) balanced diode bridge PSR. The analog multiplier PSR will be examined first.

12.2.2 The Analog Multiplier/LPF PSR

Just as a DSBSCM carrier can be made by multiplying a sinusoidal carrier by the low-frequency modulating signal, the DSBSCM signal can be demodulated by multiplying the modulated carrier by a carrier frequency reference signal of the correct phase (refer to Figure 11.1B in the preceding chapter). Let the coherent modulating signal be a low-frequency sinusoid:

$$v_m(t) = V_m \sin(\omega_m t) \tag{12.1}$$

The carrier is:

$$v_c(t) = V_c \cos(\omega_c t) \tag{12.2}$$

and the modulated carrier is:

$$y_m(t) = \left(V_m V_c/2\right)\left\{\sin\left[\left(\omega_c + \omega_m\right)t\right] + \sin\left[\left(\omega_c - \omega_m\right)t\right]\right\} \tag{12.3}$$

The reference signal is of the same frequency as the carrier but in general differs in phase by a fixed angle, $(\pi/2 + \varphi)$ radians. By trigonometric identity, this is:

$$v_r(t) = V_r \sin(\omega_c t + \varphi) \tag{12.4}$$

The analog multiplier output is:

$$v_z(t) = \left\{v_r(t)\,y_m(t)\right\}/10 = \left(V_m V_c V_r/20\right)\left\{\cos\left[\omega_m t - \varphi\right] - \cos\left[\left(2\omega_c + \omega_m\right)t + \varphi\right] + \right.$$
$$\left. \cos\left[\omega_m t + \varphi\right] - \cos\left[\left(2\omega_c - \omega_m\right)t - \varphi\right]\right\} \tag{12.5}$$

(Note that the output of a transconductance-type analog multiplier IC is the product of the inputs divided by 10.) The unity-gain low-pass filter removes the two $2\omega_c$ terms, leaving (recall that $\sin\theta$ is an odd function):

$$\overline{v_x(t)} = \left(V_m V_c V_r/20\right)\left\{\cos\left[\omega_m t - \varphi\right] + \cos\left[\omega_m t + \varphi\right]\right\} \tag{12.6}$$

From the trigonometric identity, $\{\cos\alpha + \cos\beta\} = 2\cos[\frac{1}{2}(\alpha + \beta)]\cos[\frac{1}{2}(\alpha - \beta)]$:

$$\overline{v_z(t)} = \left(V_m V_c V_r / 10\right)\cos(\omega_m t)\cos(\varphi) \tag{12.7}$$

In the preceding development, it was assumed that $0 < \omega_m \ll \omega_b \ll \omega_c$, where ω_b is the LPF's break frequency. Note that the recovered modulating signal is maximum when the reference signal is in phase with the quadrature carrier of the DSBSCM signal. Thus, an analog multiplier can form DSBSCM signals and also demodulate them, returning a signal $\propto v_m(t)$.

12.2.3   The Switched Op Amp PSR

Figure 11.13 in Chapter 11 illustrates a PSR that uses three op amps and a digitally controlled analog MOS switch to demodulate DSBSCM signals. The MOS switch, when closed, has a very low resistance. When it is open, its resistance is on the order of megohms. The switch is controlled by the function, $\operatorname{sgn}\{V_r \sin(\omega_c t)\}$, which is +1 when $\sin(\omega_c t)$ is ≥ 0 and -1 when $\sin(\omega_c t) < 0$. The output, $v_z(t)$, is a full-wave rectified $y_m(t)$, which goes negative when the sign of the modulating signal, $v_m(t)$ goes negative. It is easy to see that after low-pass filtering, $v_z(t)$ is $\propto v_m(t)$. The average (dc value) of a full-wave rectified sine wave is $\pi V_{pk}/2$. Note that the action of the switch effectively multiplies the DSBSCM input signal by a ± 1 peak value square wave of frequency $\omega_c/2\pi$ Hz.

12.2.4   The Chopper PSR

Figure 12.1(A) illustrates the circuit of an electromechanical chopper. Electromechanical choppers are basically SPDT switches commutated by a driver coil at switching frequencies from 50 to 400 Hz or so. Developed in the WWII era as modulator/demodulators for ac DSBSCM signals, they are now obsolete. The same SPDT action can be obtained using appropriately buffered MOS switches that can be commutated in the hundreds of kilohertz or by photoelectrically turning phototransistors on and off in a photoelectric chopper. The basic electromechanical chopper uses a center-tapped signal transformer to couple the DSBSCM carrier to the switch points.

Figure 12.1(B) illustrates the raw switch output, $v_z(t)$. This signal must be low-pass filtered to recover $v_m(t)$. Note that the phase shift φ causes some of the chopped signal to be negative over φ radians of the cycle. When averaged, this negative area subtracts from the output signal. It can be shown that the phase error φ in the reference signal effectively multiplies the averager output by $\cos(\varphi)$. Thus, if the reference signal is 90° out of phase, the low-pass filtered output will always be zero.

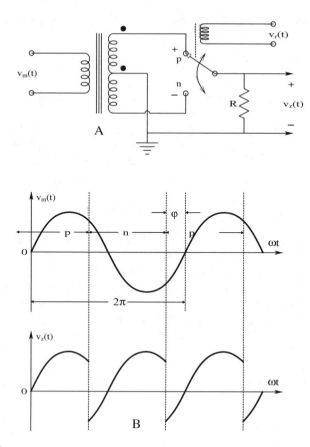

FIGURE 12.1

(A) Circuit of an electromechanical chopper phase-sensitive rectifier (PSR). (B) Upper waveform: chopper input. *p* and *n* denote the intervals the chopper switch dwells on the positive or minus contacts, respectively. Lower waveform: chopper output when the switch control sync voltage, $v_r(t)$, is out of phase with $v_m(t)$ by φ radians. Perfect full-wave rectification is not achieved.

12.2.5   The Balanced Diode Bridge PSR

Still another circuit that can be used to demodulate DSBSCM signals is the balanced diode bridge PSR, illustrated in Figure 12.2. The modulated signal, $y_m(t)$, and the reference signal, $v_r(t)$, are coupled to the diode bridge by two center-tapped transformers. The transformer on the left is called the *signal transformer* and the one on the right is the *reference transformer*.

To understand how the diode bridge PSR works, refer to Figure 12.3. Assume $v_r(t) > 0$, diodes *a* and *b* conduct current i_{r+}, and *c* and *d* are cut off (treated as open circuits). The positive signal voltage at node B causes a current, i_{ma} and i_{mb}, to flow through diodes *a* and *b*, respectively. Assume that $i_{ma} > i_{r+}$, so diode *a* continues to conduct. The currents i_{ma} and i_{mb} flow through both halves of the reference transformer secondary, combine, and flow to

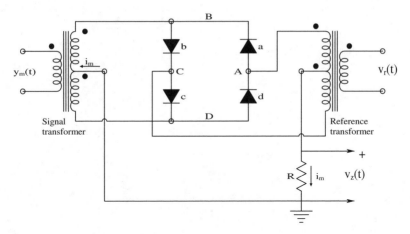

FIGURE 12.2
A balanced-bridge diode PSR.

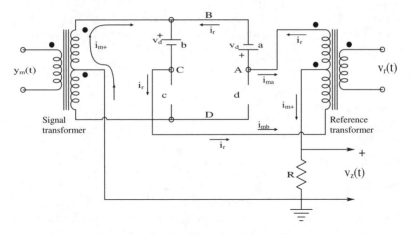

FIGURE 12.3
The diode bridge PSR when diodes *a* and *b* are conducting, and *c* and *d* are blocking current flow.

ground through the resistor R. Note that it is the top half of the signal transformer that supplies i_{m+}.

The output voltage is $v_o(t) = i_{m+}(t)R$ for positive $v_r(t)$ and positive (or negative) $v_m(t)$. During the negative half cycle of $v_r(t)$ shown in Figure 12.4, diodes c and d conduct and a and b are reverse biased. Now the lower half of the signal transformer secondary delivers signal current i_{m-} to the load R in the same direction as i_{m+}, producing phase-sensitive rectification. Note that if the phase of $y_m(t)$ changes by 180°, the sign of the rectified $v_o(t)$ also changes, giving a negative output. The output of the balanced diode bridge PSR has a relatively high output impedance and therefore must be buffered before $v_o(t)$ is sent to a low-pass filter for averaging. The permissible upper

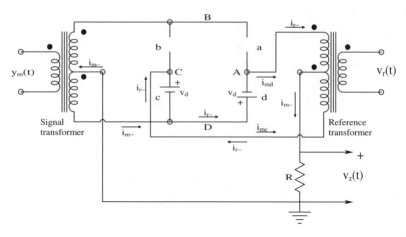

FIGURE 12.4
The diode bridge PSR when diodes *c* and *d* are conducting, and *a* and *b* are blocking current flow.

carrier frequency of the BDBPSR is determined by the types of diodes used. Schottky diodes switch extremely fast because they are majority carrier devices and there is no minority carrier storage at the junction; they will give satisfactory results in the hundreds of megahertz (Yang, 1988).

12.3 Phase Detectors

12.3.1 Introduction

A phase detector (PD) operates on two periodic signals of the same frequency and returns a dc signal voltage proportional to the phase difference between the two signals. PDs have several important applications. They are used in lock-in amplifiers to ensure the reference signal retains the correct phase relation with the input carrier for optimum demodulation (McDonald and Northrop, 1993). They are also used as an essential component in all phase-lock loops, which have many applications. Sections 12.4.5 and 12.8.3 will show that a PD is necessary in a phase-locked laser radar (LAVERA) system. PDs are also used in the impedance and autobalancing bridges used to measure body impedance or admittance. PDs can be subdivided into analog and digital designs.

12.3.2 The Analog Multiplier Phase Detector

The simplest analog phase detector (PD) is the analog multiplier followed by a low-pass filter, as shown in Figure 12.5. The input sinusoid with the phase to be measured is

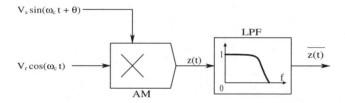

FIGURE 12.5
Block diagram of an analog multiplier phase detector.

$$v_s(t) = V_s \sin(\omega_c t + \theta) \tag{12.8}$$

The reference sinusoid is the quadrature signal,

$$v_r(t) = V_r \cos(\omega_c t + \phi) \tag{12.9}$$

and the output of the analog multiplier is:

$$z(t) = v_r(t)v_s(t)/10 \tag{12.10}$$

By trigonometric identity:

$$z(t) = \left(V_r V_s/20\right)\left\{\sin\left(2\omega_c t + \theta + \phi\right) + \sin\left(\theta - \phi\right)\right\} \tag{12.11}$$

The LPF attenuates the $2\omega_c$ frequency term; its output simply estimates the average:

$$\overline{z(t)} = \left(V_r V_s/20\right)\sin\left(\theta - \phi\right) \tag{12.12}$$

Thus, for $\left|\theta_e\right| < 15°$,

$$\overline{z(t)} \cong \left(V_r V_s/20\right)\left(\theta_c\right) \tag{12.13}$$

where $\theta_e \equiv (\theta - \phi)$ is in radians.

A systems approximation for the analog multiplier PD is shown in Figure 12.6. Note that for small phase error, the PD is linear, but exhibits periodic nonlinear behavior. Because the two coherent signals must be 90° out of phase for the AM PD to work, it is called a *quadrature PD*.

As in the case of the switched op amp PSR, it is possible to have a switched op amp or transistor PD in which the input analog signal, $v_s(t)$, given by Equation 12.8 is effectively multiplied by a ±1 reference quadrature square wave given by sgn$\{V_r \cos(\omega_c t)\}$. To demonstrate that the switched PD gives the same result as the analog multiplier PD, recall that a unity square wave

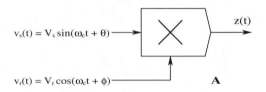

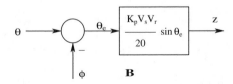

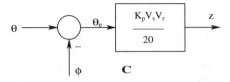

FIGURE 12.6
(A) Analog multiplier quadrature phase detector without LPF. (B) Sin(θ – ϕ) approximation to analog multiplier quadrature phase detector. (C) When $|\theta-\phi| < 15°$, then z ∝ (θ – ϕ).

can be expressed by its Fourier series. The Fourier series for a periodic time function, $f(t)$, can be written as the infinite harmonic sum (Northrop, 2003):

$$f(t) = a_0 + \sum_{n=1}^{\infty} a_n \cos(n\omega_o t) + b_n \sin(n\omega_o t) \qquad (12.14)$$

where the fundamental (or carrier) frequency is defined as:

$$\omega_o \equiv 2\pi/T \text{ r/s} \qquad (12.15A)$$

$$a_0 = \text{the average value of } f(t) \qquad (12.15B)$$

$$T = \text{period of } f(t) \qquad (12.15C)$$

The coefficients of the Fourier series are given by:

$$a_n \equiv \frac{2}{T} \int_{-T/2}^{T/2} f(t)\cos(n\omega_o t)dt \qquad (12.16)$$

$$b_n \equiv \frac{2}{T} \int\limits_{-T/2}^{T/2} f(t)\sin(n\omega_o t)dt \qquad (12.17)$$

To show that the product, $z(t) = V_s \sin(\omega_o t + \theta_e)$ **sgn**$\{V_r \cos(\omega_o t)\}$, when averaged, gives phase detection, use the fundamental frequency ($n = 1$) term in the F-series for the cosine square wave, **sgn**$\{V_r \cos(\omega_o t)\}$. The higher-order harmonics in the F-series lead to output frequencies that are multiples of ω_o and therefore filtered out. Note also for **sgn**$\{V_r \cos(\omega_o t)\}$ that $a_0 = 0$ and $b_n = 0$ because $f(t)$ is an even function. Thus, $f(t)$ is approximated by:

$$f_1(t) \cong (4/\pi)\cos(\omega_o t) \qquad (12.18)$$

Thus,

$$z(t) = (4V_s/\pi)\sin(\omega_o t + \theta_e)\cos(\omega_o t) = (2V_s/\pi)\left[\sin(2\omega_o t + \theta_e) + \sin(\theta_e)\right] \quad (12.19)$$

After low-pass filtering, the desired output is:

$$\overline{z(t)} = (2V_s/\pi)\sin(\theta_e) \cong (2V_s/\pi)(\theta_e), \; (\theta_e) \text{ in radians.} \qquad (12.20)$$

The latter term in Equation 12.20 is valid for the phase difference between input and output waves, $|\theta_e| < 15°$. Note that this PD has the same $\sin(\theta)$ nonlinearity as the pure analog multiplier PD. This type of phase detector is used in many IC phase-lock loop designs.

12.3.3 Digital Phase Detectors

Analog phase detectors based on ideal multiplication require a quadrature reference signal and a low-pass filter, and produce a nonlinear output given by $\sin(\theta_e)$. Digital phase detectors, on the other hand, accept two logic signal inputs and generally give a low-pass filtered output that is linear over some range of θ_e but periodic in θ_e.

The first digital phase detector to be examined is the exclusive NOR PD, illustrated with waveforms in Figure 12.7. This PD accepts two TTL square waves with 50% duty cycles, which have the same frequency but differ in phase by an amount, θ_e. The op amp has two functions: (1) it subtracts approximately 1.7 V from the Q waveform, so when Q has a 50% duty cycle, the average output, $\overline{V_z(t)} = 0$; (2) it low-pass filters the offset Q signal and outputs its average value. Note that $\overline{V_z(t)} = 0$ when $\theta_e = \pm k\pi/2$, k odd. Like the analog multiplier PD, the ENOR PD is also a quadrature PD. Note that the average output is linear with θ_e over a range of 0 to π radians, but is also periodic in θ_e with period 2π. The frequency of the Q output is $2/T$ pps.

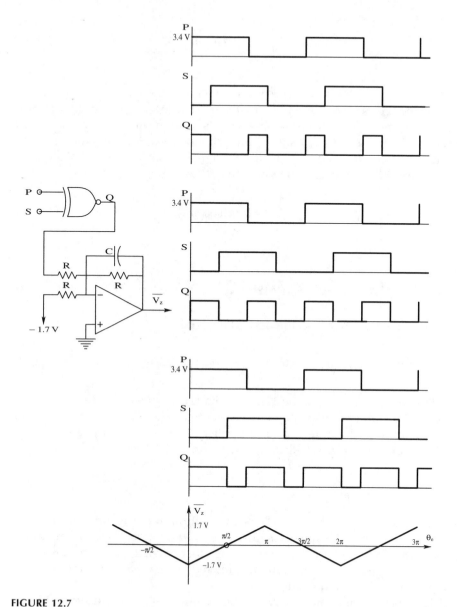

FIGURE 12.7

An exclusive NOR digital phase detector and examples of its waveforms. The bottom graph shows a plot of the (offset) average output voltage of this PD vs. the phase difference between TTL inputs P and S. Note the zeros are at odd integer multiples of $(\pi/2)$.

Another linear digital PD can be realized with a simple RS flip-flop (RSFF), as shown in Figure 12.8. Note that the RSFF PD uses the same DC offset and LPF op amp circuit as the ENOR PD. Inputs to the RSFF PD are required to be narrow complementary pulses, such as those that can be generated by the rising edges of the two TTL square waves triggering one-shot multivibrators'

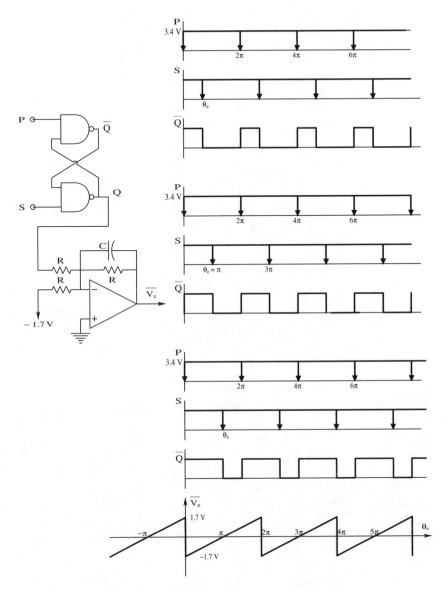

FIGURE 12.8
The RS flip-flop PD and its waveforms. The bottom graph shows a plot of the (offset) average output voltage of this PD vs. the phase difference between TTL inputs P and S. Note the significant zeros are at odd integer multiples of π.

(one-shots) complementary outputs. Note that the $\overline{V_z(t)v_s}$ θ_e characteristic is also periodic with period 2π, but the linear range extends the full $0 \leq \theta_e \leq 2\pi$ range. This PD's characteristic has no negative slope portion. The $\overline{V_z}$ (θ_e) curve has its zero at $\theta_e = \pi$, so it is not a quadrature system. The reference square wave needs only logical inversion before triggering the one-shot.

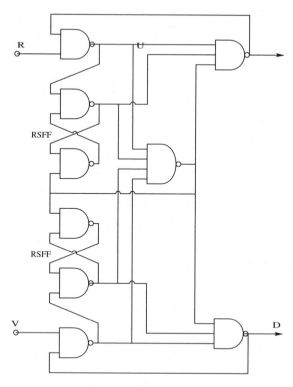

FIGURE 12.9
A combinational/sequential logic PD based on the Motorola MC4044 digital PD IC.

More complex linear digital phase detectors have been devised. One venerable design based on the Motorola MC4044 IC is shown in Figure 12.9. This PD's architecture is made up from various NAND gates. Note the two RS flip-flops in the center of the left-hand column. Figure 12.10 illustrates the input and output waveforms at nodes R, V, U, and D, respectively. The digital waveforms for V lagging R (top set) and for V leading R (middle set) are shown. Subtracting U from D by a simple op amp DA and low-pass filtering the difference to recover the average output, $\bar{V}_z$, yields a linear output voltage, v_s θ_e, over a full $\pm 2\pi$ interval, as shown in Figure 12.11.

Another logic chip-based digital PD is shown in Figure 12.12. This circuit uses a 7495 (or Fairchild 9300) four-bit, bidirectional shift register (Northrop, 1990). As a PD in a PLL, it can detect lock ($\omega_p = \omega_r$) by $Q_0 = $ LO, $Q_2 = $ HI, and Q_1 has the TTL phase signal similar to the RSFF output. If $\omega_p > \omega_r$, then $Q_0 = $ LO, $Q_1 = $ LO, and Q_2 has a duty cycle proportional to ($\omega_p - \omega_r$). If $\omega_p < \omega_r$, then $Q_1 = $ HI, $Q_2 = $ HI, and Q_0 has a duty cycle proportional to ($\omega_r - \omega_p$). Note that this phase-frequency detector's phase difference output on Q_1 is not periodic in θ_e, like other digital PDs; it saturates LO for $\omega_p > \omega_r$ and saturates HI when $\omega_p < \omega_r$. Q_1 has a 50% duty cycle when $\omega_p = \omega_r$ radians, giving $\bar{V}_z$ (θ_e) = 0. Note that the P and R inputs must be narrow complementary pulses derived from the $\bar{Q}$ outputs of one-shots.

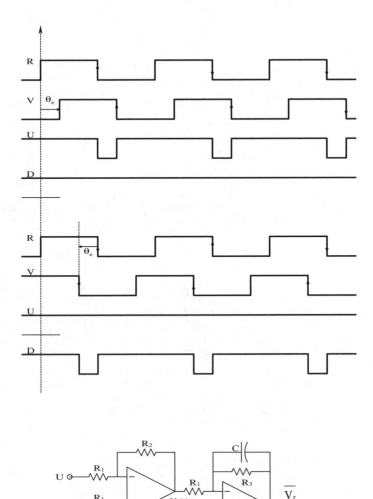

FIGURE 12.10
Top: example of the 4044 PD's waveforms for *V* lagging *R*. Middle: example of the 4044 PD's waveforms for *V* leading *R*. Bottom: op amp DA and low-pass filter used to condition the 4044 PD's outputs, *U* and *D*.

Because of their linearity, digital PhDs are useful in instrumentation schemes in which phase must be measured. Note that it is possible to run two noise-free sinusoidal signals through comparators with hysteresis to generate two digital signals that can be measured with a simple digital PD.

A microcomputer-based, frequency-independent digital phase meter with one-millidegree resolution was designed and tested by Du (1993) in the

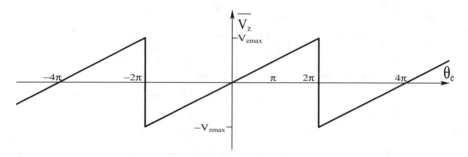

FIGURE 12.11
Average output voltage vs. input phase difference for the 4044 PD with the op amp signal conditioner. Note each linear segment spans a full $\pm 2\pi$ radians, and has zero output for zero phase difference between R and V.

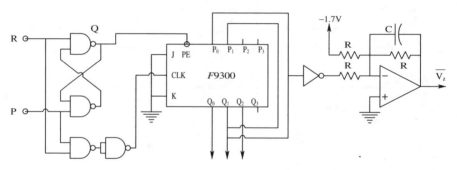

FIGURE 12.12
A shift register-based digital phase-frequency detector.

author's laboratory. The reference digital input channel was also the input to a Signetics NE564 phase-lock loop that used a divide-by 360,000 counter between its VCO and its phase detector. Thus, the VCO TTL output was phase locked to the input R signal and its output frequency was 360,000 times the input frequency, f_o.

The high level of the $\overline{Q}_R$ comparator output is NANDed with the Q_S output of the signal comparator. Any phase shift between V_R and V_S produces a narrow complementary gating pulse at the output of the NAND gate that allows the PLL output at 360,000 f_o to be counted. The count occurs once per cycle for a preset number of cycles. The total count is stored in the shift registers (74F299) and then downloaded into the PC for averaging. Each count is the phase lag between V_R and V_S in millidegrees and is independent of the frequency of the inputs.

Du's phase meter worked with input frequencies, f_o, of up to 100 Hz and gave a numerical output of θ_e and its statistics. Figure 12.13 and Figure 12.14 illustrate the architecture of the millidegree phase meter and the PLL used

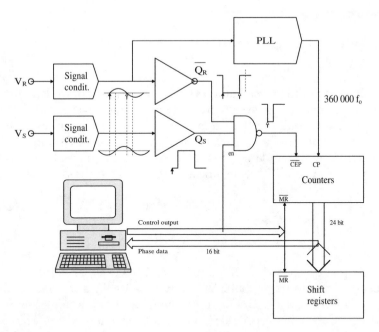

FIGURE 12.13
Architecture of the millidegree phase detector devised by Du (1993). The system is based on a phase-lock loop with a clock that runs 360,000 times faster than the input frequency.

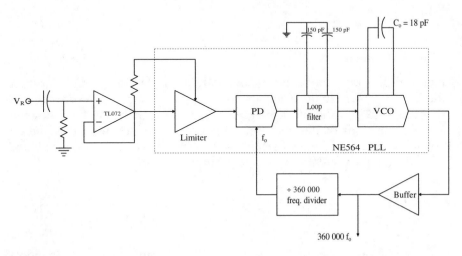

FIGURE 12.14
Detailed block diagram of Du's PLL.

as a ×360,000 frequency multiplier. Du's system was used in dielectric materials measurements where it was desired to measure minute phase shifts caused by dielectric losses at power line frequencies.

12.4 Voltage and Current-Controlled Oscillators

12.4.1 Introduction

The voltage-controlled oscillator (VCO) (or current controlled oscillator, CCO) is an important subsystem in many electronic devices and systems. It is an important component system in the phase-lock loop, as well as in certain communication and instrumentation systems. VCOs and CCOs can have sinusoidal, triangular, or TTL outputs of constant amplitude. The frequency of a VCO or CCO in its linear range can be expressed by:

$$f_o = K_V V_C + b \text{ Hz} \tag{12.21A}$$

$$f_o = K_C I_C + b \tag{12.21B}$$

The frequency constants, K_V and K_C, can have either sign, as can the intercept, b. It is desirable that a VCO have a wide linear operating range = $[(f_{omax} - f_{omin})/(f_{omax} + f_{omin})]$; low noise (phase and amplitude); low tempco $(\Delta f_o \Delta T)(1/f_o)$; and a high spectral purity (low THD) if it produces a sinusoidal output. (Many VCOs produce TTL outputs, or triangle wave outputs.)

There are many architectures for VCOs. The first examined is a "linear amplifier" oscillator in which f_o is tuned by two variable-gain elements that can be analog multipliers or multiplying digital-to-analog converters (MDACs).

12.4.2 An Analog VCO

Figure 12.15 shows the schematic of an electronically tuned VCO based on the use of linear circuit elements connected in a positive feedback loop (Northrop, 1990). The block diagram below the schematic illustrates the transfer functions of the two minor loops whose poles are set by the dc voltage V_C input to the two analog multipliers. After the two minor loops are reduced, the oscillator's loop gain can be written as:

$$A_L(s) = \frac{+s k V_C/(10RC)}{s^2 + s 2V_C/(10RC) + V_C^2/(10RC)^2} \tag{12.22}$$

From Section 5.5 on oscillators in Chapter 5, it can be seen that the root-locus diagram for this oscillator is a circle centered on the origin. The locus branches for the closed-loop poles begin at $s = -V_C (10RC)$ r/s, cross the $j\omega$ axis in the s-plane at $s = \pm j\omega_o$ when $k = 2$, and hit the positive real axis at $s = +\omega_o$. Then, one branch approaches the zero at the origin while the other branch goes toward $+\infty$ as k increases.

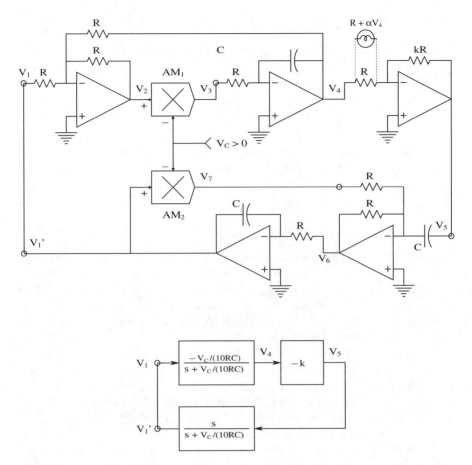

FIGURE 12.15
Schematic of a voltage-tuned oscillator using positive feedback. The tungsten filament lamp is used to limit and stabilize oscillation amplitude. A systems block diagram of the linear part of the oscillator is shown below the schematic. See text for analysis.

Using the venerable Barkhausen criterion (Millman, 1979) for oscillation on this oscillator:

$$A_L(j\omega_o) \equiv 1\angle 0° = \frac{j\omega_o k V_C/(10RC)}{-\omega_o^2 + V_C^2/(10RC)^2 + j\omega_o 2V_C/(10RC)} \qquad (12.23)$$

Clearly, the real terms in the denominator must sum to zero. This condition gives the radian oscillation frequency,

$$\omega_o = V_C/(10RC) \quad r/s, \qquad (12.24)$$

and the minimum gain for oscillation, $k = 2$. Thus, V_C can set ω_o over a wide range, e.g., $0.01 \le V_C \le 10$ V, or a 1:1000 range. For practical reasons, make $k > 2$ and use a PTC tungsten lamp instead of the input R to the third op amp. Now the overall gain of this stage is:

$$\frac{V_5}{V_4} = -\frac{kR}{R + \alpha V_4} = -2 \qquad (12.25)$$

If $k = 4$ is set, then the steady state, equilibrium value of V_4 is found to be R/α for any ω_o. Making $k = 4$ allows the oscillations to grow rapidly to the equilibrium level.

12.4.3 Switched Integrating Capacitor VCOs

Certain VCOs can simultaneously output TTL pulses, a triangle wave, and a sine wave of the same frequency. An example of this type of VCO is the Exar XR8038 waveform generator, which works over a range of millihertz to approximately 1 MHz with proper choice of timing capacitor, C_T. A newer version of the XR8038 is the Maxim MAX038 VFC, which can generate various waveforms from 1 mHz to 20 MHz.

Figure 12.16 illustrates the organization of a generic switched integrating capacitor VCO. Assume that $V_{in} > 0$. At $t = 0$, the MOS switch is in position u and the capacitor is charged by current $G_m V_{in}$, so V_T goes from 0 to $V_T = \phi_+$ when the output of the upper comparator goes HI, which makes the RS flip-flop Q output go HI, causing the MOS switch to go to position d. In position d, the capacitor C_T is discharged by a net current, $-G_m V_{in}$, causing V_T to ramp down to $\phi_- < 0$. When V_T reaches ϕ_-, the output of the lower comparator goes high, causing the RSFF Q output to go LO, which switches the MOS switch to u again, causing the capacitor to charge positively again from current $G_m V_{in}$, etc.

V_{in} is the controlling input to the two VCCSs. Note that the capacitor C_T integrates the current:

$$V_T = \left(1/C_T\right) \int i_C \, dt \qquad (12.26)$$

Thus, from the V_T triangle waveform, it is easy to find the frequency of oscillation:

$$f = 1/T = \frac{G_m V_{in}}{4 C_T \phi} \text{ Hz} \qquad (12.27)$$

In Equation 12.27, $\phi = \phi_+ = -\phi_- > 0$ was assumed.

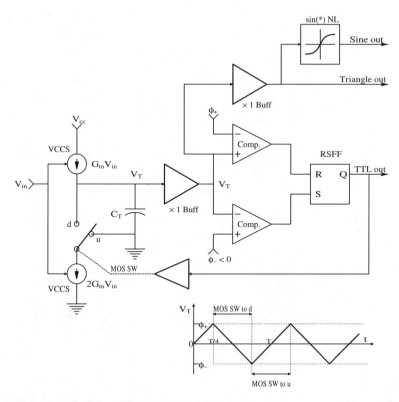

FIGURE 12.16
Block diagram of a switched integrating capacitor VCO.

Note that this VCO produces simultaneous sine, triangle, and TTL outputs. The sinusoidal output is derived from the buffered capacitor waveform, V_T, by passing it through a diode wave-shaper, sin(*) NL. This type of VCO is often used as the basis for laboratory function generators.

12.4.4 The Voltage-Controlled, Emitter-Coupled Multivibrator

Figure 12.17 illustrates the simplified schematic of another popular VCO architecture. This astable, emitter-coupled multivibrator (AMV) derives its frequency control from the transistors Q_5 and Q_6, which act as VCCSs and control the rate that C_T charges and discharges and, thus, the AMV's frequency. This architecture is inherently very fast; versions of it using MOSFETs have been used to build a VCO with an 800-MHz tuning range that operates in excess of 2.5 GHz (Herzel et al., 2001).

The heart of this VCO is the free-running, astable multivibrator (AMV), which alternately switches Q_1 and Q_2 on and off as the timing capacitor charges and discharges. Detailed analysis of this circuit can be found in

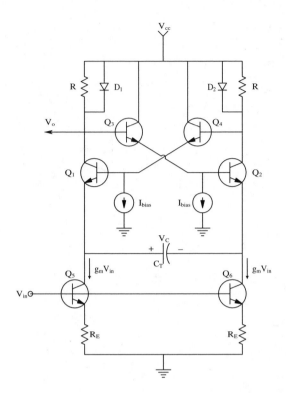

FIGURE 12.17
Simplified schematic of a *v*oltage-controlled, *e*mitter-coupled, (astable) *m*ultivibrator (VCECM).

Franco (1988) and in Gray and Meyer (1984). Analysis is helped by considering the circuit of Figure 12.18 and the waveforms of Figure 12.19. According
to analysis by Gray and Meyer:

> We calculate the period [frequency] by first assuming that Q_1 is turned
> off and Q_2 turned on. The circuit then appears as shown in [Figure
> 12.18]. We assume that current I [I_{c2}] is large so that the voltage drop IR
> is large enough to turn on diode [D_2]. Thus the base of Q_4 is one diode
> drop below V_{CC}, the emitter is two diode drops below V_{CC}, and the base
> of Q_1 is two diode drops below V_{CC}. If we can neglect the base current
> of Q_3, its base is at VCC and its emitter is one diode drop below V_{CC}.
> Thus the emitter of Q_2 is two diode drops below V_{CC}. Since Q_1 is off, the
> current I_1 [$g_m V_{in}$] is charging the capacitor so that the emitter of Q_1 is
> becoming more negative. Q_1 will turn on when the voltage at its emitter
> becomes equal to three diode drops below V_{CC}. Transistor Q_1 will then
> turn on, and the resulting collector current in Q_1 turns on [D_1]. As a result,
> the base of Q_3 moves in the negative direction by one diode drop, causing
> the base of Q_2 to move in the negative direction by one diode drop. Q_2
> will turn off, causing the base of Q_1 to move positive by one diode drop
> because [D_2] also turns off. As a result, the emitter-base junction of Q_2 is
> reverse-biased by one diode drop because the voltage on C_T cannot

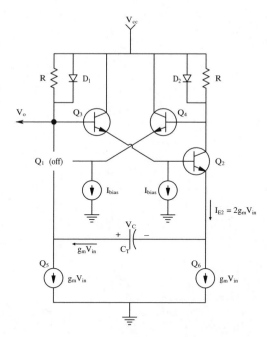

FIGURE 12.18
The VCECM charging C_T with Q_1 OFF.

change instantaneously. Current $[g_m V_{in}]$ must now charge the capacitor voltage in the negative direction by an amount equal to two diode drops before the circuit will switch back again. Since the circuit is symmetrical, the half period is given by the time required to charge the capacitor and is:

$$T/2 = Q/(g_m V_{in}) = \frac{C_T 2V_{BE(on)}}{g_m V_{in}} \tag{12.28}$$

where $Q = C_T \Delta V = C_T 2V_{BE(on)}$ is the charge on the capacitor. The frequency of the oscillator [VCECM] is thus:

$$f = \frac{1}{T} = \frac{g_m V_{in}}{C_T 4V_{BE(on)}} \tag{12.29}$$

Note the similarity between Equation 12.29 and Equation 12.27 and that the AMV is a regenerative positive feedback circuit when it is switching. The complementary state changes of Q_1 and Q_2 are made more rapid by the positive feedback.

Figure 12.20 illustrates the use of two nose-to-nose varactor diodes (also called epicap diodes by Motorola) to tune an MC1648 emitter-coupled multivibrator VCO. A varactor diode (VD) is a reverse-biased Si *pn* junction diode, characterized by a voltage-variable depletion capacitance modeled by:

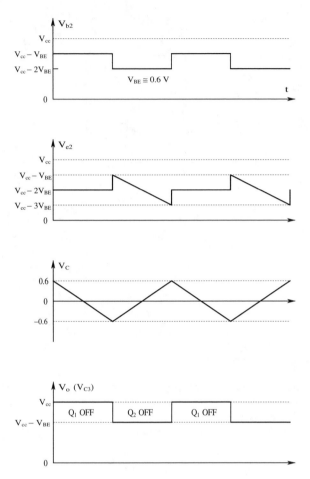

FIGURE 12.19
Relevant waveforms in the VCECM for two cycles of oscillation.

$$C_v = \frac{C_{vo}}{\left(1 - V_D/\psi_o\right)^\gamma}, \quad V_D < 0. \tag{12.30}$$

where C_{vo} is the diode's junction capacitance at $V_D = 0$, ψ_o is the "built-in barrier potential," typically on the order of 0.75 V for a Si diode at room temperature, and γ is the capacitance exponent. γ can vary from approximately 1/3 to 2, depending on the doping gradients at the junction boundary and can be shown to be $\cong 0.5$ for an abrupt (step) junction (Gray and Meyer, 1984).

The output of the MC1648 oscillator is an emitter-coupled logic (ECL) square wave; frequencies as high as 225 MHz can be obtained with this IC,

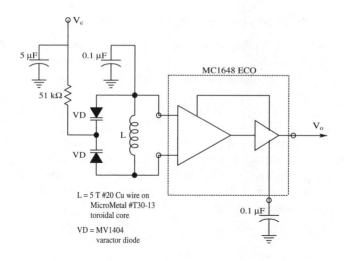

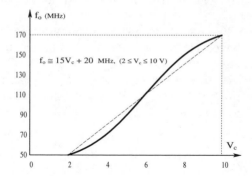

FIGURE 12.20
Top: A VCO that uses the voltage-variable capacitance of two varactor diodes to set its output frequency. Bottom: The frequency vs. dc control voltage characteristic of the varactor VCO.

which can serve as the VCO in a PLL. In the circuit shown, the tuning range lies between $V_D = -2$ to -10 V (or $2 \leq V_c \leq 10$ V). The actual $f_o(V_c)$ curve is sigmoid, but can be approximated by the linear VCO relation,

$$f_o \cong 15V_c + 20 \text{ MHz}, \tag{12.31}$$

over the range of V_c shown. Note that two VDs are used in series to halve their capacitance, seen in the resonant "tank" circuit. A Motorola MV1404 VD's capacitance goes from 160 pF at $V_D = -1$ to approximately 11 pF at $V_D = -10$ V.

12.4.5   The Voltage-to-Period Converter and Applications

The voltage-to-period converter (VPC) is a variable frequency oscillator in which the period of the oscillation, T, is directly proportional to the controlling voltage, V_c. Mathematically, this is simply stated as:

$$T = K_P V_c + b \text{ seconds} \tag{12.32}$$

Here b is a positive constant and K_P is the VPC constant in seconds per volt. Practical considerations dictate lower and upper bounds to T. Obviously, the VPC's output frequency is $1/T$ Hz. The conventional voltage-to-frequency converter (VFC) has its output frequency directly proportional to its input voltage (or current),

$$f_o = K_V V_c + d \tag{12.33}$$

K_V is the VCO constant in Hertz per volt and d is a constant (Hertz).

In several important instrumentation applications, use of a VPC (rather than a VFC) linearizes the measurement system output; several examples are described next.

Realization of VPCs. As has been shown, many IC manufacturers make VFC VCOs. Some have TTL outputs; others generate sine, triangle, and TTL outputs. No one, to this author's knowledge, markets a VPC IC. One obvious way to make a VPC is to take a VFC in which $f_o = K_V V_c + d$ and use a nonlinear analog circuit to process the input, V_1, so that the net result is a VPC. Mathematically,

$$T = K_P V_1 + b = \frac{1}{K_V V_2 + d} \tag{12.34}$$

To find the required nonlinearity, solve Equation 12.34 for $V_2 = f(V_1)$. This gives:

$$V_2 = \frac{1 - bd - d K_P V_1}{K_V \left(K_P V_1 + b\right)} \tag{12.35}$$

Considerable simplification accrues if a VFC with d = 0 is used. Now the nonlinearity needs to be:

$$V_2 = \frac{1}{K_V \left(K_P V_1 + b\right)} \tag{12.36}$$

Figure 12.21 illustrates an op amp circuit that will generate the requisite V_2 for the VFC to produce a VPC. Note that V_3 must be >0 and V_R = +0.1 V.

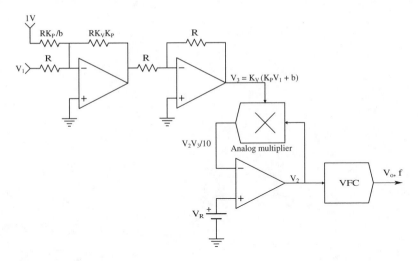

FIGURE 12.21
Schematic of a nonlinear op amp circuit used to make a voltage-to-period converter from a conventional voltage-to-frequency converter.

Another approach to building a VPC used in the author's laboratory is shown in Figure 12.22. Here the differential output of a NOR gate RS flip-flop is integrated by a high slew rate op amp. Assume output C of the FF is high. The op amp output voltage ramps up at a slope fixed by the voltage difference at the FF outputs (e.g., 4 V) times $1/RC$ of the integrator. When V_o reaches the variable threshold, V_C, the upper AD 790 comparator goes low, triggering the upper one-shot to reset the FF output C to low. Now V_o ramps down until it reaches the fixed -10-V threshold of the lower comparator. The lower comparator goes high, triggering the lower one-shot to set FF output C high again, etc. The two-input NOR gate gives a VPC output pulse at every FF state transition. The AD 840 op amp has a slew rate of 400 V/µs, or 4.E 8 V/s. It is connected as a differential integrator.

In this VPC design, V_C varies over $-9 \le V_c \le + 10$ V. Choose $R = 1$ k, $C = 850$ pF, and let the FF's $\Delta V = 4$ V. These data show that V_o ramps up or down with a slope of $m = \Delta V/RC = 4.71E6$ V/s. Now when $V_c = 0$, $T = b = 2.125E{-}6$ sec and $K_p = 2.125E{-}7$. It is easy to see that the $maxT = 20$ V 4.71E6 = 4.250E{-}6 sec and $f_{min} = 2.353E5$ Hz. Likewise, the $minT = 1$ V/4.71E6 = 2.125E{-}7 sec and $f_{max} = 4.71$ MHz.

Applications. A VFC or a VPC can be used as the signal source in a closed-loop, constant-phase velocimeter and ranging system (Northrop, 2002). However, as will be shown later and in Section 12.8.3, the use of a VPC produces a linear range output and a velocity signal independent of range, while the use of a VFC produces a nonlinear range output and a range-dependent velocity signal.

The basic architecture of a type 1 closed-loop, constant-phase laser velocimeter and ranging system is shown in Figure 12.23. This system uses narrow,

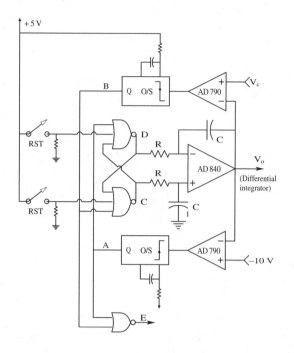

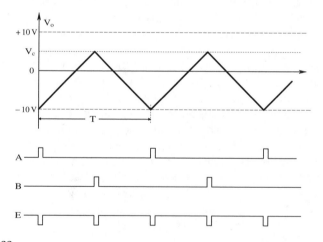

FIGURE 12.22
Top: Schematic of a hybrid VPC with digital output. Bottom: Waveforms of the hybrid VPC.

periodic pulses of IR laser light reflected from a moving target. The system's feedback automatically adjusts the pulse repetition rate so that a preset phase lag is always maintained between the transmitted and received optical pulses. The system is unique in that it simultaneously outputs voltages proportional to target range and velocity. The emitted radiation of this type of system can also be CW or pulsed sound or ultrasound, or pulsed or

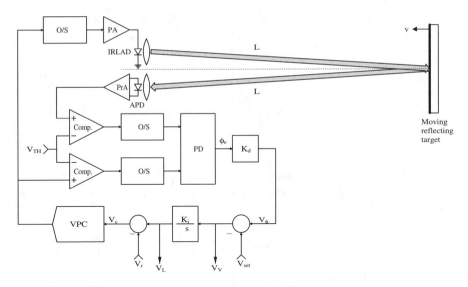

FIGURE 12.23
Block diagram of a closed-loop, constant-phase pulsed laser velocimeter and ranging system devised by the author.

amplitude-modulated microwaves, as well as photonic energy. Such systems have wide applications, ranging from medical diagnostics to weapons systems.

In the steady state, for a fixed target range, L_o, the period (or frequency) output of the VPC oscillator reaches a value so that a fixed phase lag, ϕ_m, exists between the received and transmitted signals. When $\phi_e = \phi_m$, the input to the integrator is zero and the integrator output voltage, V_L, can be shown to be:

$$V_L = K_R L_o \tag{12.37}$$

The range constant, K_R, is derived later.

If the reflecting object is moving at constant velocity, directly away from or toward the transducers, $v = \pm dL/dt = \pm \dot{L}$, then it is easy to show that the input voltage to the integrator, V_V, is given by:

$$V_V = K_S v \tag{12.38}$$

If a VPC is used, K_S is independent of L. In this example, to facilitate heuristic analysis, neglect the propagation delays inherent to logic elements and analog signal conditioning pathways. The type 1 feedback system shown in Figure 12.23 uses pulsed laser light to measure the distance L to a stationary reflective target. The nominal phase lag between received and transmitted pulses is simply:

$$\phi_e = 360 \, (2L/c)(1/T) \text{ degrees} \tag{12.39}$$

where c is the velocity of light in m/s, T is the VPC output period, and $(2L/c)$ is the round-trip time for a pulse reflected from the target. The phase detector module produces an output voltage with an average value of:

$$V_\phi = K_d\,\phi_e \tag{12.40}$$

K_d has the dimensions of volts per degree. A dc voltage, V_{set}, is subtracted from V_ϕ, so:

$$V_V = V_\phi - V_{set} \tag{12.41}$$

V_V is the input to the integrator whose output, V_L, is added to $-V_r$ to give the input to the VPC, V_C. Because the closed-loop system is type 1, in the steady state, $V_V \to 0$. Thus,

$$V_{set} = K_d\,\phi_m = K_d\big[360(2L/c)(1/T)\big] = K_d\big[360(2L/c)f\big] \tag{12.42}$$

Thus, the steady-state phase lag is simply:

$$\phi_e = \phi_m = V_{set}\,K_d \text{ degrees} \tag{12.43}$$

The VPC steady-state period is found from Equation 12.42 to be:

$$T_{ss} = K_p V_C + b = \frac{720L}{c\,\phi_{mss}} \text{ seconds} \tag{12.44}$$

From the preceding equation, the VPC input voltage is:

$$V_C = \frac{720L}{c\,\phi_{mss}\,K_P} - b/K_P \text{ volts} \tag{12.45}$$

If $V_r = b/K_P$, then V_L is directly proportional to L:

$$V_L = \frac{720}{c\,K_P\big(V_{set}/K_d\big)}L \text{ volts.} \tag{12.46}$$

Now consider the situation in which the reflecting target is approaching the transducers at constant velocity, $v \ll c$. Because $V_L = (K_i\,s)\,V_V$ and $v = \dot{L}$, it is possible to write in the time domain:

$$V_V = \dot{V}_o/K_i = v\,\frac{720\,K_d}{c\,K_P\,V_{set}\,K_i} \text{ volts} \tag{12.47}$$

Thus, a simple type 1 closed-loop, constant phase system can provide simultaneous voltage outputs that estimate target range and velocity in a linear manner.

Examine the system design with practical numbers: let $\phi_m \equiv 10°$; $K_i = 1$ and $K_p = 8.0E-6$ sec/V; and $720/c = 2.40E-6$. These numbers give a reasonable range sensitivity:

$$K_R = \frac{720}{c\, K_p\, \phi_{mss}} = 3.0E-2 \text{ V/m} \tag{12.48}$$

From Equation 12.47, the velocity sensitivity is also useful:

$$K_S = 2.40E-6 \frac{1}{K_p\, \phi_{mss}\, K_i} = 3.0E-2 \text{ V/m/s} \tag{12.49}$$

The VPC steady-state output frequency at a 1-m range is 4.17 MHz; when $L = 100$ m, it is 41.7 kHz.

12.4.6 Summary

There are a variety of architectures for voltage-controlled oscillators, including "linear" VCOs using variable gain elements, switched integrating capacitor VCOs, and emitter-coupled, astable multivibrators. Versions of the latter architecture have been made to oscillate in the gigahertz. Another VHF–UHF VCO architecture (not shown here) makes use of the varactor diode (VD). The VD is a reverse-biased *pn* junction diode in which the diode depletion capacitance is controlled by the reverse-bias voltage. This voltage-variable capacitance can be used to tune oscillators such as the familiar Hartley design and to generate NBFM by adding the modulating signal to the reverse diode bias voltage. VCOs are used in all phase-lock loops and in FM communications applications, as well as in many instrumentation systems.

The voltage-to-period converter (VPC) is a VCO in which the output oscillation's period is linearly proportional to the input voltage. The VPC is a useful circuit component in a closed-loop, constant-phase laser velocimeter and ranging system. The same closed-loop, constant-phase architecture can also be used with sound or ultrasound to measure object range and velocity simultaneously.

12.5 Phase-Locked Loops

12.5.1 Introduction

A phase-locked loop (PLL) (also called a phase-lock loop) is a closed-loop feedback system in which the phase of the PLL's periodic output is made to follow the phase of a periodic input signal. The closed-loop PLL system's

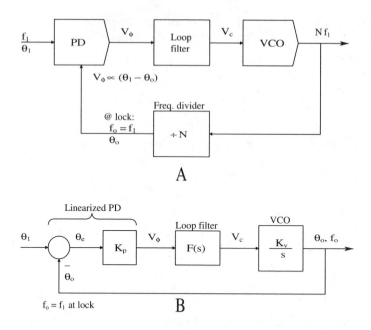

FIGURE 12.24
(A) Basic architecture of a phase-locked loop (PLL). (B) Systems block diagram of a PLL.

natural frequencies are, in general, several orders of magnitude lower than the frequency of the input signal. Phase-lock loops have many applications in communications, control systems, and instrumentation systems. They can be used to modulate and demodulate narrow-band FM (NBFM) signals; demodulate double-sideband/suppressed carrier (DSBSC) signals; demodulate AM signals; generate a frequency-independent phase shift; measure frequencies, including heart rate; synthesize signals used in digital communications systems; detect touch-tone frequencies and status signals used in telephony; control motor speed, etc.

The basic architecture of a PLL is shown in Figure 12.24(A). It includes a phase (difference) detector (PD), loop filter, VCO (VFC), and, sometimes, a frequency divider between the VCO and the PD. (Phase detectors were described in Section 12.3.) A phase detector returns an *average* voltage proportional to the phase difference between the input signal and the VCO output.

Analysis of PLL dynamics is done assuming lock, i.e., that the input and VCO frequencies are equal. When a PLL first acquires its input signal, $f_1 \neq f_o$ and the loop must attain lock through a nonlinear process known as acquisition. The time required for acquisition is important in such PLL applications as telephone touch-tone decoding and the demodulation of FSK signals. Empirical formulas for acquisition times can be found in Northrop (1990) and Gardner (1979).

12.5.2 PLL Components

As mentioned earlier, phase detectors such as those used in PLLs have already been considered in Section 12.3. Most IC PLLs use PDs in which the analog input signal is effectively multiplied by a ± 1 square wave derived from the VCO. This type of PD is a quadrature detector; the zero phase error condition requires that $\theta_1 - \theta_o = \pi/2$. Analog multiplier and exclusive OR PDs are also quadrature detectors. Only the RSFF PD and the MC 4044 PD are in-phase detectors.

All PDs produce an analog output whose average value, V_ϕ, is proportional to $\sin(\theta_e)$ or to θ_e. When $|\theta_e| < 15°$, $\sin(\theta_e)$ can be replaced with θ_e in radians. Thus, for small-signal errors at lock, the PLL can be modeled by the block diagram in Figure 12.24(B). The VCO is modeled in the frequency domain by K_v s because $\omega_o = V_c K_v$ r/s and its output phase is, in general, the integral of its output frequency, i.e., $\theta_o = \int \omega_o \, dt$. The PLL's dynamics in response to changes in θ_1 are determined in part by its closed-loop poles, which can be found from its linear loop gain using root-locus techniques. The PLL's loop gain is generally:

$$A_L(s) = \frac{K_p F(s) K_v}{s} \tag{12.50}$$

If $F(s) = K_f (s + a)/s$, then the loop gain function has a zero at $s = -a$, and two poles at the origin. Its root-locus is the well-known circle, shown in Figure 12.25. Effective design of this PLL wants the closed-loop poles at $s = -a \pm ja$. This gives a damping factor of $\xi = 0.707$ and an undamped natural frequency of $\omega_n = a\sqrt{2}$. The scalar gain product, $K_p K_f K_v$, is adjusted to obtain these closed-loop parameters. It can be shown that $K_p K_f K_v = 2a$ will put the closed-loop poles at $s = -a \pm ja$ (Northrop, 1990).

The PLL's loop filter is generally low-pass and can be of the form $F(s) = K_f (s/b + 1)$, $K_f (s + a)/s$, $K_f (s/a + 1)/(s/b + 1)$, etc. The loop filter is generally chosen to give the PLL the desired dynamic response in tracking changes in θ_1. The PLL's VCO can have a digital (TTL) or sinusoidal output. The VCO used on IC PLLs often uses the voltage-controlled, emitter-coupled astable multivibrator architecture (see above).

12.5.3 PLL Applications in Biomedicine

One application of a PLL is its use to measure heart rate. Figure 12.26 illustrates the block diagram of a 4046 CMOS PLL used as a cardiotachometer (Northrop, 1990). The loop filter's transfer function is found from the voltage-divider relation:

$$\frac{V_c}{V_\phi} = \frac{R_2 + 1/sC}{R_1 + R_2 + 1/sC} = \frac{sCR_2 + 1}{sC(R_1 + R_2) + 1} \tag{12.51}$$

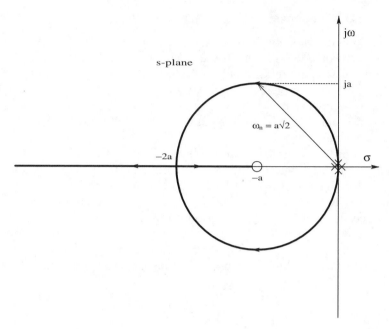

FIGURE 12.25
Root-locus diagram of a PLL having a loop filter of the form, $F(s) = K_f(s + a)/s$.

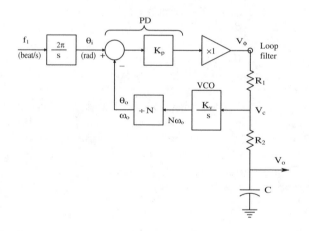

FIGURE 12.26
Block diagram of a PLL used as a heart rate monitor. V_o is proportional to the average heart rate.

Similarly, the output transfer function is:

$$\frac{V_o}{V_\phi} = \frac{1/sC}{R_1 + R_2 + 1/sC} = \frac{1}{sC(R_1 + R_2) + 1} \tag{12.52}$$

and the PLL's loop gain is:

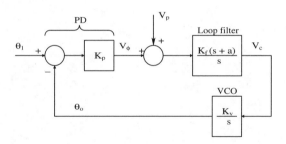

FIGURE 12.27
Block diagram of a PLL used to generate a frequency-independent phase shift. $(\theta_i - \theta_o) \propto V_p$.

$$A_L(s) = -\frac{K_p K_v (sCR_2 + 1)}{Ns[sC(R_1 + R_2) + 1]} = -\frac{K_p K_v CR_2 (s + 1/CR_2)}{NC(R_1 + R_2)s[s + 1/C(R_1 + R_2)]} \quad (12.53)$$

The PLL's transfer function is thus:

$$\frac{V_o}{f_1} = \frac{(2\pi/s)K_p}{[1 - A_L(s)][s + 1/C(R_1 + R_2)]C(R_1 + R_2)}$$

$$= \frac{2\pi N/K_v}{s^2 NC(R_1 + R_2)/K_p K_v + s[N + K_p K_v CR_2]/K_p K_v + 1} \quad (12.54)$$

The denominator of the preceding equation is of the standard quadratic form: $s^2 \omega_n^2 + s\, 2\xi\, \omega_n + 1$. Thus:

$$\omega_n = \sqrt{\frac{K_p K_v}{NC(R_1 + R_2)}} \ \text{r/s} \quad \text{and} \quad \xi = \frac{N + K_p K_v R_2 C}{2\sqrt{NC(R_1 + R_2)K_p K_v}} \quad (12.55)$$

Examine system ω_n, ξ, and dc gain given the typical circuit parameters: $K_p = 8.33$; $K_v = 3.14$; $N = 4$; $C = 1.E-5$; $R_1 = 62k$; and $R_2 = 150k$. These values yield: $\omega_n = 1.76$ r/s; $\xi = 1.45$ (overdamped); and dc gain $V_o/f_1 = 8.00$ volts/beat/sec = 0.133 V/beat/min. Note that ω_n and the damping ξ are measures of the PLL's response dynamics to *changes* in the heart rate, f_1 beats/sec.

In the second example of PLL applications, Figure 12.27 illustrates the block diagram of a PLL used to generate a frequency-independent phase shift between the input signal and the VCO output. This application is important in maximizing the output of a phase-sensitive rectifier or lock-in amplifier. The PLL's loop gain is:

$$A_L(s) = -\frac{K_p K_f K_v (s + a)}{s^2} \quad (12.56)$$

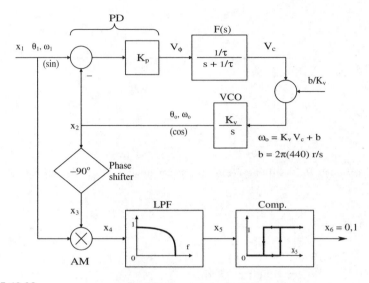

FIGURE 12.28
Block diagram of a (tuned or frequency-selective) audio tone decoder PLL.

Taking the reference phase input, $\theta_1 = 0$, the transfer function between θ_o and V_p can be written:

$$\frac{\theta_o}{V_p} = \frac{K_f K_v (s+a)}{s^2 + s K_p K_f K_v + a K_p K_f K_v} \tag{12.57}$$

The undamped natural frequency of this PLL is $\omega_n = \sqrt{a K_p K_f K_v}$ r/s; its damping factor is $\xi = \sqrt{K_p K_f K_v}\,(2\sqrt{a})$. These parameters relate to the system's response to changes in the phase-shifting voltage, V_p, and have nothing to do with the input carrier frequency, ω_1. The steady-state phase shift at lock is simply $\theta_{oss} = V_p/K_p$.

A third example of PLL applications examines a tone decoder, that is, a PLL system that outputs a logic HI when a sinusoidal signal is present at its input that has a frequency, f_1, within some $\pm \Delta f_c$. Note that $f_1/\Delta f_c$ defines a capture "Q" for the tone decoder. Figure 12.28 illustrates the block diagram of a tone decoder PLL. Note that this system uses two phase detectors of the quadrature (multiplicative) type. In the absence of a sinusoidal input signal, x_1, $V_c \to 0$ and the VCO output frequency is by design $\omega_o = b = 2\pi(440)$ r/s. Also, $x_6 = $ LO. The PLL acquires lock if the input sinusoid, $x_1 = A\sin(\omega_1 t)$, lies within the capture range of $\pm\Delta\omega_c$ around ω_1. Once the loop acquires lock, $x_2 = B\cos(\omega_1 t)$, $x_3 = B\sin(\omega_1 t)$, and $x_4 = x_3 x_1 = (AB/2)[\cos(0) - \cos(2\omega_1 t)]$. After the LPF, $x_5 = AB/2$ and $x_6 = 1$ (HI). It can be shown (Grebene, 1971) that lock occurs when the input frequency ω_1 lies in the capture range, given by:

$$\Delta\omega_c = 2\pi\Delta f_c \equiv K_T \left| F(j\Delta\omega_c) \right|, \tag{12.58}$$

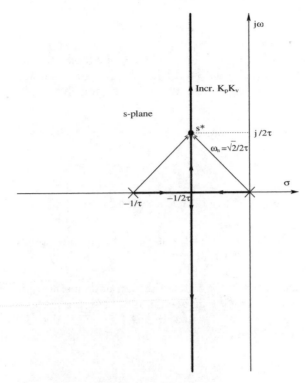

FIGURE 12.29
Root locus diagram for the PLL tone decoder.

where $|F(j\Delta\omega_c)|$ is the loop filter's gain magnitude at $\omega = \Delta\omega_c$ r/s, $F(s) = (1/\tau)/(s + 1/\tau)$, and $K_T \equiv K_p K_v F(0)$. The lock range of input frequency over which the PLL will maintain lock is given by $\Delta\omega_L = K_T > \Delta\omega_c$. Thus, the tone decoder PLL behaves like a nonlinear tuned filter.

In order to design the system to respond to A_{440} to within $\pm 1\%$, the PLL must acquire $f_1 = 440 \pm 4.4$ Hz. Thus, $\Delta f_c = 8.8$ Hz. It is also necessary that the loop damping factor be $\xi = 0.707$. The PLL's loop gain is simply:

$$A_L(s) = -\frac{K_p K_v / \tau}{s(s + 1/\tau)}$$

(12.59)

From $A_L(s)$, using the root-locus technique, one can find the value of the gain product $K_p K_v$ to put the PLL's closed loop poles at $s^* = -1/2\tau \pm j\, 2\tau$. (See Figure 12.29.) The RL magnitude criterion indicates:

$$K_p K_v / \tau = \left[\sqrt{2}/(2\tau)\right]^2$$

$\downarrow$

$$K_p K_v = 1/(2\tau) \qquad (12.60)$$

Also, from the RL geometry, $\omega_n = \sqrt{2}\,(2\tau)$. The loop filter time constant is found by substituting Equation 12.60 for $K_p\,K_v$ into Equation 12.58 and solving the resultant quadratic equation for τ^2, and thus τ.

$$\Delta\omega_c = K_p K_v \frac{1/\tau}{\sqrt{\Delta\omega_c^2 + 1/\tau^2}} \qquad (12.61)$$

$$\downarrow$$

$$\tau^4 + \tau^2/\Delta\omega_c^2 - 1/\left(4\Delta\omega_c^4\right) = 0 \qquad (12.62)$$

When $\Delta\omega_c = 2\pi(8.8) = 55.292$ r/s is substituted into Equation 12.62, $\tau = 8.231 \times 10^{-3}$ sec, $\omega_n = 85.91$ r/s, and $K_p\,K_v = K_T = 60.75$ r/s.

The NE/SE567 tone decoder PLL IC (Philips Semiconductors' linear products) data sheets contain a wealth of design and operating information in graphical form, including the greatest number of input cycles in a tone burst before the PLL acquires the input and goes high. Tone decoders are used in emergency response radios (for EMTs, firemen) to gate transmission of alert messages.

12.5.4 Discussion

PLLs are versatile systems with wide applications in communications, control, and instrumentation; this section has only scratched the surface of this topic. The interested reader is encouraged to examine the many texts dealing with the design and applications of this ubiquitous IC. See, for example, Northrop (1990, Chapter 11); Gray and Meyer (1984, Chapter 10); Blanchard (1976); Exar Integrated Systems (1979); and Grebene (1971).

12.6 True RMS Converters

12.6.1 Introduction

The analog true RMS converter is a system that provides a dc output proportional to the root-mean-square of the input signal, $v(t)$. An analog RMS operation first squares $v_1(t)$ then estimates the mean value of $v_2(t)$, generally by time averaging by low-pass filtering. Finally, the square root of the mean squared value, $\overline{v^2(t)}$, is taken.

The RMS value of a sine wave is easily seen to be its peak value divided by the $\sqrt{2}$. When one says that the U.S. residential line voltage is 120V, this means RMS volts. The average power dissipated in a resistor, R, that has a sinusoidal voltage across it is $P_{av} = (V_{RMS})^2 R$ watts. Random signals and noise can also be described by their mean-squared values or RMS values. In fact, noise voltages are characterized by measuring them with a true RMS voltmeter; it is meaningless to measure random noise with a rectifier-type ac meter.

12.6.2 True RMS Circuits

Figure 12.30 illustrates the block diagram of an explicit RMS system using analog multipliers and op amp ICs. The low-pass filter (LPF) is a quadratic Sallen and Key design. Its transfer function is:

$$H(s) = \frac{1}{s^2/\omega_n^2 + s(2\xi)/\omega_n + 1} \tag{12.63}$$

Its undamped natural frequency can be shown to be (Northrop, 1997) $\omega_n = 1/(R\sqrt{C_1 C_2})$ r/s and its damping factor is $\xi = \sqrt{(C_2 C_1)}$. The low-pass filtering action effectively estimates the mean of $v_1^2(t)/10$. The output, V_o, can be found by assuming the third op amp is ideal and writing the node equation for its summing junction:

$$\frac{\overline{v_1^2(t)}}{10R} = \frac{V_o^2}{10R} \tag{12.64}$$

Thus,

$$V_o = \sqrt{\overline{v_1^2(t)}}, \tag{12.65}$$

the RMS value of $v_1(t)$. Note that this analog square root circuit requires that $v_1^2(t) \geq 0$ and it is.

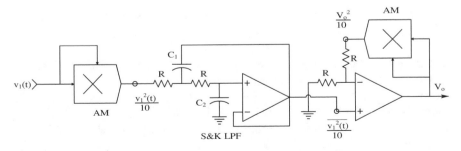

FIGURE 12.30
An analog circuit that finds the true RMS value of the input voltage, $v_1(t)$. Two analog multipliers (AM) are used.

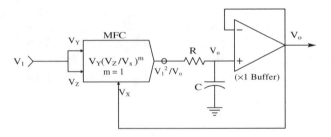

FIGURE 12.31
A true RMS conversion circuit using a multifunction converter.

Another (implicit) TRMS circuit can be made from an analog IC known as a *multifunction converter* (MFC). The MFC, such as the Burr–Brown 4302, computes the analog function,

$$V_2 = V_Y (V_Z / V_X) m, \quad 5 \ge m \ge 1, \quad 0 \le (V_x, V_y, V_Z) \le 10 \text{ V} \tag{12.66}$$

From the circuit of Figure 12.31, note that the R–C LPF acts as an averager of $V_2 = V_1^2 V_o$. Thus, the identity:

$$V_o = \overline{V_1^2 / V_o} \tag{12.67}$$

can be written and, from this, it is clear that

$$V_o^2 = \overline{V_1^2} \text{ MSV}, \tag{12.68}$$

and V_o is the RMS value of V_1.

The RMS voltage of a signal can also be found using vacuum thermocouple (VTC) elements, as shown in Figure 12.32. The vacuum thermocouple consists of a thin heater wire of resistance R_{Ho} at a reference temperature, T_A (e.g., 25°C), inside an evacuated glass envelope. Electrically insulated from but thermally intimate with R_H is a thermocouple junction (TJ) (Pallàs–Areny and Webster, 2001; Northrop, 1997; Lion, 1959). For example, the venerable Western Electric model 20D VTC has $R_H = 35 \ \Omega$ at room temperature; the nominal thermocouple resistance (Fe and constantan wires) is 12 Ω. The maximum heater current is 16 mA RMS (exceed this and the heater melts). The 20D VTC has an open-circuit DC output voltage $V_o = 0.005$ V when $I_H = 0.007$ A RMS. Because the heater temperature is proportional to the average power dissipated in the heater, or the mean squared current × R_H, this VTC produces $K_T = 0.005 / [(0.007)^2 \times 35] = 2.915$ V/W, or mV/mW. The EMF of the tesla joules is given in general by the truncated power series:

$$V_J = A(\Delta T) + B(\Delta T)^2 / 2 + C(\Delta T)^3 / 3 \cong S \Delta T \tag{12.69}$$

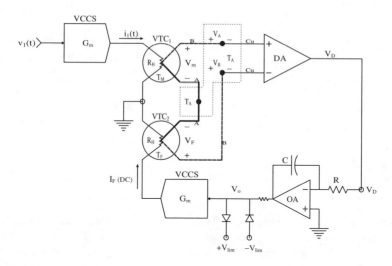

FIGURE 12.32
A feedback vacuum thermocouple true RMS voltmeter (or ammeter).

where ΔT is the difference in junction temperature above the ambient temperature, T_A. S for an iron/constantan (Fe/CN) $TC = 50 \times 10^{-6}$. In a VTC, $\Delta T = T_H - T_A$. T_H is the heater resistor temperature as the result of Joule's law heating. ΔT can be modeled by:

$$\Delta T = \overline{i_h^2} R_H \Theta \qquad (12.70)$$

The electrical power dissipated in the heater element is given by the mean-squared current in the heater times the heater resistance. The thermal resistance of the heater *in vacuo* is Θ; its units are degrees Celsius/watt. This relation is not that simple because R_H increases with increasing temperature — an effect that can be approximated by:

$$R_H = R_{Ho} (1 + \alpha\Delta T) \qquad (12.71)$$

where α is the alpha tempco of the R_H resistance wire. If the preceding equation is substituted into Equation 12.70, one can solve for ΔT:

$$\Delta T = \frac{\overline{i_1^2} R_{Ho} \Theta}{1 - \alpha\left[\overline{i_1^2} R_{Ho} \Theta\right]} \cong \overline{i_1^2} R_{Ho} \Theta\left[1 + \alpha \overline{i_1^2} R_{Ho} \Theta\right] \qquad (12.72)$$

Assuming that R_H remains constant, $\Delta T = V_J S = 0.005/(50 \times 10^{-6}) = 100°C$ from Equation 12.69. The thermal resistance of the WE 20D VTC is thus $\Theta = \Delta T/P_H = 100° (1.715 \times 10^{-3})$ W $= 5.831 \times 10^4$ °C/W. This thermal resistance is large because of the vacuum. High Θ gives increased VTC sensitivity.

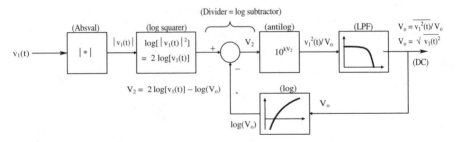

FIGURE 12.33
Simplified block diagram of Analog Devices' AD637 true analog RMS conversion IC.

In the feedback TRMS meter, the TC EMF is found by substituting Equation 12.72 into Equation 12.69. Examination of the TRMS TC feedback voltmeter of Figure 12.32 shows that it is a self-nulling system. At equilibrium, $V_F = V_m$ and it can be shown from the thermoelectric laws that $V_A - V_B = 0$, so $V_D = 0$. V_F and V_m are given approximately by:

$$V_F \cong A\left[I_F^2 R_{Ho} \Theta\right] = A\left[\left(V_o G_m\right)^2 R_{Ho} \Theta\right] = V_m \cong A\left[\overline{\left(v_1(t) G_m\right)^2} R_{Ho} \Theta\right] \quad (12.73)$$

From this equation, it can be written that

$$V_o(DC) = \sqrt{\left[\overline{v_1^2(t)}\right]} \quad (12.74)$$

i.e., V_o equals the RMS value of $v_1(t)$.

Note that this system is an even-error system. That is, the voltage V_F is independent of the sign of V_o because the same heating occurs regardless of the sign of I_F in R_H. Not shown but necessary to the operation of this system is a means of initially setting $V_o \rightarrow 0$ just before the measurement is made. Then V_o and I_F increase until $V_D \rightarrow 0$ and $V_m = V_F$.

Still another class of true RMS to DC converters is found in the Analog Devices' AD536A/636 and AD637 ICs. Figure 12.33 illustrates the block diagram of the AD637 TRMS converter IC. The front end of this system makes use of the identity:

$$v_1^2 = \left|v_1\right|^2 \geq 0 \quad (12.75)$$

Squaring is done by taking the logarithm of $\left|v_1\right|$ and doubling it. Division by V_o is accomplished by subtracting the log of the dc output voltage, V_o, from $2\log(v_1)$, giving V_2, which is antilogged to recover $v_1^2(t) V_o$. $v_1^2(t) V_o$ is low-pass filtered to produce the implicitly derived DC RMS output voltage from $v_1(t)$. Figure 12.34 illustrates the organization of the TRMS subsystems

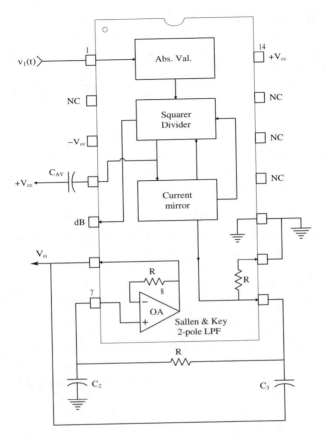

FIGURE 12.34
Block diagram of functions on the AD536 true RMS converter chip.

in the AD536 TRMS converter. A two-pole, Sallen and Key low-pass filter is used to give a smooth DC output in this configuration (Kitchin and Counts, 1983).

Note that all true RMS converters estimate the mean of the squared voltage by low-pass filtering. This means that they work well for DC inputs and for inputs whose power density spectra have harmonics well above the break frequency of the LPF. Low-frequency input signals will give ripple on V_o, making TRMS measurement difficult. The size of the LPF time constant is a compromise between meter settling time and the lowest input frequency that can be accurately measured.

Although this text has concentrated on analog electronic systems and ICs in describing TRMS conversion, the reader will appreciate that the entire process can be done digitally, beginning with analog anti-aliasing filtering followed by periodic A-to-D conversion of the signal under consideration. A finite number of samples (a data epoch) are stored in an array. Next, the converted signal is squared, sample by sample, and the results stored in a second array. The squared samples are then numerically low-pass filtered to estimate their mean. The numerical square root of the mean squared value is taken and stored for the kth epoch. The process is repeated until M epochs have been processed; then the average of M estimates of the RMS signal is finally calculated. The only components required are the anti-aliasing LPF, an ADC, some interface chips, and, of course, a PC.

12.7 IC Thermometers

12.7.1 Introduction

Temperature measurement is very important in medicine and biology. Many means have been devised to measure temperature, based on the fact that many physical phenomena vary with temperature, including, but not limited to: physical volume expansion (mercury and alcohol thermometers); resistance; EMF generated by the Seebeck (thermoelectric) effect; change in pemittivity of materials; change in reverse current through a *pn* junction; etc.

Many electronic means have been devised to circumvent use of the slow (and toxic) mercury thermometer. The fact that the resistance of metals *increases* with temperature has been the basis of one important class of electronic thermometer. The platinum resistance temperature detector (RTD) is widely used in scientific applications (Northrop, 1997). Its resistance is modeled by the truncated power series:

$$R(T) = R_o\left[1 + 3.908 \times 10^{-3}\,T - 5.8 \times 10^{-7}\,T^2\right] \qquad (12.76)$$

where R_o is the Pt RTD's resistance at 0°C and T is the RTD's temperature in degrees Celsius.

RTD resistance changes are sensed by using a Wheatstone bridge and suitable electronic amplification. Often a look-up table is used to correct for slight nonlinearity in the platinum RTD's resistance vs. T characteristic. The look-up table can be in the form of an ROM in which correction values are stored. Other metals (Ni, W, Cu, Si) can be used for RTD design, but Pt is the one most widely encountered because its $R(T)$ is fairly linear compared to other metals and it can be used at elevated (industrial) temperatures.

Thermistors are also used with Wheatstone bridges to sense temperature. Thermistors are amorphous semiconductor resistors; they are very nonlinear, but have much greater thermal sensitivity compared to metal RTDs. The resistance of a negative temperature coefficient (NTC) thermistor is modeled by the relation (Northrop, 1997):

$$R(T) = R_o \exp\left[\beta\left(1/T - 1/T_o\right)\right] \qquad (12.77)$$

If the temperature coefficient of a resistor is defined by:

$$\alpha \equiv \frac{dR(T)/dT}{R(T)} \qquad (12.78)$$

then the NTC thermistor's tempco is:

$$\alpha = -\beta/T^2 \qquad (12.79)$$

Beta is typically 4000 K and, for $T = 300$ K, $\alpha = -0.044$. By contrast, the α tempco of Pt is $+0.00392$. It should be remarked that there are also PTC thermistors. The author has used NTC thermistors to measure ΔTs on the order of $0.0001°C$ in *in-vitro* chemical assays of blood glucose using the enzyme glucose oxidase.

Other electrical/electronic means of temperature measurement use the minute DC voltages generated by thermocouples and thermocouple arrays called *thermopiles* used for photonic radiation power measurements. The interested reader should consult texts by Northrop (1997), Lion (1959), and Pallàs–Areny and Webster (2001) for further details on thermocouples and thermopiles.

Still other temperature measurement devices have been invented that measure the long-wave infrared (LIR) blackbody radiation from the eardrum. This class of fever thermometer is characterized by a fast response time (seconds), a minimally invasive implementation (inserted in the ear canal), and reasonable expense. The primary sensor is a thermopile or a pyroelectric material (PYM) such as triglicine sulfate or barium titanate. Further details on the Thermoscan™ thermometers can be found in Northrop (2002).

12.7.2 IC Temperature Transducers

Figure 12.35 illustrates a simplified schematic of the Analog Devices' AD590 temperature-controlled current source (TCCS). AD also makes the AD592 precision TCCS, which uses basically the same circuit. These ICs behave as two-terminal, 1-μA K current sources for supply voltages between $+4 \leq V_{cc} \leq +30$ V. Analog Devices (1994) gives the following circuit description for the AD590:

> The AD590 uses a fundamental property of the silicon transistors from which it is made to realize its temperature proportional characteristic: if two identical transistors are operated at a constant ratio of collector current densities, r, then the difference in their base-emitter voltages will be $(kT/q)ln(r)$. Since both k, Boltzmann's constant, and q, the charge of an electron, are constant, the resulting voltage is directly proportional to absolute temperature (PTAT). In the AD590, this PTAT voltage is converted to a PTAT current by low temperature coefficient thin film resistors.

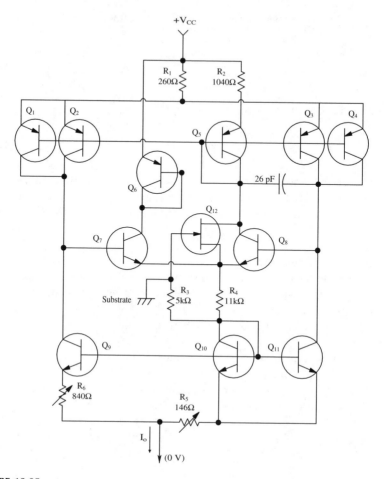

FIGURE 12.35
Simplified schematic of Analog Devices' AD590 analog temperature-controlled current source (TCCS) temperature sensor.

The total current of the device is then forced to be a multiple of this PTAT current. Referring to Figure [12.35], the schematic diagram of the AD590, Q8 and Q11 are the transistors that produce the PTAT voltage. R5 and R6 convert the voltage to current. Q10, whose collector current tracks the collector currents in Q9 and Q11, supplies all the bias and substrate leakage current for the rest of the circuit, forcing the total current to be PTAT. R5 and R6 are laser trimmed on the wafer to calibrate the device at +25°C.

The AD590 temperature-to-current transducer can operate over a −55 to +150°C range; the AD592 operates over a −25 to +105°C range. There are many applications for these electronic TCCSs. Figure 12.36 illustrates a simple op amp circuit that converts 1 μA K to 100 mV/°C. A chopper-stabilized op amp (CHSOA) is used for low dc drift tempco. The trim pots are used to

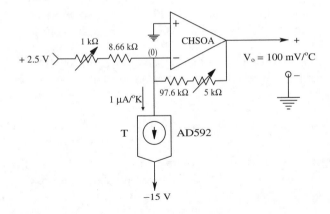

FIGURE 12.36

A simple op amp current-to-voltage converter that converts the current output of an AD592 temperature sensor to 100 mV/°C.

calibrate the amplifier exactly so that it has zero gain and offset error at the design temperature, e.g., 37°C.

Note that National Semiconductor also makes IC temperature sensors. The National LM135 series of sensors behave as temperature-controlled voltage drops (much like a zener diode). They give 10 mV/K drop with approximately 1-Ω dynamic resistance for DC currents ranging from 400 µA to 5 mA. They cover a wide, −55 to +150°C range. The National LM35 precision Celsius temperature sensor is a three-terminal device that outputs an EMF of 10 mV/°C over a −55 to +150°C range, given a supply voltage from 4 to 30 VDC.

12.8 Instrumentation Systems

12.8.1 Introduction

The previous sections of this chapter have described and analyzed the characteristics of selected ICs useful in designing biomedical instrumentation systems. This section focuses on examples of biomedical instrumentation systems taken from the research of the author and some of his graduate students. In each system, op amps are used extensively for various linear and nonlinear subsystems.

12.8.2 A Self-Nulling Microdegree Polarimeter

A polarimeter is an instrument used to measure the angle of rotation of linearly polarized light when it is passed through an optically active material. There are many types of polarimeters as well as a number of optically active substances found in living systems; probably the most important is dissolved D-glucose. Clear biological liquids such as urine, blood plasma, and the aqueous humor of the eyes contain dissolved D-glucose with a molar concentration in proportion to the blood glucose concentration (Northrop, 2002). Using polarimetry, D-glucose concentration can be measured by the simple relation:

$$\phi = [\alpha]_\lambda^T C L \text{ degrees} \tag{12.80}$$

where ϕ is the measured optical rotation of linearly polarized light (LPL) of wavelength λ passed through a sample chamber of length L containing the optically active analyte at concentration C and temperature T.

The constant $[\alpha]_\lambda^T$ is called the *specific optical rotation* of the analyte; its units are generally in degrees per (optical path length unit $\times$ concentration unit). $[\alpha]_\lambda^T$ for D-glucose in 25°C water and at 512 nm is 0.0695 milli-degrees/(cm $\times$ g/dl). Thus, the optical rotation of a 1-g/l solution of D-glucose in a 10-cm cell is 69.5 millidegrees. Note that $[\alpha]_\lambda^T$ can have either sign, depending on the analyte; if N optically active substances are present in the sample chamber, the net optical rotation is given by superposition:

$$\phi = L \sum_{k=1}^{N} [\alpha]_\lambda^{T_k} C_k \tag{12.81}$$

To describe how a polarimeter works, one must first describe what is meant by linearly polarized light. When light from an incoherent source such as a tungsten lamp is treated as an electromagnetic wave phenomenon (rather than photons), the propagating radiation is composed of a broad spectrum of wavelengths and polarization states. To facilitate the description of LPL, examine a monochromatic ray propagating in the z-direction at the speed of light in the medium in which it is traveling. This velocity in the z-direction is $v = c/n$ m/s; c is the velocity of light *in vacuo* and n is the refractive index of the propagation medium (generally >1.0). A beam of monochromatic light can have a variety of polarization states, including random (unpolarized), circular (CW or CCW), elliptical, and linear (Balanis, 1989). Figure 12.37 illustrates an LPL ray in which the **E**-vector propagates entirely in the x–z plane, and its orthogonal $\mathbf{B}_y$–vector lies in the y–z plane; **E** and **B** are in-phase and both vectors are functions of time and distance.

For the $\mathbf{E}_x(t, z)$ vector:

$$\mathbf{E}_x(t,z) = \mathbf{E}_{ox} \cos\left[\frac{2\pi c}{\lambda} t - \frac{2\pi}{\lambda} z\right] \tag{12.82}$$

Note that the **E**-vector need not lie in the *x–z* plane; its plane of propagation can be tilted some angle θ with respect to the x-axis and still propagate in

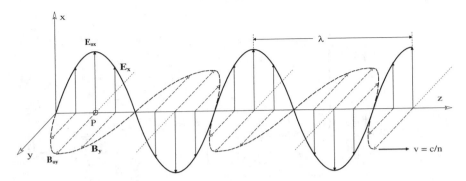

FIGURE 12.37
Diagram of a linearly polarized electromagnetic wave (e.g., light) propagating in the z direction. $B_y(t)$ is orthogonal in space to $E_x(t)$.

the z-direction (the orthogonal **B**-vector is rotated θ with respect to the y-axis). When describing LPL, examine the positive maximums of the E-vector and make a vector with this maximum and at an angle θ with the x-axis in the x–y plane.

Figure 12.38 illustrates what happens to LPL of wavelength λ passing though a sample chamber containing an optically active analyte. Polarizer P_1 converts the input light to a linearly polarized beam that is passed through the sample chamber. As the result of the interaction of the light with the optically active solute, the emergent LPL ray is rotated by an angle, θ. In this figure, the analyte is dextrorotary, that is, the emergent **E**-vector, E_2, is rotated clockwise when viewed in the direction of propagation (along the +z-axis). (D-glucose is dextrorotary.)

To measure the optical rotation of the sample, a second polarizer, P_2, is rotated until a null in the light intensity striking the photosensor is noted (in its simplest form, the photosensor can be a human's eye). This null is when P_2's pass axis is orthogonal to $E_2 \angle \theta$. Because polarizer P_1 is set with its pass axis aligned with the x-axis (i.e., at 0°) it is easy to find θ, and then the concentration of the optically active analyte, [G]. In the simple polarimeter of Figure 12.38, and other polarimeters, the polarizers are generally made from calcite crystals (Glan calcite) and have extinction ratios of approximately 10^4. (Extinction ratio is the ratio of LPL intensity passing through the polarizer, when the LPL's polarization axis is aligned with the polarizer's pass axis, to the intensity of the emergent beam when the polarization axis is made 90° (is orthogonal) to the polarizer's axis.)

To make an electronic polarimeter, an electrical means of nulling the polarimeter output is needed, as opposed to rotating P_2 around the z-axis physically. One means of generating an electrically controlled optical rotation is to use the Faraday magneto-optical effect. Figure 12.39 illustrates a Faraday rotator (FR). An FR has two major components: (1) a magneto optically active medium. Many transparent gasses, liquids and solids exhibit magneto-optical activity, e.g., a lead glass rod with optically flat ends or a glass test

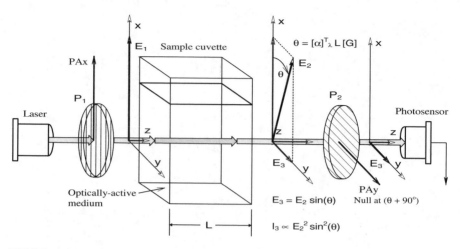

FIGURE 12.38

Diagram showing the rotation of the polarization axis of the incident $\mathbf{E}_1$ vector by passing the LPL through an optically active medium of length L. The system is a polarimeter: When the pass axis of linear polarizer P_2 is rotated by angle $\theta + 90°$, a null is observed in the output intensity, I_3. Thus, θ can be measured.

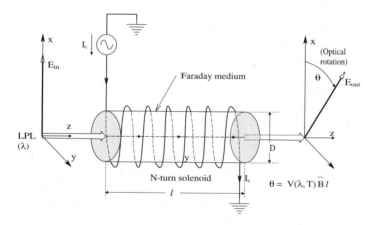

FIGURE 12.39

Diagram of a Faraday rotator (FR). The z-axis magnetic field component from the current-carrying solenoid interacts with the Faraday medium to cause optical rotation of LPL passing through the medium in the z-direction.

chamber with optically flat ends containing a gas or liquid can be used. (2) A solenoidal coil wound around the rod or test chamber that generates an axial magnetic field, **B**, inside the rod or chamber collinear with the entering LPL beam. The exiting LPL beam undergoes optical rotation according to the simple Faraday relation (Hecht, 1987):

$$\theta_m = V(\lambda, T)\bar{B}_z l \tag{12.83}$$

where θ_m is the Faraday optical rotation in degrees, $V(\lambda, T)$ is the magneto optically active material's Verdet constant, having units of degrees/(Tesla meter).

Verdet constants are given in a variety of challenging units, such as 10^{-3} min of arc/(gauss.cm). $\overline{B}_z$ is the average axial flux density collinear with the optical path and l is the length of the path in which the LPL is exposed to the axial **B** field. A material's Verdet constant *increases* with *decreasing* wavelength, and with *increasing* temperature. When a Verdet constant is specified, the wavelength and temperature at which it was measured must be given. For example, the Verdet constant of distilled water at 20°C and 578 nm is 218.3°/(Tm) (Hecht, 1987, Chapter 8). This value may appear large, but the length of the test chamber on which the solenoid is wound is 10 cm = 10^{-1} m and 1 T = 10^4 G, so actual rotations tend to be < ±5°. The Verdet constant for lead glass under the same conditions is about six times larger. Not all Verdet constants are positive; for example, an aqueous solution of ferric chloride and solid amber have negative Verdet constants.

Two well-known formulas for axial B inside a solenoid follow (Krauss, 1953). At the center of the solenoid, on its axis:

$$B_z = \frac{\mu NI}{\sqrt{4R^2 + l^2}} \text{ tesla} \qquad (12.84)$$

At either end of the solenoid, on its axis:

$$B_z = \frac{\mu NI}{2\sqrt{R^2 + l^2}} \text{ tesla} \qquad (12.85)$$

It can be shown, by averaging over l, that B_z over the length l of the solenoid is approximately:

$$\overline{B}_z \cong \frac{3\mu NI}{4\sqrt{4R^2 + l^2}} \rightarrow \frac{3\mu NI}{4l} \text{ tesla, when } l \gg 2R \qquad (12.86)$$

It should be clear that a Faraday rotator can be used to null a simple polarimeter electrically. See Figure 12.40 for an illustration of a simple dc electrically nulled polarimeter. The dc FR current is varied until the output photosensor registers a null ($E_4 = 0$). At null, the optical rotation from the FR is equal and opposite to the optical rotation from the optically active analyte. Thus:

$$V(\lambda, T)\frac{3\mu NI}{4l}l = [\alpha]_\lambda^T CL \qquad (12.87)$$

and the concentration of OA analyte is:

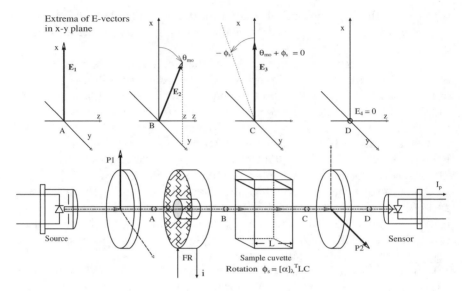

FIGURE 12.40
A simple electrically nulled polarimeter. The optical rotation from the FR is made equal and opposite to the optical rotation of the sample to get a null.

$$C = \frac{3V\mu NI}{4[\alpha]L} \tag{12.88}$$

Note that C is dependent on three well-known parameters (N, I, and L) and two that are less well known and temperature dependent (V and $[\alpha]$). This type of operation yields accuracy in the tenths of a degree.

Figure 12.41 illustrates an improvement on the static polarimeter shown in Figure 12.40. Now an ac current is passed through the FR, causing the emergent polarization vector at point B to rock back and forth sinusoidally in the x–y plane at audio frequency $f_m = \omega_m 2\pi$ Hz. The maximum rocking angle is θ_{mo}. This rocking $\mathbf{E_2}$ vector is next passed through the optically active sample where, at any instant, the angle of $\mathbf{E_2}$ has the rotation ϕ_s added to it, as shown at point C. Next, the asymmetrically rocking $\mathbf{E_3}$ vector is passed through polarizer P_2, which only passes the y-components of $\mathbf{E_3}$ as $\mathbf{E_{4y}}$ at point D. Thus $E_{4y}(t)$ can be written:

$$E_{4y}(t) = E_{4yo} \sin\left[\phi_s + \theta_{mo} \sin(\omega_m t)\right] \tag{12.89}$$

The sinusoidal component in the sin[*] argument is from the audio-frequency polarization angle modulation. The instantaneous intensity of the light at D, $i_4(t)$, is proportional to $E_{4y}^2(t)$:

$$i_4(t) = E_{4yo}^2\left[c\varepsilon_o/2\right]\sin^2\left[\phi_s + \theta_{mo} \sin(\omega_m t)\right] \text{ Watts/m}^2 \tag{12.90}$$

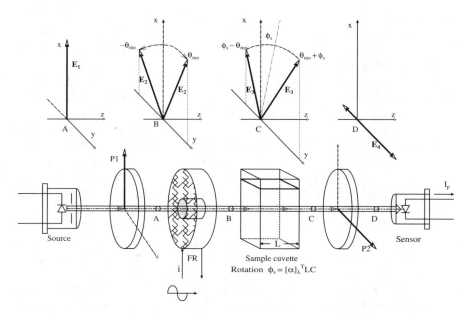

FIGURE 12.41

An open-loop Gilham polarimeter. The input polarization angle is rocked back and forth by $\pm\theta_{mo}$ degrees by passing ac current through the FR. See text for analysis.

Now, by trigonometric identity, $\sin^2(x) = \frac{1}{2}[1 - \cos(2x)]$, yielding:

$$i_4(t) = E_{4yo}^2\left[c\varepsilon_o/2\right]\frac{1}{2}\left\{1 - \cos\left[2\phi_s + 2\theta_{mo}\sin(\omega_m t)\right]\right\} \qquad (12.91)$$

Because the angle argument of the cosine is small, i.e., $\left|2(\phi_s + \theta_{mo})\right| < 3°$, the approximation $\cos(x) \cong (1 - x^2/2)$ may be used. Assume the instantaneous photosensor output voltage, $v_p(t)$, is proportional to $i_4(t)$, so:

$$v_p(t) = K_P\,i_4(t) \qquad (12.92)$$

$$\cong K_P\left\{E_{4yo}^2\left(c\varepsilon_o/2\right)\frac{1}{2}\left\{1 - \left[1 - \frac{4\phi_s^2 + 4\theta_{mo}^2\sin^2(\omega_m t) + 8\phi_s\theta_{mo}\sin(\omega_m t)}{2}\right]\right\}\right.$$

$$\downarrow$$

$$v_p(t) = K_V\left[\phi_s^2 + \theta_{mo}^2\,\frac{1}{2}\left(1 - \cos(2\omega_m t)\right) + 2\phi_s\theta_{mo}\sin(\omega_m t)\right] \qquad (12.93)$$

where $K_V = K_P\,E_{4yo}^2\,(c\,\varepsilon_o\,2)$.

Thus the photosensor output voltage contains three components: (1) a dc component of no interest; (2) a double-frequency component with no information on ϕ_s; and (3) a fundamental frequency sinusoidal term whose peak amplitude is proportional to ϕ_s. By using a high-pass filter, the dc components can be blocked; by using a phase-sensitive rectifier synchronized to the FR modulating current sinusoid at ω_m, a dc signal proportional to ϕ_s can be recovered while rejecting the $2\omega_m$ sinusoidal term.

By feeding a dc current proportional to ϕ_s back into the FR, the system can be made closed loop and self-nulling. The first such feedback polarimeter was invented by Gilham in 1957; it has been improved and modified by various workers since then (Northrop, 2002; Cameron and Coté; 1997, Coté, Fox, and Northrop, 1992; Rabinovitch, March, and Adams, 1982). Instruments of this sort can resolve ϕ_s to better than ±20 microdegrees.

Browne, Nelson, and Northrop (1997) devised a feedback polarimetry system that has microdegree resolution and is designed to measure glucose in bioreactors. The system is illustrated in Figure 12.42. Before its design and operation are described, it is necessary to understand how a conventional Gilham-type closed-loop polarimeter works.

A conventional closed-loop polarization angle-modulated Gilham polarimeter is shown in Figure 12.43. The dc light source can be a laser or laser diode. (A 512-nm (green) diode laser was used.) The light from the laser is passed through a calcite Glan-laser polarizer, P_1, to improve its degree of polarization, and then through the Faraday rotator. Two things happen in the FR: (1) the input LPL is polarization angle-modulated at frequency f_m. θ_{mo} is made about 2°. After passing through the sample, the angle modulation is no longer symmetrical around the y-axis because the optically active analyte's rotation has been added to the modulation angle. As shown previously, this causes a fundamental frequency sinusoidal voltage to appear at the output of the high-pass filter (HPF) whose peak amplitude is proportional to the desired ϕ_s. The phase-sensitive rectifier and LPF output a dc voltage, V_L, proportional to ϕ_s.

(2) V_L is integrated and the dc integrator output, V_o, is used to add a dc nulling current component to the FR ac input. This nulling current rotates the angle-modulated output of the FR so that, when it passes through the sample, no fundamental frequency term is in the photosensor output, V_d. Thus, the system is at null and the integrator output, V_o, is proportional to − ϕ_s. Integration is required to obtain a type 1 control system that has zero steady-state error to a constant input (Ogata, 1990). (The integrator is given a zero so that it will have a proportional plus integral (PI) transfer function to make the closed-loop system stable.)

Now, a return to the system of Browne et al. (1997) reveals that it is the same as the polarimeter system of Figure 12.43, with the exception that the FR and the sample cuvette are replaced with a single cylindrical chamber around which is wound the solenoid coil. The 10-cm sample chamber contains D-glucose dissolved in water, and other dissolved salts, some of which may be optically active. The solenoid current is supplied from a 3-op amp precision VCCS (see Section 4.4 in Chapter 4). The reason for using a VCCS to drive the coil is because the Faraday magnetorotatory effect is proportional to the axial **B** field, which in turn depends on the current through the coil.

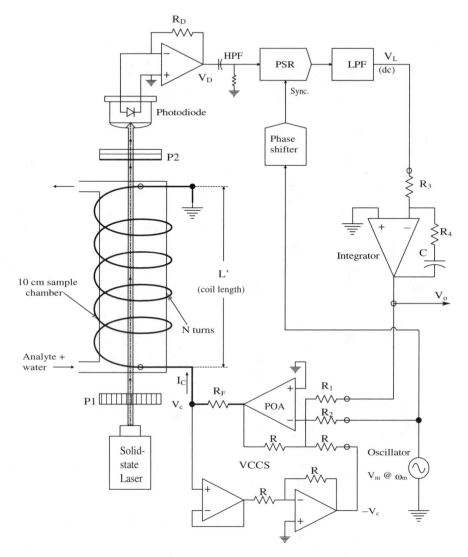

FIGURE 12.42

A system devised by the author to measure the concentration of dissolved glucose. It is a self-nulling Gilham-type polarimeter in which the external FR has been replaced by the Faraday magneto-optical effect of the water solvent in the test chamber. Glucose is the optically active medium (analyte) dissolved in the water.

Because the coil is lossy, it gradually heats from the power dissipated by the ac modulation excitation and the dc nulling current. As the coil wire temperature increases, its resistance goes up. Thus, if a voltage source (op amp) were used to drive the coil, **B** would be a function of temperature as well as the input voltage, V_c. The **B** temperature dependence is eliminated by using the VCCS.

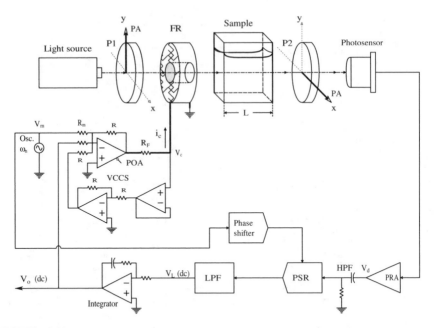

FIGURE 12.43
A conventional self-nulling Gilham-type polarimeter. A VCCS is used to drive the external FR's coil, which carries the ac modulation signal and the dc nulling current. A PSR/LPF is used to sense null.

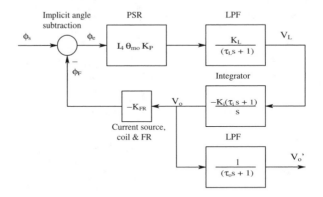

FIGURE 12.44
A block diagram describing the dynamics of the novel polarimeter of Figure 12.42.

    The FR can be eliminated because the water solvent in the chamber has a Verdet constant and, when subject to ac and dc magnetic fields, causes optical rotation of the transmitted LPL. The glucose solute is optically active, so, in the same path length, Faraday rotation occurs because of the action of **B** on the water and optical rotation occurs because of the dissolved D-glucose.

    It is possible to summarize the operation of this interesting system by a block diagram, shown in Figure 12.44. The input to the measurement system is the physical angle of rotation of the polarization vector, ϕ_s, caused by passing the LPL through the optically active analyte. The negative feedback of the system output voltage, V_o, leads to a Faraday counter-rotation of the LPL, ϕ_F, forming a net (error) rotation, ϕ_e. The dc counter-rotation, ϕ_F, is simply:

$$\phi_F = V\overline{B}L' = V(3/4)\frac{\mu N}{L'}L'I_c = \left[V(3/4)\mu N\right]\left[-\frac{V_oR}{R_1R_F}\right] = -K_{FR}V_o \quad (12.94)$$

Clearly, $K_{FR} = V(3/4)\mu N R/(R_1R_F)$ degrees/volt. The closed-loop response of the system is found from the block diagram:

$$\frac{V_o}{\phi_s}(s) = \frac{-I_4\theta_{mo}K_PK_LK_i(\tau_is+1)}{s^2\tau_L + s\left[1+\tau_iI_4\theta_{mo}K_PK_LK_iK_{FR}\right]+I_4\theta_{mo}K_PK_LK_iK_{FR}} \quad (12.95)$$

It is of interest to consider the dc or steady-state response of this closed-loop polarimeter to a constant ϕ_s. This can be shown to be:

$$\frac{V_o}{\phi_s} = \frac{-1}{K_{FR}} \quad (12.96)$$

Equation 12.96 is a rather serendipitous result, revealing that the system's calibration depends only on K_{FR}, which depends on the transconductance of the VCCS, the dimensions and number of turns of the coil, the Verdet constant, and the permeability (μ) of water. The dc gain is independent of the light intensity (I_4), the depth of polarization angle modulation (θ_{mo}), the frequency of modulation (ω_m), and the system's gain parameters (K_P, K_L, and K_i) and time constants (τ_L and τ_i).

The prototype system built and tested by Browne et al. (1997) was evaluated for D-glucose concentrations (**x**) from 60 to 140 mg/dl. By least mean-square error curve fitting, the output voltage (**y**) was found to follow the linear model,

$$\mathbf{y} = 0.0544\,\mathbf{x} + 0.0846 \quad (12.97)$$

with $R^2 = 0.9986$. System resolution was 10.1 $\mu°$/mV out, at 27°C with a 10-cm cell, and the glucose sensitivity was 55.4 mV/mg%. Noise in V_o was reduced by low-pass filtering (not shown in Figure 12.42).

Note that, in this instrument, op amps were used exclusively for all active components, including the photodiode current-to-voltage converter (transresistor) (see Section 2.6.4 in Chapter 2); the phase-sensitive rectifier (see Section 12.2.3 in Chapter 12); the low-pass filter (see Section 7.2 in Chapter 7); the PI integrator (see Section 6.6 in Chapter 6); the oscillator (see Section 5.5 in Chapter 5); and the VCCS (see Section 4.4 in Chapter 4).

12.8.3   A Laser Velocimeter and Rangefinder

Many conventional laser-based velocimeters are based on a time-of-flight rangefinder principle in which laser pulses are reflected from a reflective (cooperative) target back to the source position and the range is found from the simple relation:

$$L = c \, \Delta t \, 2 \text{ meters} \tag{12.98}$$

If the target is moving toward or away from the laser/photosensor assembly, the relative velocity can be found by approximating $v = \dot{L}$ by numerically differentiating the sequence of return times for sequential output pulses, $Dt = \sum \Delta t_k$. In 1992, Laser Atlanta made a vehicular velocimeter that used this principle.

The *laser velocimeter and rangefinder* (LAVERA) system described in this section uses quite a different principle to provide simultaneous velocity and range output. The LAVERA system was developed by Northrop (1997) and reduced to practice by a graduate student (Nelson, 1999) for his MS research in biomedical engineering at the University of Connecticut. The motivation for developing the system was to make a walking aid for the blind that could be incorporated into a cane.

The system uses sinusoidally amplitude-modulated CW light from an NIR laser diode (LAD). The beam from the LAD is reflected from the target object and then travels back to the receiver photosensor where its intensity is converted to an ac signal whose phase lags that of the transmitted light. The phase lag is easily seen to be:

$$\Delta\phi = (2\pi)(\Delta t/T) = (2\pi)(2L/c)/T \text{ radians} \tag{12.99}$$

where, as discussed previously, Δt is the time it takes a photon to make a round trip to the target; T is the period of the modulation; and c is the speed of light.

The system developed is a closed-loop system that tries to keep $\Delta\phi$ constant regardless of the target range, L. This means that, as L decreases, T must decrease and, conversely, as L increases, T must increase to maintain a constant phase difference. Figure 12.45 illustrates the functional architecture of the LAVERA system. Start the analysis by considering the voltage-to-period converter (VPC), which is an oscillator in which the output period is proportional to V_p. Thus:

$$T = 1/f = K_{VPC} \, V_p + b \text{ seconds} \tag{12.100}$$

By way of contrast, the output from a conventional voltage-to-frequency oscillator is described by:

$$f = K_{VCO} \, V_C + d \text{ Hz} \tag{12.101}$$

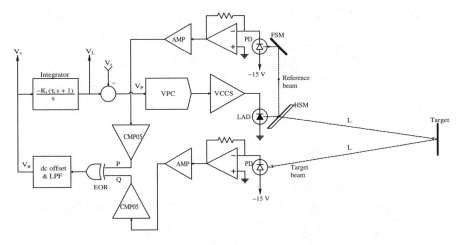

FIGURE 12.45
Block diagram of the LAVERA system developed by Nelson (1999). Sinusoidal modulation of the laser beam's intensity was used because less bandwidth is required for signal conditioning than for a pulsed system. The system simultaneously measures target range and velocity.

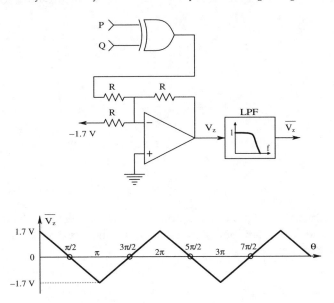

FIGURE 12.46
The EOR phase detector used in the LAVERA system, and its transfer function.

Next, consider the phase detector. This subsystem measures the phase difference between the transmitted modulated signal intensity and the delayed, reflected modulated signal intensity. An analog multiplier can be used directly to measure this phase difference; however, in this system, the analog sine waves proportional to light intensity are passed through comparators to convert them to TTL waves with a phase difference sensed by an exclusive or (EOR) gate phase detector (PD). The EOR PD is a quadrature detector, i.e., its output duty cycle is 50% when one input lags (or leads) the other by odd multiples of $\pi/2$. Figure 12.46 (adapted from Northrop, 1990) illustrates the EOR PD's waveforms and transfer function. The op amp inverts the TTL output of the EOR gate and subtracts a dc level so that V_z swings ±1.7 V.

For a heuristic view of how the system works, the PD output can be written as:

$$V_\phi = \overline{V_z} = V_v = -(3.4/\pi)\phi + 1.7 \text{ volts} \tag{12.102}$$

In the steady-state with fixed L, $V_v = 0$ in a type 1 feedback loop. For $V_v = 0$, $\phi_{ss} = \pi/2$. However, it has already been established that the phase lag for a returning modulated light beam is:

$$\phi = (2\pi)(2L/c)(1/T) \text{ radians} \tag{12.103}$$

If Equation 12.103 for ϕ is solved for T and T is substituted into the VPC equation,

$$T_{ss} = (2\pi)(2L/c)(1/\phi_{ss}) = K_{VPC}V_{Pss} + b \tag{12.104}$$

$$\downarrow$$

$$8L/c = K_{VPC}[V_{Lss} - V_r] + b \tag{12.105}$$

If $V_r \equiv b/K_{VPC,}$ the final expression for V_{Lss} is obtained:

$$V_{Lss} = 8L/(cK_{VPC}) \tag{12.106}$$

The steady-state V_L is indeed proportional to L. Going back to the VPC equation, one finds that, for a stationary target, the steady-state VPC output frequency is given by:

$$f_{ss} = 1/T_{ss} = c/(8L) \text{ Hz.} \tag{12.107}$$

At $L = 1$m, $f_{ss} = 37.5$ MHz; when $L = 30$ m, $f_{ss} = 1.25$ MHz, etc.

Now suppose the target is moving away from the transmitter/receiver at a constant velocity, $v = \dot{L}$. V_v is no longer zero, but can be found from the integrator relation:

$$V_v = -\dot{V_L}/K_i = \frac{-8\dot{L}}{K_i K_{VPC} c} \tag{12.108}$$

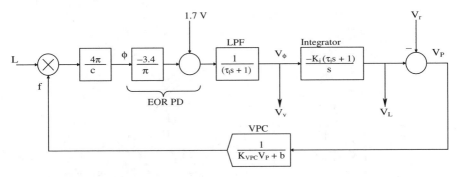

FIGURE 12.47
Systems block diagram of the LAVERA system of Figure 12.45.

Notice the sign of V_v is negative for a receding target; also, as the target recedes, the VPC output frequency drops. Clearly, practical considerations set a maximum and a minimum for L. The limit for near L is the upper modulation frequency possible in the system; the limit for far L is the diminishing intensity of the return signal, and noise.

To appreciate the closed-loop dynamics of the LAVERA system, it is possible to make a systems block diagram as shown in Figure 12.47. Note that this system is nonlinear in its closed-loop dynamics. It can be shown (Nelson, 1999) that the closed-loop system's undamped natural frequency, ω_n, and damping factor are range dependent, even though the steady-state range and velocity sensitivities are independent of L. The undamped natural frequency for the LAVERA system of Figure 12.47 can be shown to be:

$$\omega_n = \sqrt{\frac{4(3.4)cK_iK_{VPC}}{64\tau_iL_o}} \ r/s \tag{12.109}$$

The closed-loop LAVERA system's damping factor can be shown to be:

$$\xi = \frac{1}{2}\left[\frac{64L_o}{4(3.4)cK_iK_{VPC}} + \tau_i\right]\sqrt{\frac{4(4.3)cK_iK_{VPC}}{64\tau_iL_o}} \tag{12.110}$$

Finally, to illustrate the ubiquity of the op amp in electronic instrumentation, refer to Figure 12.48 — the complete prototype LAVERA system built by Nelson (1999). Op amp subsystems will be discussed, beginning clockwise with the voltage-controlled current source (VCCS). The VCCS is used to drive the laser diode with a current of the form:

$$i_{LD}(t) = I_{LDo} + I_{Dm}\sin(\omega t), \ I_{LDo} > I_{Dm}. \tag{12.111}$$

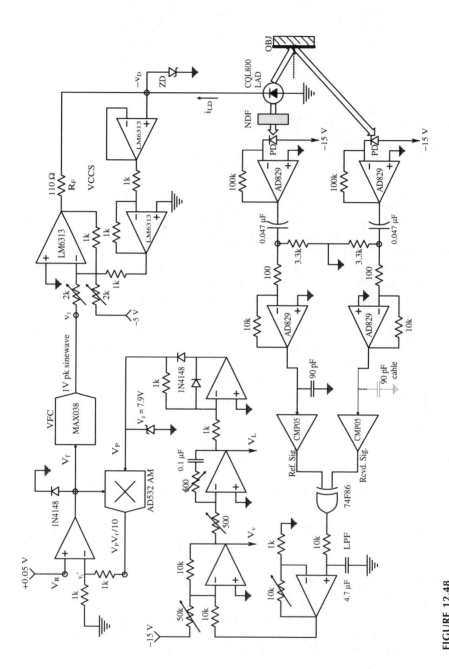

FIGURE 12.48
Simplified schematic of the LAVERA system showing the ubiquitous use of op amps.

This 3-op amp circuit was analyzed in detail in Section 4.4 in Chapter 4. At mid-frequencies, it was shown that $i_{LD}(t) = -v_1(t) \, G_M = -v_1(t)/110$ amps. The zener diode is to protect the LAD from excess forward or reverse voltage.

A Philips CQL800, 675-nm, 5-mW laser diode (LAD) was used. A small fraction of its modulated light was directed in a very short path (approximately 1 cm) through a neutral density filter (NDF) to the reference photodiode (PD). The PDs were Hammamatsu S2506-02 PIN photodiodes with spectral response from 320 to 1100 nm, with a peak at 960 nm. PD responsivity was approximately 0.4 A/W at 660 nm. The reference and received signal channels were made identical to avoid phase bias between channels; the receiver PD viewed the target through a collimated, inexpensive telescope. The photocurrents from the PDs were proportional to the light intensities striking their active areas and amplified by AD829 high-frequency op amp transresistors.

The AD829 has an $f_T = 120$ MHz, a slew rate of $\eta = 230$ V/μs, and $e_{na} = 2$ nV/√Hz. The voltage outputs from the AD829 transresistors were passed through a simple R–C high-pass filter to block dc. The HPF corner frequencies were 10 kHz. The high-pass filtered signals were then amplified by AD829 inverting amplifiers with gains of –100. A 90-pF capacitance to ground was placed at the input of the reference channel comparator to compensate for the measured 90-pF capacitance of the shielded cable coupling the receiver channel AD829 to its comparator. PMI CMP05 amplitude comparators were used to convert the sinusoidal signals at the outputs of the AD829 amplifiers to TTL digital signals, which were then input to the exclusive OR gate used as a quadrature phase detector. The EOR output was low-pass filtered, and amplified; then a negative voltage of approximately 1.7 V was added to make $V_v = 0$ when the phase difference was 90° between the reference and received channels (see Figure 12.46).

The nearly dc V_v is then integrated by the PI integrator. (The zero from the PI integrator is required for good closed-loop LAVERA system dynamic response.) As shown previously, V_v is proportional to target velocity, $\dot{L}$. The integrator output, V_L, is proportional to target range L. V_L is conditioned by a precision half-wave rectifier circuit to prevent the input to the VPC circuit from going negative, which locks up the system. The 7.9 V zener is also used to limit the input to the VPC, V_P.

The voltage-to-period converter (VPC) uses a Maxim MAX038 wide-range VFC that has a 0.1-Hz to 20-MHz operating range and a sinusoidal output. A nonlinear op amp circuit is used to convert V_P to V_f so that $V_P \rightarrow v_1$ has an over-all VPC characteristic. To examine how the nonlinear circuit works, assume the op amp is ideal and write a node equation on its summing junction (note that $V_i' = V_R$):

$$V_R \, G + (V_R - V_P \, V_f \, 10)G = 0 \tag{12.112}$$

$$\downarrow$$

$$2V_R = V_P V_f \, 10 \tag{12.113}$$

If $V_R = 1/20 = 0.05$ V, then it is clear that

$$V_f = 1/V_P \tag{12.114}$$

The VFC output frequency is approximately

$$f = K_f\, V_f = K_f\, V_P \text{ Hz} \tag{12.115}$$

or

$$T = 1/f = V_P\, K_f = K_{VPC}\, V_P \tag{12.116}$$

The sinusoidal output of the MAX038 VFC, v_1, is a 1-V peak sine wave that is used to drive the LAD.

Nelson (1999) reported a prototype CW LAVERA system with a linear V_L vs. L characteristic over $1\ m \le L \le 5\ m$ range with an $R^2 = 0.998$. A linear V_v vs. L was observed over 0.5 to 2 m/s. Wider dynamic ranges were limited by practical considerations, not by the circuit.

A problem to be solved in order to develop a practical system is how to use the velocity and range output voltages from the system to generate an audible or tactile signal that can warn a blind person of moving objects that may present a hazard. V_v goes positive for a moving target approaching the system, negative for a receding target, and zero for a stationary target. Thus, V_v might be used to control the pitch of an audio oscillator (not shown) around some zero-velocity frequency, e.g., 550 Hz. An approaching target would raise the audio pitch to as high as 10 kHZ; a receding target might lower the velocity pitch to 30 Hz minimum. But how is the range coded? Range is always positive and close objects should demand more attention, so another VPC circuit (not shown) can be used to generate "click" pulses that can be added to the velocity tone signal. Thus, a rapidly approaching constant velocity vehicle would generate a high, steady sinusoidal tone plus a click rate of increasing frequency as the range decreases. If the vehicle stops nearby, e.g., at a traffic light, the sinusoidal tone would drop to the 0-V frequency (550 Hz), but the click rate would remain high, e.g., 20/sec for a 2-m L.

12.8.4   Self-Balancing Impedance Plethysmographs

One way to measure the volume changes in body tissues is by measuring the electrical impedance of the body part being studied. As blood is forced through arteries, veins, and capillaries by the heart, the impedance is modulated. When used in conjunction with an external air pressure cuff that can gradually constrict blood flow, impedance plethysmography (IP) can provide noninvasive diagnostic signs about abnormal venous and arterial blood flow. Also, by measuring the impedance of the chest, the relative depth and rate of a patient's breathing can be monitored noninvasively. As the lungs inflate and the chest expands, the impedance magnitude of the chest increases; air is clearly a poorer conductor than tissues and blood.

For safety's sake, IP is carried out using a controlled ac current source of fixed frequency. The peak current is generally kept less than 1 mA and the frequency used typically is between 30 to 75 kHz. The high frequency is used because human susceptibility to electroshock, as well as physiological effects on nerves and muscles from ac, decreases with increasing frequency (Webster, 1992). The electrical impedance can be measured indirectly by measuring the ac voltage between two skin surface electrodes (generally ECG- or EEG-type, AgCl + conductive gel) placed between the two current electrodes. Thus, four electrodes are generally used, although the same two electrodes used for current injection can also be connected to the high-input impedance, ac differential amplifier that measures the output voltage, V_o. By Ohm's law, the body voltage is: $V_o = I_s Z_t = I_s [R_t + j B_t]$.

At a fixed frequency, the tissue impedance can be modeled by a single conductance in parallel with a capacitor; thus, it is algebraically simpler to consider the tissue admittance, $Y_t = Z_t^{-1} = G_t + j\omega C_t$. G_t and C_t change as blood periodically flows into the tissue under measurement. The imposed ac current is carried in the tissue by moving ions, rather than electrons. Ions such as Cl^-, HCO_3^-, K^+, Na^+, etc. drift in the applied electric field (caused by the current-regulated source); they have three major pathways: (1) a resistive path in the extracellular fluid electrolyte; (2) a resistive path in blood; and (3) a capacitive path caused by ions that charge the membranes of closely packed body cells.

Ions can penetrate cell membranes and move inside cells, but not with the ease with which they can travel in extracellular fluid space and in blood. Of course, many, many cells are effectively in series and parallel between the current electrodes. C_t represents the net equivalent capacitance of all the cell membranes. Each species of ion in solution has a different mobility. The mobility of an ion in solution is $\mu \equiv v/E$, where v is the mean drift velocity of the ion in a surrounding uniform electric field, E. Ionic mobility also depends on the ionic concentration, as well as the other ions in solution. Ionic mobility has the units of $m^2\ sec^{-1}\ V^{-1}$. Returning to Ohm's law, one can write in phasor notation:

$$V_o = I_s/Y_t = I_s \frac{G_t - j\omega C_t}{G_t^2 + \omega^2 C_t^2} = I_s \left[Re\{Z_t\} - j\,Im\{Z_t\}\right] \qquad (12.117)$$

where $Re\{Z_t\} = G_t/(G_t^2 + \omega^2 C_t^2)$ is the real part of the tissue impedance and $Im\{Z_t\} = B_t = -\omega C_t\ (G_t^2 + \omega^2 C_t^2)$ is the imaginary part of the tissue impedance. Note that $Re\{Z_t\}$ and $Im\{Z_t\}$ are frequency dependent and that V_o lags I_s.

There are several ways of measuring tissue Z_t magnitude and angle. In the first method, described in detail later, an ac voltage, V_s, is applied to the

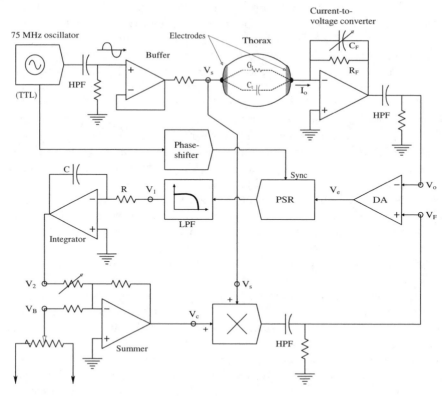

FIGURE 12.49
Block diagram of the author's self-nulling admittance plethysmograph.

tissue. The amplitude is adjusted so that the resultant current, I_o, remains less than 1 mA. I_o is converted to a proportional voltage, V_o, by an op amp current-to-voltage converter circuit. In general, V_o and V_s differ in phase and magnitude. A self-nulling feedback circuit operates on V_o and V_s. At null, its output voltage, V_c, is proportional to $|Z_t|$.

A second method uses the ac current source excitation, I_s; the output voltage described previously, V_o, is fed into a servo-tracking two-phase lock-in amplifier, which produces an output voltage, $V_z \propto |Z_t|$, and another voltage, $V_\theta \propto \angle Z_t$. A self-nulling plethysmograph designed by the author is illustrated in Figure 12.49. A 75-kHz sinusoidal voltage, V_s, is applied to a chest electrode. An ac current phasor, I_o, flows through the chest to virtual ground and is given by Ohm's law:

$$I_o = V_s [G_t + j\omega C_t] \tag{12.118}$$

This current is converted to ac voltage, V_o, by the current-to-voltage op amp:

$$\mathbf{V_o} = -\frac{\mathbf{I_o}}{G_F + j\omega C_F} \tag{12.119}$$

$$\downarrow$$

$$\mathbf{V_o} = -\mathbf{I_o}\frac{G_F - j\omega C_F}{G_F^2 + \omega^2 C_F^2} = -\mathbf{V_s}\left[G_t + j\omega C_t\right]\frac{G_F - j\omega C_F}{G_F^2 + \omega^2 C_F^2} \tag{12.120}$$

$$\downarrow$$

$$\mathbf{V_o} = -\mathbf{V_s}\frac{G_t G_F - j\omega C_F G_t + j\omega C_t G_F + \omega^2 C_t C_F}{G_F^2 + \omega^2 C_F^2} \tag{12.121}$$

With the patient exhaled and holding his breath, C_F is adjusted so that $\mathbf{V_o}$ is in phase with $\mathbf{V_s}$. That is, C_F is set so that the imaginary terms in Equation 12.121 $\rightarrow 0$. That is,

$$C_F = C_{Fo} \equiv C_{to}/(R_F G_{to}). \tag{12.122}$$

Then,

$$\mathbf{V_o} = -\mathbf{V_s}\frac{G_{to}G_F + \omega^2 C_{to}C_{Fo}}{G_F^2 + \omega^2 C_{Fo}^2} \rightarrow -\mathbf{V_s}\left(R_F/R_{to}\right) \tag{12.123}$$

Now when the patient inhales, the lungs expand and the air displaces conductive tissue, causing the parallel conductance of the chest, G_t, to *decrease* from G_{to}. Substitute $G_t = G_{to} + \delta G_t$ and $C_t = C_{to} + \delta C_t$ into Equation 12.121 and also let $R_F C_F = C_{to} R_{to}$ from the initial phase nulling. After a considerable amount of algebra,

$$\frac{\mathbf{V_o}}{\mathbf{V_s}}(j\omega) = \frac{-R_F}{\left[1 + \omega^2\left(R_F C_F\right)^2\right]}\Big[G_{to}\left(1 + \delta G_t/G_\omega\right) + \omega^2\left(R_F C_F\right)^2 G_{to}\left(1 + \delta C_t/C_{to}\right) +$$

$$j\omega C_{to}\left(\delta C_t/C_{to} - \delta G_t/G_{to}\right)\Big] \tag{12.124}$$

This relation reduces to Equation 12.123 for $\delta C_t = \delta G_t \rightarrow 0$. If it is assumed that $\delta C_t \rightarrow 0$ only, then Equation 12.124 can be written:

$$\frac{\mathbf{V_o} + \delta\mathbf{V_o}}{\mathbf{V_s}}(j\omega) \cong -R_F G_{to} - \frac{\delta G_t R_F}{\left[1 + \omega^2\left(R_F C_F\right)^2\right]} \tag{12.125A}$$

where

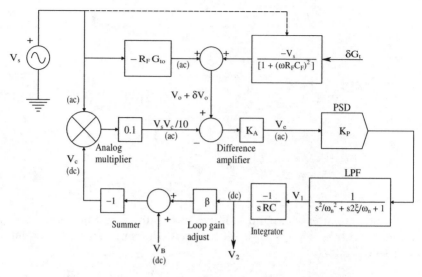

FIGURE 12.50
Systems block diagram describing the dynamics of the self-nulling plethysmograph.

$$\mathbf{V_o} = \left(-R_F G_{to}\right)\mathbf{V_s} \tag{12.125B}$$

$$\delta\mathbf{V_o} = -\frac{\left(\delta G_t\right)R_F}{\left[1+\omega^2\left(R_F C_F\right)^2\right]}\mathbf{V_s} \tag{12.125C}$$

Note that $\delta G_t < 0$ for an inhaled breath.

Figure 12.50 illustrates a systems block diagram for the author's self-balancing plethysmograph, configured for the condition where $\delta C_t \to 0$. The three RC high-pass filters in Figure 12.49 are used to block unwanted dc components from $\mathbf{V_s}$, $\mathbf{V_o}$, and $\mathbf{V_F}$. In the first case, $\delta G_t \to 0$. In the steady state, $\mathbf{V_e} \to 0$, so:

$$\mathbf{V_s}V_c/10 = -\mathbf{V_s}R_F G_{to} \tag{12.126}$$

Thus,

$$V_c = -10R_F G_{to} = -\left(V_B + \beta V_2\right), \tag{12.127}$$

and the dc integrator output, V_2, is proportional to G_{to}:

$$V_2 = \left(10R_F G_{to} - V_B\right)/\beta \tag{12.128}$$

V_B, G_{to}, and $\mathbf{V_s}$ do not change in time, so this steady-state analysis is valid. Using superposition, the system's response to a time varying, δG_t, can be examined. The transfer function, $\delta V_2 \, \delta G_t$, can be written:

$$\frac{\delta V_2}{\delta G_t}(s) = \frac{V_s K_A K_P \Big/ \left\{ RC\left[1 + \left(\omega R_F C_F\right)^2\right]\right\}}{s\left(s^2/\omega_n^2 + s2\zeta/\omega_n + 1 + V_s \beta K_A K_P/(10RC)\right)} \qquad (12.129)$$

The damping of the cubic closed-loop system is adjusted with the attenuation β. The dc steady-state incremental gain is:

$$\frac{\delta V_2}{\delta G_t} = \frac{10}{\left[\left(1 + \left(\omega R_F C_F\right)^2\right]\beta\right]} \quad \text{volts/siemen} \qquad (12.130)$$

A prototype of this system was run at 75 kHz and tested on the chests of several volunteers after informed consent was obtained. Both $\delta V_2 \propto \delta G_t$ and $V_1 \propto \delta G_t$ were recorded. System outputs followed the subjects' respiratory volumes, as expected.

A second type of IP makes use of a novel self-balancing, two-phase, lock-in amplifier (LIA) developed by McDonald and Northrop (1993); the system is described in Northrop (2002). A lock-in amplifier is basically nothing more than a synchronous or phase-controlled full-wave rectifier followed by a low-pass filter. Its input is generally a noisy amplitude-modulated or double-sideband-suppressed carrier ac signal. The LIA output is a dc voltage proportional to the peak height of the input signal; the low-pass filter averages out the noise and any other zero-mean output component of the rectifier. Signal buried in as much as 60 dB of noise can be recovered by an appropriately set-up LIA.

Figure 12.51 illustrates how the LIA is connected to the voltage across the tissue, $\mathbf{V_o}$, where $\mathbf{V_o} = \mathbf{I_s}(R_t + jB_t)$, ($B_t = -1/\omega C_t$). Note that if the angle of $\mathbf{I_s}$ is taken as zero (reference), then the angle of $\mathbf{V_o}$ is $\theta_s = \tan^{-1}(B_t R_t)$. The ac reference voltage, $\mathbf{V_r}$ in phase with $\mathbf{I_s}$ is used to control the LIA's synchronous rectifier. $\mathbf{V_r}$ also allows one to monitor $\mathbf{I_s}$ because $\mathbf{V_r} = \mathbf{I_s} R_F$. The self-nulling quadrature LIA outputs a dc voltage, V_φ, proportional to the phase difference between $\mathbf{I_s}$ and $\mathbf{V_o}$ and a dc voltage, V_p, proportional to the magnitude of the impedance, $|\mathbf{Z_t}|$, of the tissue under study. V_p and V_φ follow the slow physiological variations in Z_t caused by blood flow and/or breathing. The modulation of R_t and B_t by pulsatile blood flow or lung inflation can have diagnostic significance.

12.8.5 Respiratory Acoustic Impedance Measurement System

Acoustic impedance in this section is defined as the vector (phasor) ratio of pressure (e.g., dynes/cm²) to the volume flow (e.g., cm³ sec) caused by that

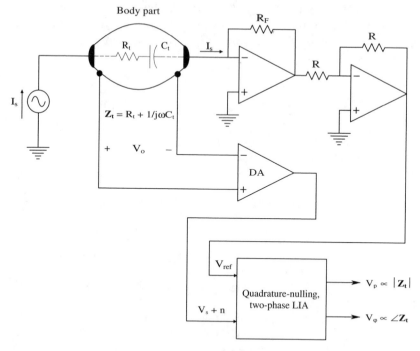

FIGURE 12.51

An impedance plethysmograph in which a constant ac current is passed through the body part being studied. A self-nulling, two phase lock-in amplifier is used to output voltages proportional to the impedance magnitude and angle. These voltages can be used to generate a polar plot of Z_t.

pressure at a given sinusoidal frequency. Acoustic impedance has been used experimentally to try to diagnose obstructive lung diseases, as well as problems with the eardrum and middle ear (Northrop, 2002). This section describes the electronic circuitry associated with a simple prototype acoustic impedance measurement system. Figure 12.52 illustrates an electric circuit that is an analog of the acoustic system used to measure the complex acoustic impedance vector looking into the respiratory system through the mouth. Note that phasor sound pressure levels P_1 and P_2 are analogous to voltages; acoustic resistance, R_{ac}, and complex acoustic impedance, $Z_{ac}(j\omega)$, are analogous to electrical resistance and impedance; and the complex volume flow rate, $\dot{Q}_2(j\omega)$, is analogous to the phasor electrical current, $I_2(j\omega)$. Thus, by the "acoustical Ohm's law":

$$\dot{Q}_2(j\omega) = (P_1 - P_2)/R_{ac} = P_2/Z_{ac}(j\omega) \tag{12.131}$$

Thus,

$$Z_{ac}(j\omega) = \frac{P_2 R_{ac}}{(P_1 - P_2)} \text{ cgs acoustic ohms} \tag{12.132}$$

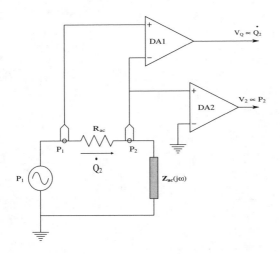

FIGURE 12.52
Electric circuit analog of the system used by the author to measure the acoustic impedance, $Z_{ac}(f)$, of the respiratory system. In the circuit, voltage is analogous to pressure and current is analogous to volume flow.

Assume that a microphone output voltage is proportional to the incident acoustical sound pressure, i.e., $V_2 = K_m P_2$, $V_1 = K_m P_1$. Thus, the vector $\mathbf{Z}_{ac}(j\omega)$ can be found by substituting the conditioned microphone voltages into Equation 12.132.

Figure 12.53 illustrates the system devised by the author to measure $\mathbf{Z}_{ac}(j\omega)$ in polar form — i.e.,

$$V_\theta \propto \angle \mathbf{Z}_{ac}(j\omega) = -\angle(\mathbf{V}_1 - \mathbf{V}_2),\tag{12.133}$$

and

$$\left|\mathbf{Z}_{ac}(j\omega)\right| \propto \frac{|\mathbf{V}_2| R_{ac}}{|\mathbf{V}_1 - \mathbf{V}_2|}\tag{12.134}$$

where the angle of $\mathbf{V}_2$ is taken as 0 (reference).

Note that the angle between $\mathbf{V}_1$ and $\mathbf{V}_2$ (P_1 and P_2) is measured by passing these sinusoidal voltages into voltage comparators serving as zero-crossing detectors producing 50% duty cycle TTL waves with the same phase difference as the analog $\mathbf{V}_1$ and $\mathbf{V}_2$. The TTL phase difference is sensed by a digital phase detector of the MC4044 type (see Section 12.3.3), giving a dc output, V_θ. Simultaneously, the ac voltages ($\mathbf{V}_1 - \mathbf{V}_2$) and $\mathbf{V}_2$ are converted to their dc RMS values, V_Q and V_P, respectively. V_θ, V_P, and V_Q are sampled and converted to digital format and passed through a computer interface. The computer calculates and displays:

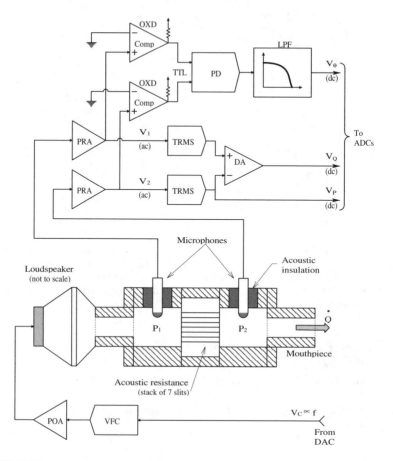

FIGURE 12.53
Block diagram of the RAIMS system developed by the author. Infrasound pressure between 0.3 to 300 Hz was introduced into the trachea and lungs through the mouth. Output signal processing by computer allowed display of $\mathbf{Z_{ac}}(f)$ in polar form over this frequency range.

$$\left|\mathbf{Z_{ac}}(j\omega)\right| = K_z \frac{\left|\mathbf{V}_2\right| R_{ac}}{\left|\mathbf{V}_1 - \mathbf{V}_2\right|} \tag{12.135}$$

and

$$\angle \mathbf{Z_{ac}}(j\omega) = -K_\theta \angle(\mathbf{V}_1 - \mathbf{V}_2) \tag{12.136}$$

as a polar plot for the range of frequencies used.

An 8-in. loudspeaker drove the acoustic resistance chamber. The loudspeaker was driven by a power amplifier with sinusoidal input from a VFC. The VFC, in turn, got its dc input voltage, V_C, from an 8-bit DAC with input from the computer.

A critical part of the design was the acoustic resistance, R_{ac}, across which the sound pressure drop was assumed to be without phase shift over the operating frequency range of the instrument, i.e., R_{ac} was real over the frequency range. Many "pure" acoustical resistances, such as those used in pneumotachs, etc., are made from many parallel capillary tubes. Capillary tubes' acoustic resistance is real up to some frequency at which they begin looking inductive due to the acoustic inertness of the tubes (Olson, 1940). To extend the range of real R_{ac}, a stack of (parallel) thin slits with rectangular cross sections was used. It can be shown (Northrop, 2002) that the R_{ac} of slits remains real to a frequency significantly higher than that for an equivalent R_{ac} made from capillary tubes. This RAIMS system was designed to operate from 0.3 to 300 Hz. An earlier system described by Pimmel et al. (1977) that used a commercial capillary-tube pneumotach for R_{ac} had a high frequency limit of 16 Hz before the pneumotach turned significantly reactive.

The prototype RAIMS system described here worked well with phantom acoustic lung impedances and normal volunteers in the lab, but was not investigated clinically.

12.9 Chapter Summary

Four diverse examples were chosen to illustrate the use of analog electronic circuit ICs in biomedical instrumentation system design:

1. The microdegree polarimeter represents an instrument that has evolved from a manually nulled instrument, with limited sensitivity to the optical rotation angle caused by polarized light passing through an optically active medium, to a closed-loop optoelectronic system with microdegree sensitivity. The optical rotation is used to measure D-glucose concentration in clear liquids. In the author's design, an expensive Faraday rotator was eliminated; instead the water solvent of the test solution was used for the Faraday medium.

2. Also developed was a closed-loop laser velocimeter and ranging system in which a CW laser beam was sinusoidally amplitude modulated (instead of using pulsed laser light and measuring nanosecond delays in the return reflection). The frequency of the amplitude modulations was automatically adjusted so that the phase difference between the transmitted and received modulations was held constant. This LAVERA system gave two simultaneous analog outputs proportional to target range and velocity; it was designed as a prototype aid for blind persons.

3. The third system described was a self-balancing impedance plethysmograph designed to measure small changes in volume as changes

in admittance in certain anatomical regions, such as the chest or legs. This system operated at a constant 75 kHz and used feedback to null an error voltage between the applied voltage and a voltage proportional to the body part's admittance at a standard condition. It was used to detect respiration and heartbeat simultaneously in an experimental context.

4. The fourth system was a **respiratory acoustic impedance measurement system** (RAIMS) — a prototype instrument intended to detect obstructive lung disease by comparison with "normal" records. The acoustic driving point impedance was defined and the acoustic equivalent of the voltmeter–ammeter method of measuring electrical impedance was described. An acoustic pressure source (analogous to a voltage) from a loudspeaker forced acoustic volume flow through a real acoustic resistance and then the unknown acoustic impedance of the respiratory system (pharynx, trachea, bronchial tubes, and alveoli). Specially modified microphones were used to sense the driving-point pressure at the mouth, P_2, and the volume flow proportional to pressure difference to across the acoustical resistance, $\dot{Q}_2 = (P_1 - P_2)/R_{ac}$. Instrument display was in polar form: $|Z_{ac}(f)|$ vs. $\angle Z_{ac}(f)$ over $0.3 \leq f \leq 300$ Hz.

References

Allen, P.E. and D.R. Holberg. 2002. *CMOS Analog Circuit Design*. Oxford University Press, New York.

Analog Devices. 1994. *Design-In Reference Manual*. Analog Devices, Norwood, MA.

Angelo, E.J., Jr. 1969. *Electronics: BJTs, FETs and Microcircuits*. McGraw–Hill, New York.

ARRL Staff. 1953. *The Radio Amateur's Handbook*. American Radio Relay League, W. Hartford, CT.

Aseltine, J.A. 1958. *Transform Method in Linear System Analysis*. McGraw–Hill, New York.

Balanis, C.A. 1989. *Advanced Engineering Electromagnetics*. John Wiley & Sons, New York.

Barnes, J.R. 1987. *Electronic System Design: Interference and Noise Control Techniques*. Prentice–Hall, Englewood Cliffs, NJ.

Blanchard, A. 1976. *Phase-Locked Loops*. John Wiley & Sons, New York.

Boylstead, R. and L. Nashelsky. 1987. *Electronic Devices and Circuit Theory*, 4th ed. Prentice–Hall, Englewood Cliffs, NJ.

Browne, A.F., T.R. Nelson, and R.B. Northrop. 1997. Microdegree polarimetric measurement of glucose concentrations for biotechnology applications, in *Proc. 23rd Ann. Northeast Bioengineering Conf.* J.R. Lacourse, Ed. UNH/Durham 5/21,22/97, pp. 9–10.

Cameron, B.D. and G.L. Coté. 1997. Noninvasive glucose sensing utilizing a digital closed-loop polarimetric approach. *IEEE Trans. Biomed. Eng.* 44(12): 1221–1227.

Chen, W.-K. 1986. *Passive and Active Filters: Theory and Implementation*. John Wiley & Sons, New York.

Chirlian, P.M. 1981. *Analysis and Design of Integrated Electronic Circuits*. Harper & Row, New York.

Clarke, K.K. and D.T. Hess. 1971. *Communication Circuits: Analysis and Design*. Addison–Wesley, Reading, MA.

Coté, G.L., M.D. Fox, and R.B. Northrop. 1992. Noninvasive optical polarimetric glucose sensing using a true phase measurement technique. *IEEE Trans. Biomed. Eng.* 39(7): 752–756.

Deliyannis, T., Y. Sun, and J.K. Fiddler. 1998. *Continuous-Time Active Filter Design*. CRC Press, Boca Raton, FL.

Dorf, R.C. 1967. *Modern Control Systems*. Addison-Wesley, Reading, MA.

Du, Z. 1993. A Frequency-Independent, High Resolution Phase Meter. MS dissertation in Biomedical Engineering, University of Connecticut, Storrs (R.B. Northrop, major adviser).

Eisner Safety Consultants. 2001. *Overview of IEC60601-1 Medical Electrical Equipment*. http:www.EisnerSafety.com.

Exar Integrated Systems, Inc. 1979. *Phase-Locked Loop Data Book*. Sunnyvale, CA.

Franco, S. 1988. *Design with Operational Amplifiers and Integrated Circuits.* McGraw–Hill, New York.

Gardner, F.M. 1979. *Phaselock Techniques.* 2nd ed. John Wiley & Sons, New York.

Ghaussi, M.S. 1971. *Electronic Circuits.* D. Van Nostrand Co., New York.

Gilham, E.J. 1957. A high-precision photoelectric polarimeter. *J. Sci. Instrum.* 34: 435–439.

Goldwasser, S.M. 2001. *Diode Lasers.* 103 pp. Web article (Sam's Laser FAQ). http://www.laserfaq.com/laserdio.htm.

Gray, P.R. and R.G. Meyer. 1984. *Analysis and Design of Analog Integrated Circuits.* John Wiley & Sons, New York.

Grebene, A.B. 1971. The monolithic phase-locked loop — a versatile building block. *IEEE Spectrum.* March, 38–49.

Guyton, A.C. 1991. *Textbook of Medical Physiology,* 8th ed. W.B. Saunders, Philadelphia.

Hannaford, B. and S. Lehman. 1986. Short-time Fourier analysis of the electromyogram: fast movements and constant contraction. *IEEE Trans. Biomed. Eng.* 33(12): 1173–1181.

Hecht, E. 1987. *Optics,* 2nd ed. Addison–Wesley, Reading, MA.

Herzel, F., H. Erzgräber, and P. Weger. 2001. Integrated CMOS wideband oscillator for RF applications. *Electron. Lett.* 37(6).

Hodgkin, A.L. and A.F. Huxley. 1952. A quantitative description of membrane current and its application to conduction and excitation in nerve. *J. Physiol.* (London). 117: 500–544.

Huelsmann, L.P. 1993. *Active and Passive Analog Filter Design: An Introduction.* McGraw–Hill, New York.

James, H.J., N.B. Nichols, and R.S. Philips. 1947. *Theory of Servomechanisms.* McGraw–Hill, New York.

Kanai, H., K. Noma, and J. Hong. 2001. Advanced spin-valve GMR-head. *Fujitsu Sci. Tech. J.* 37(2): 174–182.

Kandel, E.R., J.H. Schwartz, and T.M. Jessel. 1991. *Principles of Neural Science,* 3rd ed. Appleton and Lange, Norwalk, CT.

Katz, B. 1966. *Nerve, Muscle and Synapse.* McGraw-Hill, New York.

Kitchin, C. and L. Counts. 1983. *RMS to DC Conversion Application Guide.* Analog Devices Inc., Norwood, MA.

Kollár, I. 1986. The noise model of quantization. *Proc. IMEKO TC4 Symp., Noise Electric. Measurements.* Como, Italy. June 19–21, 1986. OMIKK-Technoinform, Budapest, 1987, 125–129.

Krauss, J.D. 1953. *Electromagnetics.* McGraw–Hill, New York.

Kuo, B.C. 1982. *Automatic Control Systems,* 4th ed. Prentice–Hall, Englewood Cliffs, NJ.

Lancaster, D. 1996. *Lancaster's Active Filter Cookbook,* 2nd ed. Butterworth–Heinemann, Oxford, U.K.

Lavallée, M., O.F. Schanne, and N.C. Hébert. 1969. *Glass Microelectrodes.* John Wiley & Sons, New York.

Lion, K.S. 1959. *Instrumentation in Scientific Research: Electrical Input Transducers.* McGraw-Hill, New York.

McDonald, B.M. and R.B. Northrop. 1993. Two-phase lock-in amplifier with phase-locked loop vector tracking, in *Proc. Euro. Conf. Circuit Theory and Design.* Davos, Switzerland, 30 Aug.–3 Sept. 6 pp.

Mentelos, R.M. 2003. Electrical Safety in PC Based Medical Products. App. Note. AN-10. RAM Technologies LLC, Guilford, CT. http://www.ramtechno.com

Merck Manual of Diagnosis and Therapy, 17th ed. (Centennial ed.). M.H. Beers and R. Berkow, Eds. http://www.merck.com/pubs/mmanual/section20/chapter277/277a.htm.

Millman, J. 1979. *Microelectronics.* McGraw–Hill, New York.

Nanavati, R.P. 1975. *Semiconductor Devices: BJTs, JFETs, MOSFETs, and Integrated Circuits.* Intext Educational Publishers, New York.

Nelson, T.R. 1999. Development of a Type 1 Nonlinear Feedback System for Laser Velocimetry and Ranging. MS dissertation in Biomedical Engineering, University of Connecticut, Storrs (R.B. Northrop, major adviser).

Newport Photonics. 2003. *Laser Diode Testing.* A tutorial. http://www.newport.com.

Nise, N.S. 1995. *Control Systems Engineering.* Benjamin Cummings, Redwood City, CA.

Northrop, R.B. and E.F. Guignon. 1970. Information processing in the optic lobes of the lubber grasshopper. *J. Insect Physiol.* 16: 691–713.

Northrop, R.B. and H.J. Grossman. 1974. An integrated-circuit pulse-height discriminator with multiplexed display. *J. Appl. Physiol.* 37(6): 946–950.

Northrop, R.B. 1990. *Analog Electronic Circuits: Analysis and Applications.* Addison–Wesley, Reading, MA.

Northrop, R.B. 1997. *Introduction to Instrumentation and Measurements.* CRC Press, Boca Raton, FL.

Northrop, R.B. 2000. Endogenous and Exogenous Regulation and Control of Physiological Systems. CRC Press, Boca Raton, FL.

Northrop, R.B. 2001. *Introduction to Dynamic Modeling of Neuro-Sensory Systems.* CRC Press, Boca Raton, FL.

Northrop, R.B. 2002. *Non-Invasive Instrumentation and Measurements in Medical Diagnosis.* CRC Press, Boca Raton, FL.

Northrop, R.B. 2003. *Signals and Systems Analysis in Biomedical Engineering.* CRC Press, Boca Raton, FL.

Ogata, K. 1990. *Modern Control Engineering,* 2nd ed. Prentice–Hall, Englewood Cliffs, NJ.

Olson, H.F. 1940. *Elements of Acoustical Engineering.* D. Van Nostrand Co., New York.

Ott, H.W. 1976. *Noise Reduction Techniques in Electronic Systems.* John Wiley & Sons, New York.

Pallàs-Areny, R. and J.G. Webster. 2001. *Sensors and Signal Conditioning,* 2nd ed. John Wiley & Sons, New York.

Perkin-Elmer. 2003. *Avalanche Photodiodes: A User's Guide.* http://optoelectronics.perkinelmer.com/library/papers/tp5.htm.

Phillips, C.L. and H.T. Nagle. 1994. *Digital Control System Analysis and Design.* 3rd ed. Prentice–Hall, Englewood Cliffs, NJ.

Pimmel, R.L. et al. 1977. Instrumentation for measuring respiratory impedance by forced oscillations. *IEEE Trans. Biomed. Eng.* 24(2): 89–93.

Plonsey, R. and D.G. Fleming. 1969. *Biolelectric Phenomena.* McGraw–Hill, New York.

Proakis, J.G. and D.G. Manolakis. 1989. *Introduction to Digital Signal Processing.* Macmillan, New York.

Rabinovitch, B., W.F. March, and R.L. Adams. 1982. Noninvasive glucose monitoring of the aqueous humor of the eye. I. Measurements of very small optical rotations. *Diabetes Care* 5(3): 254–258.

Schaumann, R. and M.E. Van Valkenburg. 2001. *Design of Analog Filters.* Oxford University Press.

Schilling, D.L. and C. Belove. 1989. *Electronic Circuits: Discrete and Integrated,* 3rd ed. McGraw-Hill College Division, New York.

Soltani, P.K., D. Wysnewski, and K. Swartz. 1999. Amorphous selenium direct radiography for industrial imaging. Paper 22. Proc. Conf. Computerized Tomography for Industrial Applications and Image Processing in Radiology. 15–17 March, Berlin, 123–132.

Stapleton, H. and A. O'Grady. 2001. Isolation techniques for high-resolution data acquisition systems. *EDN*. 1 Feb.

Stark, H., F.B. Tuteur, and J.B. Anderson. 1988. *Modern Electrical Communications,* 2nd ed. Prentice-Hall, Englewood Cliffs, NJ.

Stark, L. 1988. *Neurological Control Systems*. Plenum Press, New York.

van der Ziel, A. 1974. *Introductory Electronics*. Prentice-Hall, Englewood Cliffs, NJ.

Webster, J.G., Ed. 1992. *Medical Instrumentation*, 2nd ed. Houghton–Mifflin, Boston.

West, J.B., Ed. 1985. *Best and Taylor's Physiological Basis of Medical Practice*, 11th ed. Williams & Wilkins, Baltimore.

Wilson, W.L., Jr. 1996. A Sensitive Magnetoresistive MEMS Acoustic Sensor. Final Report. Contract #961004. Rice University, Houston, TX.

Yang, E.S. 1988. *Microelectronic Devices*. McGraw–Hill, New York.

Ziemer, R.E. and W.H. Tranter. 1990. *Principles of Communications: Systems, Modulation, and Noise*, 3rd ed. Houghton–Mifflin, Boston.

Index

* Pages with boldface numbers have figures illustrating the topic.